DISCARD

Standards-Based Physical Education Curriculum Development

Second Edition

Written and Edited by

Jacalyn Lund, PhD
Associate Professor
Georgia State University

Deborah Tannehill, PhD
Senior Lecturer
University of Limerick

Castleton State College

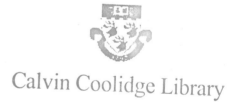

Calvin Coolidge Library

JONES AND BARTLETT PUBLISHERS
Sudbury, Massachusetts
BOSTON   TORONTO   LONDON   SINGAPORE

613.7071
St24

World Headquarters
Jones and Bartlett Publishers
40 Tall Pine Drive
Sudbury, MA 01776
978-443-5000
info@jbpub.com
www.jbpub.com

Jones and Bartlett Publishers
 Canada
6339 Ormindale Way
Mississauga, Ontario L5V 1J2
Canada

Jones and Bartlett Publishers
 International
Barb House, Barb Mews
London W6 7PA
United Kingdom

Jones and Bartlett's books and products are available through most bookstores and online booksellers. To contact Jones and Bartlett Publishers directly, call 800-832-0034, fax 978-443-8000, or visit our website, www.jbpub.com.

Substantial discounts on bulk quantities of Jones and Bartlett's publications are available to corporations, professional associations, and other qualified organizations. For details and specific discount information, contact the special sales department at Jones and Bartlett via the above contact information or send an email to specialsales@jbpub.com.

Copyright © 2010 by Jones and Bartlett Publishers, LLC

All rights reserved. No part of the material protected by this copyright may be reproduced or utilized in any form, electronic or mechanical, including photocopying, recording, or by any information storage and retrieval system, without written permission from the copyright owner.

Production Credits
Acquisitions Editor: Shoshanna Goldberg
Senior Associate Editor: Amy L. Bloom
Editorial Assistant: Kyle Hoover
Production Manager: Julie Champagne Bolduc
Production Assistant: Jessica Steele Newfell
Associate Marketing Manager: Jody Sullivan
V.P., Manufacturing and Inventory Control: Therese Connell
Composition: Publishers' Design and Production Services, Inc.
Cover Design: Kate Ternullo
Cover Image: © Joe Tree/Alamy Images
Printing and Binding: Malloy, Inc.
Cover Printing: Malloy, Inc.

Library of Congress Cataloging-in-Publication Data
Standards-based physical education curriculum development / edited by Jacalyn Lund, Deborah Tannehill., — 2nd ed.
    p. cm.
    Includes bibliographical references and index.
    ISBN 978-0-7637-7159-1 (pbk. : alk. paper)
    1. Physical education and training—Curricula. 2. Curriculum planning. 3. Education—Standards.
I. Lund, Jacalyn Lea, 1950– II. Tannehill, Deborah.
    GV363.S73 2010
    613.7'071—dc22
                                                                                    2009021915
6048

Printed in the United States of America
13 12 11 10 09   10 9 8 7 6 5 4 3 2 1

For Jeff and Nick with much love.

In memory of mom, Betty-Lee Tannehill.

For the teachers who are doing things well, addressing the standards, and offering innovative and meaningful programs to children and youth.

BRIEF CONTENTS

CONTENTS

CHAPTER 7   **The Skill Theme Approach to Physical Education**   **193**
Shirley Holt/Hale

CHAPTER 8   **Adventure Education in Your Physical Education Program**   **219**
Ben Dyson and Mike Brown

CHAPTER 13   Fitness Education   367

Karen McConnell

Section III Keeping Your Curriculum Dynamic

CHAPTER 14   It's Not Business as Usual   391

Deborah Tannehill and Jacalyn Lund

Daryl Siedentop, PhD, Professor Emeritus,
The Ohio State University

It is clear that standards-based curricula are now common for most subjects taught in American schools. In many subject areas, standards adopted by states are most often those developed by the national organization that represents the subject field. Thus, the physical education standards developed by the National Association for Sport and Physical Education (NASPE) are the standards most frequently adopted by states to inform teachers of the primary outcomes to be achieved in physical education at each grade level.

The dominant movement in public education today will likely be known as the era of "standards-based education." Both federal and state policy require that schools and teachers become aware of the state standards in their subject matters and that teachers plan learning experiences so students gradually move toward the mastery of those standards. How timely, therefore, that this curriculum text in physical education is developed wholly around the theme of the NASPE standards for K–12 physical education.

The NASPE standards, however, are somewhat different than standards in other subject areas; most science or math standards identify exactly what students should be learning in the 5th, 7th, or 9th grades. The NASPE standards do not tell us when—or even if—a student should learn a specific pass in volleyball, to traverse a horizontal climbing wall, or to reach a specific level of cardiovascular fitness. Thus, choosing the activities that compose a school physical education curriculum under NASPE standards is left open.

Many school districts approve a "district syllabus" for each school subject. Most district physical education syllabi include a large number of potential activities because teachers are at risk if they teach an activity that is not included in the district syllabus. In some districts, and even in a very few states, outcomes and syllabi in physical education have narrowed in order to focus on what has come to be called "health-related physical education" (HRPE). In good physical education programs, students experience a thoughtful variety of activities with sufficient time and progression in each activity to allow them to achieve the NASPE standards for a particular grade level. Sadly, other students will experience a hodgepodge of activities with insufficient time in any of them to become proficient, a result of which can be that they fail to meet any NASPE standards.

In *Standards-Based Physical Education Curriculum Development, Second Edition*, Jacalyn Lund and Deborah Tannehill wisely suggest that a good strategy to design a curriculum that both excites students and optimizes the chances of meeting NASPE standards is to consider "main theme" curricula as the organizing principle for curriculum planning. They have enlisted experts in each of the identified curricular models to describe the model and how to implement the model to achieve NASPE standards. Each chapter describes a main theme model, written by experts who have helped to develop the model and have experience implementing it. Some of the models, such as Fitness Education and Adventure Education, define the activities appropriate to the model; one is not likely to find a table tennis unit in either of these curricula. Other models, such as Personal and Social Responsibility and Sport Education, do not delineate particular activities but do require a particular pedagogy; Sport Education has been used for dance, fitness, outdoor, and sport activities, but the pedagogical model includes forming small, mixed-ability "teams" and having students learn all the roles necessary to implement the activity (e.g., compete, referee, keep score, organize equipment).

In examining the model theme curricula, readers will become aware that several have a distinct pedagogical approach that is part of the curriculum; some of the curriculum models define a specific pedagogy that is necessary for successful implementation of the model. This would be especially true for Personal and Social Responsibility, Sport Education, and Adventure Education. Readers would have to be comfortable with that pedagogical approach in order to implement that curricular theme.

The chapters are designed to help readers see what would be required to implement the themes in a school setting. Lund and Tannehill argue for a multi-model approach to curriculum, where several of the thematic models might be used in a school program. With reasonable time allotted for K–12 physical education, I can envision how a school district might decide to plan a Skill Theme model for Grades K–3, a Teaching Games for Understanding model in Grades 4–6, a Fitness Education model for middle school, and a Sport Education model for high school.

I have long believed that high school students should be provided choices from among attractive courses. Thus, several of the models might be appropriate for high school students, particularly the Fitness, Adventure, and Sport Education approaches. One of the primary benefits of this text is that it will require readers to think seriously about these issues and allow them to get to know models that fit their own predispositions.

Finally, this text is quite strong on assessment as one might expect from an approach committed to standards-based curricula. Put simply, organizing a curriculum to achieve standards requires ongoing assessment appropriate to the standards. The primary authors have a wealth of experience and expertise in assessment, and this is demonstrated throughout the text. *Standards-Based Physical Education Curriculum Development, Second Edition*, is a welcome addition to the resources that physical education teachers can use to develop and sustain high-quality physical education programs that are responsive to national standards as well as that provide learning opportunities for students through which students come to value the physically active lifestyle. This text also is a wonderful resource for teacher educators in physical education as they prepare the next generation of teachers to develop high quality physical education programs in schools.

Reference

Siedentop, D., Hastie, P. A., & Van der Mars, H. (2004). *Complete guide to sport education.* Champaign, IL: Human Kinetics.

While some people are wary of change, others view it as an opportunity. *Standards-Based Physical Education Curriculum Development, Second Edition*, is written to help those of you about to undertake a project to develop a new physical education curriculum for your school or district. This is an exciting time for your physical education program because you have the opportunity to create a curriculum designed to deliver a unique and satisfying physical education experience to the next generation of your community. An excellent physical education program has the potential to improve both the quality and quantity of life for its participants.

Updates to the Second Edition

In the *Second Edition* of this book, you will find several changes as the result of suggestions from our reviewers. Overall changes include the order of the chapters (grouping them in different ways from the first edition), updated references throughout the chapters, and a list of resources at the end of each chapter that students and teachers should find helpful as they seek additional information on the curriculum models discussed. We spend more time in Chapter 2 expanding on unpacking the NASPE standards, infusing technology, and the step-by-step process of building a curriculum.

A new introduction to the Main Theme Curriculum Models explains and differentiates between curricular and instructional models as well as provides an example of a multimodel curriculum. Chapter 4 has been reorganized to promote a better understanding of the assessment process as well as a revised section on developing rubrics for physical education. Doris Watson has joined with Gay Timken to write Chapter 5. Together they weave ideas from several new references into a powerful chapter on diversity. The Skill Themes chapter (Chapter 7) is now foregrounded with discussion of Developmental Physical Education before providing more concrete applications of the Skill Themes model as one example of developmental. Chapter 8 has been revised to include additional instructional ideas to expand the Adventure Curriculum model. When examining the Teaching Games for Understanding, the reader will note in Chapter 10 that the authors have clarified the progressive and sequential learning to better assist you in understanding how to begin and how to progress.

More detail is provided in Chapter 11 on how to actually plan a Sport Education season. The chapter also provides numerous examples of assessment tools to be used during a season. The Cultural Studies chapter has been revised to include examples of "real" programs that use this model and assignment examples that have been effective with young people. This text concludes with Chapter 14, which explains how a physical education curriculum can move from very good to great.

Arrangement of *Standards-Based Physical Education Curriculum Development*

Before beginning the process of writing curricula, individuals must have a basic knowledge and understanding of what they are about to undertake. Section I gives the reader a brief introduction to the curriculum process and explains how the standards movement has changed the rules for doing business in education. Developing a philosophy for the curriculum will provide the lens for making decisions about the curriculum model(s) that will be adopted as well as the activities used to implement those models. This philosophy must be compatible with the goals established for the program as well as mesh with educational goals for the district and state. Since curriculum development requires the melding of the ideas and philosophies of the individuals who develop it, the final product represents a series of compromises and midpoints between several different perspectives.

Writing a curriculum is hard work. To make sure that the hard work represents a product of the highest quality, there is still much to be done. Chapter 3 offers a means for evaluating the worth of your physical education curriculum. No matter how good a curriculum is, it can always be improved. This chapter explains the process for looking at the current status of the program and obtaining information that will help you make meaningful changes where they are needed. Curriculum evaluation should be an ongoing process that continually strives for excellence rather than a process that a district implements for an accreditation visit. We offer several suggestions for conducting evaluations and ways to measure the worth of your program from the perspectives of all those involved.

Assessment is a key component of developing a standards-based curriculum. Also included in Section I is a brief overview of the various types of assessments commonly used in physical education and a discussion about the role of assessment in a standards-based curriculum. The final chapter in Section I is designed to make you think differently about curriculum choices before venturing into Section II. A curriculum should meet the needs of all students, from the athletically gifted to those who are motor-challenged. All too often, curricular choices are made because of teachers' preferences rather than on the needs of the students. School populations represent the communities that surround them. Our goal in this text is for the reader to create a curriculum designed to instill a love for activity in all children and young people. In order to accomplish this, those developing a curriculum must consider the diverse perspectives that students bring with them. It is said that the hardest part of any journey is the first step. Section I is designed to help you take the first step on the road to developing a standards-based physical education curriculum.

The curriculum models presented in Section II provide the basis with which to teach toward the important learning goals (standards) and to do so in ways that provide unique opportunities for students to meet their own needs and desires in realistic and meaningful ways. We might think of the curriculum models as vehicles for delivering a philosophy: Your task will be to fit the curriculum model to the student, the setting, and the programmatic goals you have identified to meet state and national standards. Keep in mind that while each of the curriculum models addresses numerous national standards, none of them addresses them all (Siedentop & Tannehill, 2000). The following table visually represents our view of the contributions the various curricular models make with the NASPE content standards for physical education.

Curriculum Model	Standards					
	1	2	3	4	5	6
Cultural Studies			m		m	m
Personal and Social Responsibility	M	m	m	M	M	M
Teaching Games for Understanding	M	M			m	M
Skill Themes	M	M	M	M	M	M
Adventure Education	M	M	M		M	M
Outdoor Education	M	m	m	M	M	M
Sport Education	M	M	M	m	M	M
Fitness Education	m	M	M	M	m	M

Legend: M indicates a major focus on the standard; m suggests a minor focus.

Each of the chapters in Section II has been written by a recognized expert(s) in the respective curriculum model. The authors have 1) developed the model, 2) conducted research on its application, 3) provided workshops to teachers and school districts on how to implement it, and/or 4) written about it extensively. As you study each of the curriculum chapters, pay close attention to the philosophy the authors present and the unique characteristics that make the model appropriate to reach the standards. The authors provide insight into the main theme, characteristics of the model, and implications for teaching and learning.

This text concludes with Section III and thoughts on doing things differently. We borrowed the words of our friend and mentor, Daryl Siedentop, when we titled Chapter 14 "It's Not Business as Usual." We have spent a lifetime trying to promote the virtues of having physically educated youth as well as trying to improve the quality of physical education teaching. Here, we present ideas from students and colleagues—as well as our own thoughts—about how you can avoid the educational rut of teaching the same thing in the same way year after year. Change can be exciting, and we encourage you to use the ideas presented in Section III as fodder for making your physical education program better than you ever dreamed possible.

Reference

Siedentop, D., & Tannehill, D. (2000). *Developing teaching skills in physical education* (4th ed.). Palo Alto, CA: Mayfield.

Editors

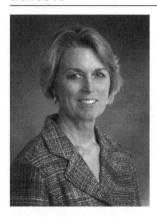

Jacalyn Lund is an Associate Professor and Chair of the Kinesiology and Health Department at Georgia State University. An educator for 38 years—after teaching in Colorado secondary schools for 16 years—she completed her doctoral degree at The Ohio State University. Other university teaching appointments have been with the University of Louisville and Ball State University. Currently, she is an adjudicator for NASPE/NCATE, the NASPE representative to the AAHPERD Board of Govenors, and a Past-President of NASPE. A member of the team that wrote the 1995 standards, she helped author the first edition of *Moving into the Future: National Standards for Physical Education*. Jackie has conducted workshops and made more than 100 presentations at the state, district, national, and international levels, including an invited presentation at the 2002 Asian Games in Busan, Korea. Current research interests involve assessment practices and curriculum development in physical education. She has published numerous articles on rubrics and assessment, including a book co-authored with Mary Fortman Kirk titled *Performance-Based Assessment for Middle and High School Physical Education*, and she has served as the Editor of the NASPE Assessment Series. Jackie has chaired committees to develop assessments for elementary and middle school physical education content standards for the state of Indiana as well as the committee to develop the Georgia Physical Education Content Standards. Favorite pastimes include spending time with her husband, Bill; sons, Jeff and Nicholas; dancing; and obedience-training dogs.

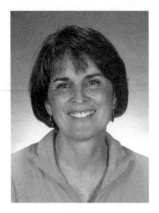

Deborah Tannehill is a Senior Lecturer in the Department of Physical Education and Sport Sciences at the University of Limerick, Ireland (UL). She is Course Director for the Graduate Diploma in Education–Physical Education and Co-Director of the Physical Education, Physical Activity, and Youth Sport (PE PAYS) Research Center. Before joining the faculty at UL, Deborah was Professor and Assistant Dean in the School of Physical Education at Pacific Lutheran University (PLU). Prior to PLU, Deborah taught and conducted research on teaching and teacher education at The Ohio State University for 12 years. She taught physical education at the middle school level for 10 years and coached track and field at the collegiate level for 6 years. Active in state, district, and national professional organizations, Deborah served as Editor of the National Association of Sport and Physical Education (NASPE) Assessment Series, Publications Coordinator for NASPE, Chair of the NASPE National Beginning Teaching Standards, Chair of the NASPE/NCATE Teacher Education Program Guidelines, and Chair of the NASPE Task Force for revision of the K–12 Content Standards. Deborah is Past Co-Editor of the *Journal of Teaching in Physical Education*, served on the editorial board of Quest, and is currently a reviewer for the *Journal of Physical Education, Recreation, and Dance*. In recognition of her professional service, Deborah was awarded the Joy of Effort Award from NASPE, was inducted as a Research Fellow into the AAHPERD Research Consortium, received the NASPE Presidential Citation, and, in March 2009, received the NASPE Curriculum and Instruction Academy Honor Award. Deborah has conducted research on teaching, supervision/mentoring, and teacher education in physical education, and she publishes frequently in both scholarly and applied journals. She has published more than 45 articles, 15 book chapters, and co-authored a textbook titled *Developing Teaching Skills in Physical Education* with Daryl Siedentop. Currently her work is focused on curriculum development and assessment and the continuing professional development of practicing teachers. Deborah enjoys reading mystery novels, cooking, and walking her whippet.

Contributors

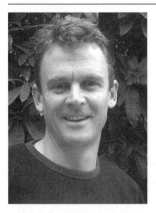

Mike Brown, PhD, teaches and completes research in the Department of Sport and Leisure Studies at the University of Waikato, New Zealand. He has worked in both academic and outdoor instructing contexts in Australia and New Zealand. His research interests include outdoor and adventure education pedagogy with a particular emphasis on place-based approaches to outdoor education and how sociocultural learning theory can inform current practice. He is a regular reviewer for several outdoor education journals and has written a number of book chapters and journal articles on various aspects of outdoor adventure practice and theory. His recreational interests include sea kayaking, cycling, and triathlons.

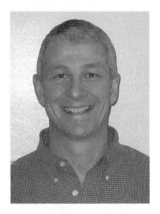

Ben Dyson is an Associate Professor in the Department of Health and Sports Sciences at the University of Memphis. He completed his PhD at The Ohio State University before taking up academic positions at McGill University, the University of New Hampshire, and the University of Memphis. His research focuses on innovative curriculum and instruction in physical education, including Adventure Education, Cooperative Learning, student perspectives, assessment, and students' physical activity in schools. In his classes he teaches and models a number of instructional models, including Cooperative Learning, Adventure Education, and experiential learning. Ben is a member of the National Task Force for Assessment in Physical Education. The Task Force has developed physical education assessments for elementary students, which were tested in schools throughout the United States and are now currently available as the PE Metrics from NASPE. With the American Heart Association, he worked to improve the amount of physical education and physical activity required in Tennessee schools. Ben currently serves on the Tennessee and southeastern-affiliate Advocacy Boards for the American Heart Association. He has presented at local, state, national, and international conferences and published professional and peer-reviewed journal articles regarding Adventure Education, Cooperative Learning, students' perspectives, and physical activity. He is a strong advocate for allowing children to have more access to "free play" opportunities; children today have too many structured activities and need more adventurous experiences in their lives. Ben is married with two children, and, when he can, he likes to participate in outdoor activities (kayaking, skiing, and hiking). He has competed in the Memphis in May Triathlon the last six years and the St. Jude's half-marathon the last seven years.

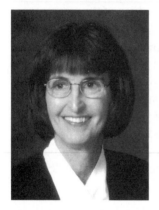

Shirley Ann Holt/Hale is an elementary physical education teacher at Linden Elementary School, Oak Ridge, Tennessee. She is the author of *On the Move* and the co-author of *Children Moving* with George Graham and Melissa Parker. Shirley serves as a consultant on curriculum, assessment, and curriculum mapping in elementary physical education. She was on the task force for the development of the National Physical Education (Content) Standards and chaired the NBPTS Committee for the development of the National Physical Education Teaching Standards. She is a former National Elementary Physical Education Teacher of the Year and has served as President of the NASPE and the American Alliance of Health, Physical Education, Recreation, and Dance.

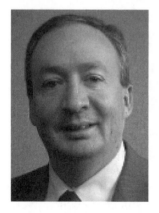

Gary D. Kinchin is a Senior Lecturer in Physical Education at the University of Southampton, England. He has held a number of positions of responsibility within the School of Education, most recently serving as the Deputy Head of School. A former head of physical education in public schools in England, Gary completed his master's degree and PhD at The Ohio State University. He has held academic appointments at De Montfort University, England, and Illinois State University. His research interests focus on sport education and more recently on physical education teacher education. Gary currently serves on the editorial board of Physical Education and Sport Pedagogy and the Physical Education Initial Teacher Training and Education (PE ITTE) Network Advisory Board. Gary has served as External Examiner for the physical education teacher education programs at Edinburgh University, Loughborough University, and Manchester Metropolitan University. An avid follower of rugby and cricket, Gary is married to Valerie, and they enjoy spending time with their two young daughters, Aimee and Ashleigh—particularly when body boarding in the north Cornwall surf!

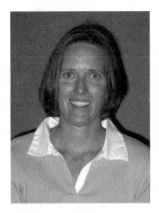

Karen McConnell is an Associate Professor in the School of Education and Movement Studies at Pacific Lutheran University (PLU) and serves as Associate Dean for the Department of Movement Studies and Wellness Education. She joined PLU in 1998 after completing her doctorate in Curriculum and Instruction in Exercise and Wellness at Arizona State University. Karen's interdisciplinary wellness background is applied to both her research and service activities. A focus on women's health issues—specifically educating others about eating disorders, body image, and weight related behaviors—is of particular interest. In addition, Karen has served as a consultant to the Comprehensive Health Education Foundation and the State Office of the Superintendent of Public Instruction in the development and implementation of the Essential Academic Learning Requirements, and the Washington Assessment of Student Learning in Health and Fitness. She is a co-author of the *Fitness for Life* curriculum (5th edition), which remains the number-one-selling high school fitness curriculum in the nation, and is a contributing author to the second edition of the *Physical Best Activity Guide: Middle and High School Levels*. Karen is a regular presenter at state, regional, and national conferences. She served on the advisory and editorial boards of the Women in Sport and Physical Activity Journal and sits on numerous department and university committees. She has been recognized as the Washington Alliance for Health, Physical Education, Recreation, and Dance University Professional of the Year (2001), and she was a recipient of the prestigious Arthur Broten Young Scholars Recognition Program Award (2001).

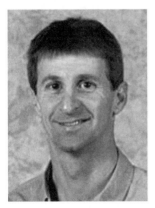

Steve Mitchell is a Professor and Coordinator of Graduate Programs in the School of Exercise, Leisure, and Sport at Kent State University. Individually and in collaboration with colleagues, he has written numerous books, chapters, articles, and coaching manuals focusing on tactical games teaching. An avid games player, Steve plays competitive soccer and tennis and recreational (not to mention, bad) golf. Just for fun, Steve also coaches a high school team. Steve's wife, Carolyn, and children, Katie and Matthew, also are enthusiastic game players.

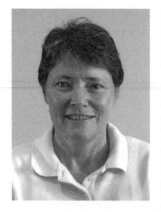

Having recently retired, Judy Oslin is a Professor Emeritus at the School of Exercise, Leisure, and Sport at Kent State University. She is currently working with local teachers to design and deliver professional development initiatives, teaching PETE modules at the University of West Indies, Trinidad/Tobago, and presenting standards-based in-service through the NASPE PIPEline project. She continues to work on numerous research projects that examine the effects of the tactical games approach on teaching and learning and serves as a volunteer substitute teacher for local physical educators. When not "working," Judy enjoys traveling, golfing, hiking, cycling, and kayaking with friends and family.

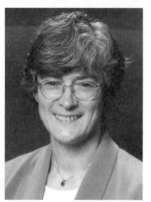

Mary O'Sullivan is currently Dean of the Faculty of Education and Health Sciences at the University of Limerick, Ireland (UL). She also is a fellow of the American Academy of Kinesiology and Physical Education (AAKPE) and has been engaged with the Research Consortium and the Curriculum and Instruction Academy of AAHPERD over the years. She is a former co-editor of the *Journal of Teaching in Physical Education* and associate editor of *Theory into Practice*, and she currently serves on the editorial boards of the *Journal of Teaching in Physical Education* and *Sport Education and Society*. She is a Vice President of the AIESEP Board of Directors (International Association for Physical Education in Higher Education). Mary has focused her recent attention to building research interest and research capacity around teacher education, physical education and youth sport in Ireland and is Co-Director with Deborah Tannehill of the Physical Education and Youth Sport Research Centre (PE PAYS) at UL. Her most recent writing has focused on teacher education and professional development as well as the impact of current educational and public health policies on physical education and youth. She likes to hike and read biographies.

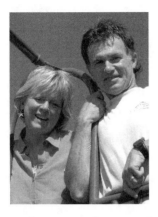

For the past 8 years, Jim Stiehl and Missy Parker have taught together at the University of Northern Colorado; however, their professional relationship spans over 15 years. They first became acquainted through a shared interest in personal and social responsibility, arriving at that point from different pathways. Jim was inspired and guided by the late Muska Mosston and Missy by Kate Barrett. Although their mentors were very different from each other, they both shaped Jim's and Missy's respective lives and careers by encouraging them to pursue what they themselves believed to be worth doing. After working together, Jim and Missy subsequently discovered a mutual interest in outdoor education, again from different paths: Missy via a fellow graduate student at The Ohio State University, which led to graduate study in that area; Jim via a colleague at the University of Colorado who persuaded him to learn more about the backcountry in which he was spending so much of his time. Their most compelling similarity is a shared belief that all education should offer change, challenge, and choice.

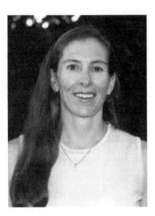

Gay L. Timken is an Assistant Professor of Physical Education Teacher Education at Western Oregon University. She supervises student teachers and teaches theoretical courses in methodology and curriculum as well as holds activity courses for preservice teachers focused on Games for Understanding, Sport Education, and Outdoor and Adventure Education. Her research interests are in the areas of teacher education and development. Gay enjoys reading, cycling, kayaking, and playing with her daughter, husband, and dogs.

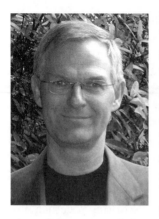

Hans van der Mars received his doctoral degree from The Ohio State University in 1984. Before joining the faculty at Arizona State University as Professor, Hans taught at Oregon State University in the professional physical education teaching licensure program. He formally held faculty positions at Arizona State University and the University of Maine at Orono. He has been an active researcher in sport pedagogy for more than 25 years. He has authored or co-authored more than 60 research and professional papers and book chapters. A frequent presenter at international, national, regional, and state level conferences, Hans also delivers workshops for K–12 teachers in physical education. He co-authored the *Complete Guide to Sport Education* and *Introduction to Physical Education, Fitness, and Sport*. He is former co-editor of the *Journal of Teaching in Physical Education* and chaired the NASPE Task Force that developed the NASPE/NCATE Advanced Physical Education Standards for Teachers. In his free time, he enjoys spending time with his family, playing golf, jogging, listening to music, and urging on his beloved New York Mets.

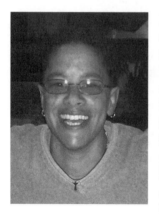

Doris Watson is an Associate Professor and Graduate Coordinator in the Department of Sports Education Leadership at the University of Nevada at Las Vegas. She joined the faculty in 2005, having previously taught at the University of Utah. She teaches at both the undergraduate and graduate levels in teaching methods and analysis of teaching. Her research interests include community-based programming for youth development and facilitation of a caring physical education environment through personal and social responsibility. Her personal interests include hiking/trekking, traveling, reading, and all things jazz.

Ancillary Materials

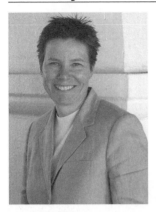

Kathryn LaMaster is Associate Dean in the College of Professional Studies and Fine Arts and a faculty member in the school of Exercise and Nutritional Sciences at San Diego State University. Her area of expertise is teacher education in physical education, and her research has focused on technology integration to impact teaching effectiveness, student learning, and assessment. Kathy works closely with the City Heights Educational Collaborative to impact quality daily physical education in local public schools. Her interests include digital photography, fly fishing, cross-country skiing, and hiking.

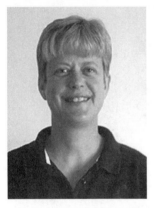

Connie Collier is an Associate Professor in the School of Exercise, Leisure, and Sport at Kent State University. She joined the faculty in 1997, having previously taught at Miami University and having spent 9 years in the public schools in Ohio. She received her BS from Defiance College and her MA and PhD from The Ohio State University. Connie's scholarship focus is the preparation and professional development of physical education teachers with an emphasis on the development of pedagogical practices and curricula that are responsive to issues of social justice. Her recent research examines and critiques innovative curricular approaches in Physical Education, in particular games teaching and sport education. She serves on the editorial board of the *Journal of Teaching in Physical Education* and is a member of the writing team responsible for the design of benchmarks and indicators for Ohio's standards based curriculum. She also is a member of AAHPERD, NASPE, AIESEP, AERA, and BERA.

The Curriculum Process

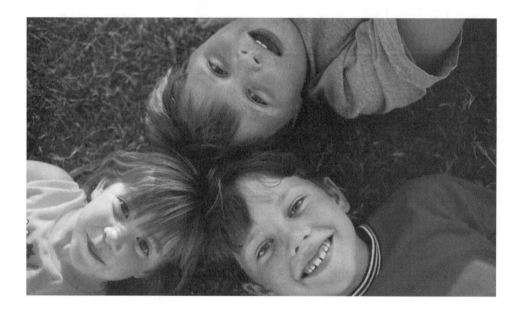

When faced with the task of designing a new curriculum, many people comment that they do not know where to begin. To gain a vision of the curriculum development process, one could compare it to building a new house: Just as one would not begin building a house without basic knowledge of design, carpentry, plumbing, and electrical wiring, one should not begin to build a curriculum before acquiring some fundamental knowledge about curriculum design. Section I is designed to give the curriculum writer information that will be useful in the process of developing a curriculum.

A vision of the outcome—knowing what the final product will look like—is critical for curriculum development. Just as a builder draws the blueprint of what the structure will eventually look like, a curriculum development team should develop a philosophy that presents a picture of the desired outcomes that will result when students are educated using this curriculum. Just as the builder must take into account factors such as the climate, the features of the land, and the size of the structure, there are several factors that a curriculum writing team should consider after determining their vision for the physical education program. Chapter 1 explains the development of a programmatic philosophy and points out several factors to consider while developing a curriculum.

After the house is envisioned, construction of a house begins with laying a foundation and building the framework on to which all the other materials will be connected. Chapter 2 explains the development of a structure for a curriculum with the unpacking of the standards. In a sense, the standards are the foundation of the curriculum and the unpacking process gives those standards meaning, becoming the framework on which all else is attached. Although standards are seen throughout the curriculum, standards look different for different grades and with different curriculum models. The framework delineates these differences and identifies an age-appropriate sequence for teaching these standards. Because this book is used in a variety of states, the National Association for Sport and Physical Education (NASPE) Physical Education Content Standards are used as the foundation. (For readers from other countries, a supplement is available in the ancillary materials comparing the standards from other countries with the NASPE standards.)

When building a house, there are various codes that a builder must meet to determine the quality of the structure. The inspection does not only occur at the end when the house is complete; there are several inspections as the house is built. Similarly, a good curriculum should have an evaluation procedure in place to regularly assess the level of quality and to help point out ways to improve the various aspects of the process. In a sense, a curriculum should have a "home remodeler" on hand, constantly looking for ways to improve the quality of the "house." An evaluation process tells the curriculum designers when change is needed. Chapter 3 presents several different types of evaluation that can be used for the various stakeholders for a curriculum while Chapter 4 presents ways to evaluate what students learn while participating in the curriculum. Both types of information are essential before any "remodeling" should occur.

The final chapter in Section I, Chapter 5, is devoted to challenging people to think inclusively about physical education and to develop a program that is sensitive to the needs of all individuals. Choice of activities can present subtle barriers for children, preventing them from learning to enjoy being active for a lifetime. Our goal is for readers to create curricula designed to instill a love of activity in all children and young people. A quality physical education program has the potential to make one's life more meaningful: Section I provides the information necessary to develop curricula designed to do just that.

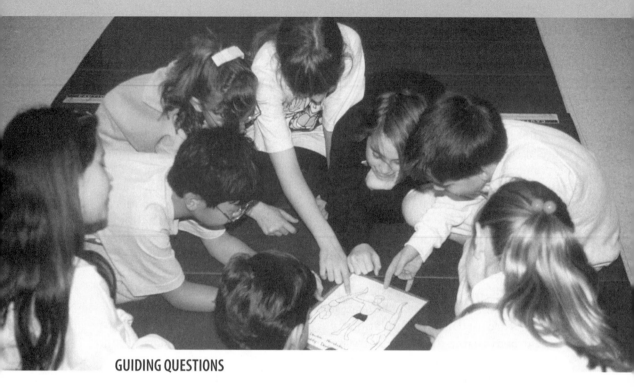

GUIDING QUESTIONS

1 What is curriculum?
2 What is standards-based curriculum?
3 How does a standards-based curriculum differ from a traditional curriculum?
4 Why have we gone to using a standards-based curriculum?
5 How has educational reform impacted schools and the way they do business?
6 What other factors have influenced curriculum development?
7 How does planning differ with traditional and standards-based curricula?
8 What role does assessment play in a standards-based curriculum?
9 How are activities selected in a standards-based curriculum?

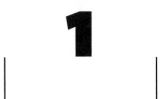

Introduction to Standards-Based Curriculum Development

Jacalyn Lund, Georgia State University
Deborah Tannehill, University of Limerick

What makes a good program good? What are its main characteristics? . . . First, it is clear that a good program accomplishes something . . . physical education must accomplish tangible outcomes to gain acceptance by students, faculty, administrators, and parents.

—Siedentop, Mand, and Taggart, 1986, p. 311

What does your physical education program stand for? Can you articulate clearly what your program is attempting to accomplish? Can you communicate this to students, parents, and administrators? Could you produce tangible evidence that this is happening? Physical education programs today are repeatedly being required to answer these and other questions. Educational reform and the move to standards-based education are changing the way educators do business.

Picture the graduate of your physical education program—how would you want this person to act? What would you want them to know and be able to do? Many physical educators would reply that they want their graduates to choose to participate in physical activity, have sufficient skill and knowledge to do so successfully, and lead an active lifestyle. Participation can manifest itself in a wide variety of forms—from square dancing with a local group, to playing softball with a recreational team, to hiking in state or national parks. An active lifestyle contributes to physical health, as well as social and mental well-being.

Having graduates participate in physical activity on a regular basis is not an automatic outcome of a physical education program, as our national health statistics confirm (Burgeson et al., 2003). Choosing to be physically active is the result of experiencing a solid curriculum that allows students to develop the skills and knowledge necessary for success, along with making them aware of activity venues within the community in which to participate (Rink, 2000). People tend to participate in activities during which they experienced success. The challenge for physical educators is twofold: first to give students the skills and knowledge they need to be successful; and second, to introduce them to activity venues where they can participate in these activities long after they graduate from high school.

As stated previously, educational reform is changing the way schools operate. The move toward standards-based education is an attempt to clarify what schools and teachers are trying to accomplish. This book is designed to help you make the journey of developing a standards-based physical education program. Since knowing where to start is often the most difficult part, this chapter is designed to help you begin by defining what a curriculum includes, describing how the standards-based movement began, and explaining the significance of this movement so that you will know the important components of developing a quality, standards-based physical education program.

What Is Curriculum?

Curriculum includes all knowledge, skills, and learning experiences that are provided to students within the school program. This encompasses even those activities that are typically offered beyond the school day such as band, student clubs, intramurals, and after school sports teams. From our perspective, curriculum includes the planned and sequenced learning experiences that allow students to reach significant goals that teachers have determined worthwhile for students to achieve. Ultimately, a curriculum represents the plan that guides delivery of learning experiences and instruction. Although it is difficult to separate instruction from the curriculum and assessment, we will attempt to do so to better clarify the latter pieces of the triad. In this text, we will narrow our description of curriculum development to include only those experiences that are delivered within the physical education class typically offered within the school day, although we recognize that the curriculum actually includes much more than that.

curriculum   Includes all knowledge, skills, and learning experiences that are provided to students within the school program.

Curriculum writing is the process of developing a sequence of activities, and/or selecting an appropriate curriculum model that will enable students to meet desired goals at the conclusion of their school experience. The curriculum outlines the big picture for this process, develops assessments that are given at various points allowing students to demonstrate success toward meeting these goals, and identifies activities that allow graduates to meet curricular goals. In the past, curricular goals were determined largely by the school district developing the curriculum. Most school districts relied on teachers within the system to write the curricular goals. Educational reform has now provided external guidelines that schools are required to follow. States have developed **standards**, which are statements describing what students should know and be able to do. Instead of developing their own goals, most states are now requiring districts to meet standards that are common throughout the state.

What Is a Standards-Based Curriculum?

Standards-based curriculum represents a huge paradigm shift for many teachers currently in the field (Doolittle, 2003). In the past, curricula were usually written to include a variety of activities traditionally included in a physical education program. The focus was on developing skill competence for students in these sports or activities. In other words, teachers taught students the skills necessary to play volleyball, soccer, tennis, dance, or swim, for example, and the only goal was for students to be able to play or perform the activity. Activities were selected because they were typically played by one gender or the other (e.g., boys wrestled and girls danced), were commonly played in a certain region (e.g., ice hockey was common in a Minnesota physical education program), teachers were competent performers in the sport or activity and/or they enjoyed teaching the unit, or due to tradition—certain sports have always been included in physical education and not including them would almost be an act of heresy (e.g., basketball). As new sports or activities emerged they might be included in the curriculum if facilities, equipment, and personnel were available (e.g., inline skating, ultimate, team handball, etc.). Other activities might

standards Curriculum goals established at the national, state, or district level that identify the skills, knowledge, and dispositions that students should demonstrate.

standards-based curriculum A curriculum that is developed by looking at the standards (district, state, or national); identifying the skills, knowledge, and dispositions that students should demonstrate to meet these standards; and identifying activities that will allow students to reach the goals stated in the standards.

be eliminated for a variety of reasons (e.g., trampoline units were eliminated largely for liability reasons).

Developing a standards-based curriculum begins by looking at the standards; recognizing the skills, knowledge, and dispositions that students should demonstrate to meet these standards; and selecting a curriculum model and/or activities that will allow students to reach the outcomes stated in the standards. Time is limited, so teachers must carefully choose content and activities that will allow students to reach the standards. Some activities may be eliminated from a program because of their minimal contribution to meeting standards.

Curricular assessments are also necessary in standards-based curricula so that students will be able to track their success, and teachers and school districts can determine whether the curriculum will allow students to meet the standards. If students are falling short of meeting district or state standards, the reason(s) why must be determined. In some cases, new approaches to teaching or different activities must be included in the program. In other instances, additional time is needed for students to achieve the standards. For example, 30 minutes per week in elementary school is not sufficient for children to learn and become competent in all the standards. When physical education is only offered for one year at the high school level, there is no opportunity for most youth, especially the slow developer, to gain the skills necessary to achieve all the standards. In these instances, schools need to identify additional ways to give students the opportunity to reach the standards, or teachers must make choices about which standards their students will meet. If physical education is not part of the state testing mandate, and school districts do not take responsibility for ensuring that the standards are met, it is unlikely that all students will reach the standards.

Due to a misunderstanding of what it is, some teachers object to a standards-based curriculum because they feel it infringes on their right to choose what students should learn. Other teachers who run recreational programs where little instruction and, consequently, little student learning occurs, dislike standards-based curricula because their programs do not allow students to meet the standards. Some teachers are so concerned that students enjoy physical activity that they sacrifice skill competency so that students can engage in game play for the majority of their class time without considering the role that skill competency has in the level of student enjoyment. Other teachers who object to standards-based curricula have traditionally taught only team sports, and tend to repeat them at every grade level and sometimes within the year. Some teachers *have* come to appreciate the standards for the guidance they provide, how they have contributed to improving what is done in the name of physical education, and how they have improved the status of our profession (Petersen, Cruz, & Amundson, 2002).

In actuality, most physical education activities can be included to assist students in meeting the standards if instruction is focused on student learning. Although we are proponents of sport when it is taught well, we also recognize that not all standards can be achieved through sport alone . . . or dance alone, climbing walls alone, or fitness alone. Dance, outdoor pursuits, body control activities (gymnastics), individual sports, fitness activities, and racquet sports have much to contribute to the development of a physically educated person. Omitting them from a curriculum does the student a serious injustice. The "key" is to provide meaningful options through variety. To help achieve this variety, many school districts have adopted main theme curriculum models, which are covered in Section II of this book.

Why Have We Gone to a Standards-Based Curriculum?

Have you ever stopped to consider what a high school diploma represents? Prior to the standards movement, for too many schools, a diploma had come to represent "seat time" (Guskey, 1996). In other words, a student attended school for a given number of years, sat at a desk for a required number of days, and thus earned a diploma. Although some students achieved competence in several subjects, this could not be said for all students. The standards movement sought to bring an end to this by stating what a graduate of a program should *minimally* know and be able to do.

What Is Educational Reform?

In 2001, federal legislation was passed in the United States that required states and their respective school districts to report student progress on reaching academic performance goals established by the state. Schools are required to report results publicly as to whether students are making adequate yearly progress toward these state mandates. This legislation, referred to as the No Child Left Behind (NCLB) Act of 2001, has resulted in schools spending many precious resources (time and money) to meet these goals. The intent of NCLB is for every child to achieve a minimal level of competency in several academic areas. To date, physical education is excluded as a core subject from this legislation and in some ways has become the forgotten subject as schools struggle to meet the expectations outlined in NCLB. This legislation is really part of a reform effort that began in the mid-1980s as the United States sought to catch up to the performance levels exhibited by many other countries around the world. The following section will briefly discuss some of the important events that led to the call for educational reform.

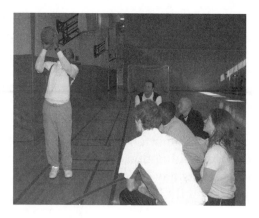

What Triggered Educational Reform?

In many respects a school is a reflection of society. Early educational systems were based on classical European models, designed for the upper class (Siedentop, 1998). As the United States became less of an agricultural society and more industrial, schools assumed more of a vocational role rather than providing a liberal arts education for a few.

Compulsory education laws caused students with less scholastic ability to stay in school. This trend, coupled with the population boost from the Baby Boomer generation, put increased demands on the structure of schools. As class sizes increased, students were less likely to receive individual attention. At the same time that schools were dealing with a more diverse population of students with a wide variation in ability, as well as larger sized classes, knowledge increased exponentially. Teachers tried to cover what they had traditionally taught along with this new information. The net result was that not all students were learning necessary skills and knowledge by the time they graduated from high school.

A similar metamorphosis impacted physical education. Physical education classes in the early 1900s found students engaged in physical training which consisted largely of calisthenics and fitness activities. Today's physical education classes may cover a variety of team and individual sports, and recreational activities, along with aerobics, hiking, disk games, dance, swimming, and fitness activities. Teachers have more to teach, less time to teach it, larger classes, and greater variation in physical ability, ethnic background, and culture.

The standards movement actually originated from the world of business as leaders began calling for educational reform. Business leaders wanted to ensure that their future workers were capable of performing the tasks necessary for success. Employers who hired graduates wanted to make sure that those holding a high school diploma had mastered at least a minimum set of skills and acquired a basic level of knowledge. Educators were called upon to identify what students should know and be able to do. This set of skills and knowledge was referred to as standards.

Because states have control of their own educational system, each state is responsible for developing its own standards. The standards movement required people to look at the graduate to define the desired knowledge base or exit skills. From there, educators could go through a process referred to as **backward design** (Jacobs, 1997), which means to design toward the ultimate goal/end, to decide what students needed to know at each grade level to enable them to successfully achieve the exit outcomes.

Many cognate areas began developing subject area standards to assist states and provide guidance. The National Association for Sport and Physical Education released physical education content standards in 1995. The NASPE Standards were based on the document *Outcomes of Quality Physical Education* (NASPE, 1992), which defined a physically educated person (see Figure 1.1). Although each state is responsible for developing its own content standards, many states have adopted the NASPE National Physical Education Content Standards (1995), as did the International Council for Health, Physical Education, Recreation, Sport, and Dance (ICHPERSD), an international physical education organization.

Although some people look at educational reform and the standards movement as being problematic, in some respects it can be looked upon as an opportunity for educational renewal. Because of the expansion of knowledge, the emphasis has changed from knowing minute facts and details to a more conceptual approach to learning (Erickson, 2002). In many instances the standards provide a lens through which to focus learning. Philosophical conversations about how to address these standards can be challenging for those willing to engage in the debate while clarifying and sharpening program goals. In physical education, a standards-based approach to curriculum development forces teachers to select activities and justify their contribution to meeting the standards rather than selecting activities by teacher preference or tradition. Recent articles (Peterson et al., 2002; Veal, Campbell, Johnson, & McKethan, 2002) have indicated positive results while moving to a standards-based approach to designing and implementing units.

backward design Intentional planning in which the teacher begins with the exit goals and designs the curriculum toward those goals; from high school down to elementary school.

> *To pursue a lifetime of healthful physical activity, a physically educated person:*
> - has learned skills necessary to perform a variety of physical activities
> - knows the implications of and the benefits from involvement in physical activities
> - participates regularly in physical activity
> - is physically fit
> - values physical activity and its contributions to a healthful lifestyle

Figure 1.1 Outcomes of Quality Physical Education Programs, which define a physically educated person. *Source:* National Association for Sport and Physical Education. (1992). *Outcomes of quality physical education programs.* Reston, VA: Author.

The NASPE content standards (2004) are the basis for the model of curriculum development proposed in this book. These standards are:

- Standard 1: Demonstrates competency in motor skills and movement patterns needed to perform a variety of physical activities.
- Standard 2: Demonstrates understanding of movement concepts, principles, strategies, and tactics as they apply to the learning and performance of physical activities.
- Standard 3: Participates regularly in physical activity.
- Standard 4: Achieves and maintains a health enhancing level of physical fitness.
- Standard 5: Exhibits responsible personal and social behavior that respects self and others in physical activity settings.
- Standard 6: Values physical activity for health, enjoyment, challenge, self-expression, and/or social interaction.

NASPE standards might be best thought of as a framework defining our subject matter. They provide benchmarks for achieving these standards for grades K–2, 3–5, 6–8, and high school. This framework can be adopted, revised, or adapted to meet the needs of each state and the contextual and political factors each faces. In South Carolina, state standards and performance benchmarks are more specific and aligned with what is possible for children and youth to achieve at specific grade levels, within the amount of time they have available (Rink et al., 2002). Wyoming, on the other hand, has developed state standards using the national standards as a framework (Deal, Byra, Jenkins, & Gates, 2002).

It is important to recognize that, unlike other disciplines, physical education does not have a national curriculum. Instead, we have a set of competencies that define the skills and knowledge that students are expected to learn through physical education (NASPE, 2004). These competencies have been labeled *content standards*, and specify what a student should know and be able to do as a result of participating in a quality physical education program. Although these content standards describe what students are expected to know and be able to do, they do not define what is considered an acceptable level of performance. That is the role of *performance standards*. NASPE suggests that a performance standard describes the levels of achievement that students are expected to attain to meet the content standards. The second edition of *Moving into the Future: National Standards for Physical Education* (2004) does not include performance standards because performance expectations will depend on the number of days per week that a child has physical education, class size, and resources (space and equipment) availability. NASPE has undertaken a large assessment project called P. E. Metrics that will provide assessments to measure student performance for each of the NASPE standards (Fisette et al., 2009).

What Other Factors Have Influenced Curriculum Development?

Although educational reform has changed the focus of curriculum development, other factors have led to the changes in physical education curriculum content. These factors are a direct result of our changing society and, more importantly, changes in the way that education is considered. This next section will discuss the impact that societal interests, mobility, choice, educational accountability, and content of teacher preparation programs have on curriculum development.

Societal Interests

Several games and activities that, in the past, were the focus of after school and weekend "play" in local parks are now popular additions to physical education programs. Physical activity trends have appropriately become curricular choices. Ultimate, inline skating, and pickleball are three examples of popular activities that have recently been added to physical education programs. When students master the basic skills of physical activities, they can learn new activities as adults. If students had developed a sidearm throw, balance, and striking skills, then the previously mentioned activities would be relatively easy to learn as adults, even though they had not previously experienced them. Physical education curricula must provide a variety of activities and skills to allow success while learning new activities as adults, even if these activities are not directly taught in physical education.

Mobility

Society today is much more mobile than in the past. Instead of living in a single community for one's entire life, people today are much more likely to work in a variety of geographical settings because of job and personal changes. An individual growing up in Florida might end up working in Colorado where skiing, hiking, and mountain climbing abound. Someone from North Dakota might settle in California and have access to beaches, beach volleyball, and surfing. Curricula need to be diverse enough to allow for the changes in the living environment that adulthood may bring.

Accessibility

Sports and physical activity are popular outlets for enjoying one's free time. As a result, many facilities have made new activities more accessible. Someone living in a major city might never visit a mountain, yet can enjoy wall climbing at a local YMCA or sport center. Some homes include exercise rooms so that busy owners can work out when it fits into their schedules. For these individuals it is important to understand training principles so they can develop their own exercise regimens. The needs of youth are varied in a physical education program. Curricula that align with the standards will identify conceptual learning, and provide youth with ways to stay physically active throughout a lifespan.

Choice

Despite what we know about the importance of physical activity and leading a physically active lifestyle, we live in a sedentary society. Too many people select sedentary activities because they have greater appeal than more physical ones. Physical education programs must have a major focus on helping children and youth choose to be physically active, and provide them with the skills and knowledge to design their own physical activity and fitness plans to carry them through adulthood. Success and enjoyment of our programs as they move through school is one way to facilitate this effort, because we tend to choose to take part in the things we enjoy.

Accountability

As stated earlier, one of the biggest components of educational reform has been the idea of accountability. In 1983, Placek found that many physical education teachers planned lessons primarily to keep students busy, happy, and "good." Although these are factors of a strong program, they are not enough alone—learning and achievement must also be an outcome. In some schools, physical education was marginalized and administrators didn't care about what students learned in physical education, as long as the classes were under control. In these schools, physical education often turned into recreation programs, with large numbers of students engaged in game play rather than instruction. In other schools, physical education became a setting where students could choose to just sit and watch others participate. In still other schools, a few days were devoted to instruction but the majority of time was spent in game play. Since learning didn't need to be documented, some administrators didn't pay much attention to what was happening in physical education. Times have changed, and the accountability movement is as important for physical education as it is for reading or mathematics.

Time

Today, because of the No Child Left Behind legislation (2001) time is a precious commodity in schools. Teachers in subjects that are tested in state-wide assessment programs are under pressure to document student learning. Physical education must become part of this accountability system if we are to keep our programs and make them viable. In states where physical education is not part of the accountability formula, some administrators have cut time available for physical education so that students can spend additional time on subjects that are tested, despite there being no documented evidence that this practice improves test scores on a long-term basis (Wechsler, 2008). If physical education is going to continue to be part of the school curriculum, teachers must find a way to connect with the educational goals of a school, and document their contribution to meeting these goals. Schools are being held accountable for student learning, and physical education is not exempt from this accountability.

How Does Planning Differ for Traditional Standards-Based Curricula?

The process of curriculum development with a standards-based format is different from the process used in planning traditional curricula. Whereas traditional curriculum development begins with identifying activities for students, a standards-based curriculum does not. The major difference between the two is that a standards-based curriculum requires those developing the curriculum to look first at what they are trying to accomplish before identifying activities that will help students attain those standards. In states where there is strong accountability (i.e., rewards and sanctions based on whether students meet standards), districts pay closer attention to whether their students are able to meet the standards.

In a standards-based curriculum, once teachers have decided what students should know and be able to do, they must decide on the level of performance. National content standards talk about competency in motor skills and movement patterns to perform a variety of physical activities. What number does "a variety" represent? What level of performance does "competency" represent? Identifying performance levels for standards helps define the standards. This process also can be part of educational renewal as teachers discuss their expectations about how good is "good enough" to satisfy the intent of the standards. These and other discussions occur as curriculum writers "unpack the standards," a process that is explained in detail in Chapter 2.

The Role of Assessment in a Standards-Based Curriculum

The second part of the paradigm shift with standards-based curricula involves the use of assessment. Assessments are a key part of the standards-based curriculum process as those developing curricula must decide what they are going to accept as evidence that students have met the standards. Additionally, they must decide at what point(s) students are going to demonstrate competence. Because exit outcomes are assessed when students have taken their last physical education class, in some districts, this may be as early as 9th grade. Teachers and school districts will also usually assess students prior to this final evaluation to see whether they are making adequate progress toward the exit outcomes. Some states have mandated when students will be assessed. In states where there are no state mandates, districts make these decisions.

The types of assessments used for a standards-based curriculum must be aligned with the standards. Although this might seem like a simplistic statement, in some cases there is a disconnect between the standards and the assessments. For example, if the state adopted standards similar to the national content standards, a paper and pencil test would not be an adequate measure for Standard 1 (competency in motor skills and movement patterns to perform a variety of physical activities). Many states have been reluctant to implement *performance-based assessments* because they are costly to administer and evaluate. It is also difficult to hire evaluators who can visit a site and administer the assessments (which is the way the United Kingdom holds programs accountable). South Carolina addresses this dilemma by requiring teachers to videotape student performance and submit 20% of the tapes for review by a panel of experts at the state level. New York is also working to develop a state accountability system in physical education. Other states have directed school districts to develop assessment systems that measure student learning and achievement of standards. The challenge of assessing physical education performance is an issue that will need to be resolved when adding physical education to a state-testing mandate.

Selecting Activities in a Standards-Based Curriculum

A standards-based curriculum calls for a careful selection of activities with adequate time provided for students to strive toward and master them. When viewing an entire standards-based program, it would appear that fewer sports and activities are offered, and instructional units tend to be extended for longer periods of time. This reflects the "less is more" principle and is built on students gaining competency in many activities, and even mastering a few. It is also intended that as students become knowledgeable with one activity they will be able to transfer that knowledge to other activities with similar characteristics. The "exposure curriculum" of the more traditional multi-activity programs simply does not allow this depth of knowledge and transfer.

Teachers often feel they are on a teeter-totter when they plan for and deliver a curriculum in physical education. On one hand, a primary function of education is to provide students with the skills and information that they will need to be active as adults. Participation patterns for adults are very different from those of youth. Physical education programs need to take these differences into consideration as they prepare students to be active adults. On the other hand, we know that if students are going to choose to be physically active as adults they must enjoy physical activity as youth. A wonderful article in *Educational Researcher,* "Lessons from Skateboarders" (Sagor, 2002), highlights the time, energy, sweat, and injury many youth will go through just to master a skateboarding skill, yet when they get to school they are unmotivated and lack interest in learning. Although what we teach should not be dictated by what the students want, we must find ways to pull them in, motivate them to persevere, and provide them with what is important, relevant, and worth their time and energy to master. This also might mean that our programs offer activities that are taking place in the community after school and on weekends and encourage students to participate in them beyond the physical education class.

Although providing options is a key to meeting the standards, activities included in the curriculum must be evaluated in terms of their contribution. For instance, golf is a great lifetime sport, but its contribution to fitness is minimal. Gymnastics contributes to the aesthetics as well as the flexibility component of fitness, but it is not something in which older adults usually participate. Activities must be selected not only for their individual contribution, but also for their impact on the overall education of the child. Just as a jigsaw puzzle needs all the pieces to show the correct picture, a curriculum needs to have all the pieces (activities) necessary for a child to be physically educated. The curriculum must have a balance between activities for the present and those for the future.

Teachers also must remember that students are very different in their activity preferences. All students are not alike—some enjoy backpacking, whereas others prefer the aesthetics that dance and gymnastics provide. Additionally, different activities are popular in different regions. Imagine trying to teach ice hockey in Alabama, and trying not to teach it in upstate New York! Clogging is a very important dance form in North Carolina, but few (if any) people in

New Mexico go clogging on a regular basis. When deciding how to meet the intent of the national content standards, each of the previously mentioned activities has its place and contribution. Teachers must select a variety of activities that will allow students to meet the standards, while respecting the participation preferences regarding physical activity in their region of the country.

One alternative is to have a main theme as the organizing center or central thrust of a program around which content is developed to meet specific goals or standards (Siedentop & Tannehill, 2000). A variety of activities presented through main theme models (e.g., net, invasion, and target games in sport education; hiking, fishing, and camping in outdoor education; trust, cooperative games, and low-level initiatives in adventure education; and basic motor skills in developmental education) will increase opportunities for students to reach these goals or standards to their fullest extent. The standards reform initiative has forced schools and school districts to think differently about what is taught, and why it is included in the curriculum.

Summary

A standards-based curriculum is complex and requires a great deal of thought to develop and implement. Writing clear goals and purposes for a physical education curriculum, and then developing assessments to measure these goals, are the first steps when creating a standards-based curriculum. A variety of curricular models may be adopted that provide interesting lenses through which to create a program. The curricular models will be explained in later chapters found in Section II. Physical education programs can be exciting and provide challenging learning opportunities for students. Additionally, they make a positive contribution to the health and well-being of those who participate in and complete the program. Although some individuals are resistant to the standards movement, we see it as an opportunity to redesign the way we think about physical education. Developing a standards-based curriculum is seen as a vehicle for educational renewal, as well as the first step toward building a quality physical education program.

References

Burgeson, C., Wechsler, H., Brener, N., Young, J., & Spain, C. (2003). Physical education and activity: results from the school health policies and programs study 2000. *Journal of Health, Physical Education, and Recreation, 74*(1), 20–36.

Deal, T., Byra, M., Jenkins, J., & Gates, W. (2002). The physical education standards movement in Wyoming: an effort in partnership. *Journal of Physical Education, Recreation, and Dance, 73*(3), 25–28.

Doolittle, S. (2003). *Assessment programs in New York State: a whole village's effort.* Paper presented at the National Conference for the American Alliance for Health, Physical Education, Recreation, and Dance, Philadelphia, PA.

Erickson, H. L. (2002). *Concept-based curriculum and instruction: teaching beyond the facts.* Thousand Oaks, CA: Corwin Press.

Fisette, J., Placek, J., Avery, M., Dyson, B., Fox, C., Franck, M., Graber, K., Rink, J., & Zhu, W. (2009). Developing quality physical education through student assessments. *Strategies, 22*(3), 33–34.

Guskey, T. (1996). *Alternative ways to document and communicate student learning.* Read by author. Cassette recording no. 296211. Alexandria, VA: Association for Supervision and Curriculum Development.

Jacobs, H. H. (1997). *Mapping the big picture.* Alexandria, VA: Association for Supervision and Curriculum Development.

National Association for Sport and Physical Education. (1992). *Outcomes of quality physical education programs.* Reston, VA: Author.

National Association for Sport and Physical Education. (1995). *Moving into the future: national standards for physical education.* Reston, VA: Author.

National Association for Sport and Physical Education. (2004). *Moving into the future: national standards for physical education* (2nd ed.). Reston, VA: Author.

Peterson, S., Cruz, L., & Amundson, R. (2002). The standards impact on physical education in New York State. *Journal of Health, Physical Education, Recreation and Dance, 73*(4), 15–18, 23.

Placek, J. (1983). Concepts of success in teaching: busy, happy and good? In T. Templin & J. Olson (Eds.), *Teaching in physical education* (pp. 46–56). Champaign, IL: Human Kinetics.

Rink, J., Mitchell, M., Templeton, J., Barton, G., Hewitt, P., Taylor, M., & Dawkins, M. (2002). High stakes assessment in South Carolina. *Journal of Health, Physical Education, Recreation and Dance, 73*(3), 21–24.

Rink, J. (2000 July). *Linking physical activity and fitness.* Presented at the National Conference sponsored by the National Association of Sport and Physical Education on Content Standards 3 and 4. Baltimore, MD.

Sagor, R. (2002). Lessons from skateboarders. *Educational Leadership, 60*(1), 34–38.

Siedentop, D. (1998). *Introduction to physical education, fitness, and sport* (3rd ed.). Mountain View, CA: Mayfield.

Siedentop, D., Mand, C., & Taggart, A. (1986). *Physical education: teaching and curriculum strategies for grades 5–12.* Palo Alto, CA: Mayfield.

Siedentop, D., & Tannehill, D. (2000). *Developing teaching skills in physical education* (4th ed.). Mountain View, CA: Mayfield.

Veal, M. L., Campbell, M., Johnson, D., & McKethan, R. (2002). The North Carolina PEPSE Project. *Journal of Health, Physical Education, Recreation and Dance, 73*(4), 19–23.

Wechsler, H. (2008). *Physical education in the United States: a status report from the CDC's 2006 school health policies and programs study.* Presentation made at NASPE's general session at the 2008 AAHPERD national convention in Ft. Worth, TX.

Additional Resources

Bulger, S., Housner, L., & Lee, A. (2008). Curriculum alignment: a view from physical education teacher education. *Journal of Physical Education, Recreation, and Dance, 79*(7), 44–49.

Carr, J., & Harris, D. (2001). *Succeeding with standards: linking curriculum, assessment, and action planning.* Alexandria, VA: Association for Supervision and Curriculum Development.

Castelli, D., & Beighle, A. (2007). The physical education teacher as school activity director. *Journal of Physical Education, Recreation, and Dance, 78*(5), 25–28.

Cooper Institute. (2002). *FITNESSGRAM test administration manual* (2nd ed.). Champaign, IL: Human Kinetics.

Corbin, C., & McKenzie, T. (2008). Physical activity promotion: a responsibility for both K–12 physical education and kinesiology. *Journal of Physical Education, Recreation, and Dance, 79*(6), 47–50.

Eisner, E. (1995). Standards for American schools: help or hindrance? *Phi Delta Kappan, 76,* 758–764.

Hirsch, S., & Killion, J. (2009). When educators learn, students learn: eight principles of professional learning. *Phi Delta Kappan, 90,* 465–469.

Kirk, D., Penney, D., Burgess-Limerick, R., Gorley, T., & Maynard, C. (2002). *A-level physical education: the reflective performer.* Champaign, IL: Human Kinetics.

Lambert, L. (2000). The new physical education. *Educational Leadership, 57*(6), 34–38.

Landers, D., & Kretchmar, S. (2008). Focus and folk knowledge. *Journal of Physical Education, Recreation, and Dance, 79*(6), 51–56.

Lawson, H. (2007). Renewing the core curriculum. *Quest, 59*, 219–243.

Lee, A., & Solmon, M. (2007). School programs to increase physical activity. *Journal of Physical Education, Recreation, and Dance, 78*(5), 22–24, 28.

Lewis, A. (1995). An overview of the standards movement. *Phi Delta Kappan, 76*, 744–750.

Locke, L. (2008). Three examples of kinesiology in physical education: why, how, and for whom? *Journal of Physical Education, Recreation, and Dance, 79*(7), 50–54.

Locke, L. (1990). Why motor learning is ignored: a case of ducks, naughty theories, and unrequited love. *Quest, 59*, 346–357.

Lynn, S. (2007). The case for daily physical education. *Journal of Physical Education, Recreation, and Dance, 78*(5), 18–21.

McCullick, B., & Chen, A. (2008). Introduction: *Journal of Physical Education, Recreation, and Dance, 79*(6), 46, 55–56.

Napper-Owen, G., Marston, R., Volkinburg, P., Afeman, H., & Brewer, J. What constitutes a highly qualified physical education teacher? *Journal of Physical Education, Recreation, and Dance, 79*(8), 26–30.

National Alliance for Nutrition and Activity. (n.d). *Model school wellness policies.* Retrieved December 17, 2008, from http://www.schoolwellnesspolicies.org

No Child Left Behind Act of 2001. Pub.L. No. 107-110, 20 U. S. C. section 6301 (2001).

President's Council on Physical Fitness and Sports. (2002). *The president's challenge.* Washington, DC: President's Council on Physical Fitness and Sports.

Thomas, J., Thomas, K., & Williams, K. (2008). Motor development and elementary physical are partners. *Journal of Physical Education, Recreation, and Dance, 79*(7), 40–43.

Tyler, R. (1949). *Basic principles of curriculum and instruction.* Chicago: University of Chicago Press.

Welk, G., Wood, K., & Morss, G. (2003). Parental influences on physical activity in children: an exploration of potential mechanisms. *Pediatric Exercise Science, 15*, 19–33.

Wiegand, R., Bulger, S., & Mohr, D. (2004). Curricular issues in physical education teacher education. *Journal of Physical Education, Recreation, and Dance, 75*(8), 47–55.

Woods, A. M., Graber, K. (2007). Stepping up to the plate: physical educators as advocates for wellness policies—part 1. *Journal of Physical Education, Recreation, and Dance, 78*(5), 17, 21.

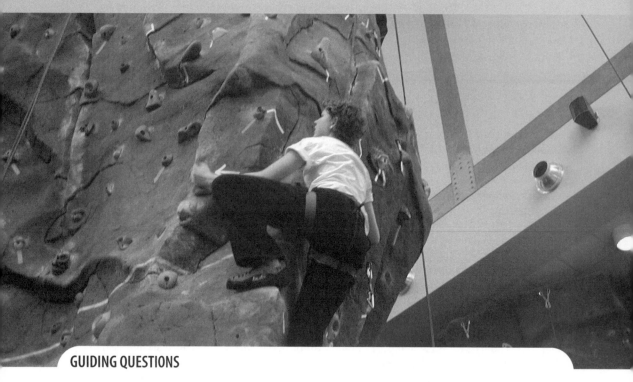

GUIDING QUESTIONS

1 What does it mean to suggest that a program "stands for something important"?

2 When we "unpack the standards," what are we doing and what are the implications?

3 What is a philosophy, and how do you develop it?

4 What do you consider to be the "goods" of physical education?

5 What is meant by a teacher's "value orientation," and why is this important in the curriculum development process?

6 Describe the emphasis of each value orientation (physical education content, the needs and interests of individual learners, and/or the goals of society) and what they might look like in practice. How do they impact curricula?

7 How are a teacher's values and expectations for student learning linked to the standards?

8 Why will the curricular decisions teachers make necessarily be different?

9 Who are the stakeholders in the curriculum process?

10 What is the relationship between enjoyment and learning (gaining competence)?

11 Describe the instructional alignment triad. How does this impact teaching and learning?

12 What aspects of the community influence curricular decisions?

13 What is the formula for calculating the amount of time available for physical education? What is the relationship between time and student learning?

14 What scheduling options are available to provide sufficient time for learners to interact with physical education content?

15 How might scope and sequence be viewed differently when teaching toward standards?

16 How might technology advances impact curricular decisions in physical education?

17 How do educational and political forces influence curricular decisions?

18 What is meant by "backward design"?

Building a Quality Physical Education Program

Deborah Tannehill, University of Limerick
Jacalyn Lund, Georgia State University

Curriculum development is about designing **quality programs**, programs that mean something, are built on a philosophy that reflects the values and beliefs of teachers, and have important goals, assessments aligned with those goals, and instructional practices and learning experiences that facilitate student learning. In this chapter, we will examine what we believe makes a quality physical education program, and then proceed to the process of creating a district and building curriculum. We will discuss issues that influence curriculum decisions, and the impact of these decisions for instructional design. To conclude the chapter, we will provide a list of questions to guide teachers in developing the physical education curriculum within a school district framework.

A Quality Program Stands for Something

The experiences that students have in the name of physical education should amount to something significant, something worthwhile, and something worth their time and energy to achieve. Physical education should be taught using effective teaching strategies that have been shown to improve student learning. Learning experiences should be exciting and serve

quality programs Programs that mean something; are built on a philosophy that reflects the values and beliefs of teachers; and have important goals, assessments aligned with those goals, and instructional practices that move students from the goal to a demonstration of learning.

to motivate students to choose to be active, to take responsibility for their own physical activity experiences, and to challenge them to gain competence. These experiences must be integrated with methods of assessing student progress as a means of their demonstrating and recognizing success, achievement, and learning. These assessments will also serve the teacher in the redesign of the instruction and student experiences to better facilitate students' achieving success. Unfortunately, these aspects of the teaching learning cycle are not always present because students frequently experience little articulation of a sound, sequential, or coherent physical education program across K–12 where they have the opportunity to be successful. Activities are often taught year after year, in the same way, with little emphasis on new skills, more complex applications, or transfer to different sports or settings. Part of the problem is teachers who fail to define what their program stands for, and what they want students to know and be able to do upon completion of their physical education experience. Another part of the problem is the lack of district-wide planning intended to develop a coherent program that stands for something important.

With the continuing focus on standards and high stakes assessments, districts have redesigned curricula toward students achieving a set of standards for which they are held accountable. But, what does this mean? Standards do not identify the content to be taught. Standards do not identify how content is delivered. **Standards** do identify what has been deemed worth students' knowing and being able to do (National Association for Sport and Physical Education [NASPE], 2004, 2009c). From this perspective, standards might be thought of as a set of meaningful learning goals to guide curriculum development. Teachers must be able to interpret the standards and make choices about how to reach them based on their own philosophies, those of their colleagues, and those of the students whose needs the curricula are designed to meet.

Unpacking the Standards

How do we move from the more global national or state standards, to a district and building programmatic philosophy, to a specific curriculum that is aligned to foster student learning? The "key," of course, is student learning, and must be the focus of our curricula:

- What is worthy of student learning?
- What is worth student time and effort?
- What is meaningful and relevant to the lives of students?

standards   What students will know and be able to do as a result of participating in a quality physical education program.

If our goal is student learning, rather than simply covering content, these are the questions we must ask. To answer them, as a group of teaching colleagues we will look to the standards that have been identified, which represent at a minimal level what we, as a profession, believe is worth students' knowing and being able to do in physical education. Again, keep in mind that the standards are merely guidelines, and must be defined by teachers based on their own values, beliefs, and philosophies.

When teachers define the standards, they **unpack the standards** to clarify what they mean, in order to determine how they might best be achieved and student success measured. In a sense, the performance indicators that accompany the standards are a sample of unpacking the standards. Teachers need to do the same thing for their programs, their needs, and their students. The standards must be unpacked on two levels (Figure 2.1). First, they must be unpacked conceptually. This might be done by asking such questions as what is the intent of the standard, how has the standard evolved, how might it be interpreted? The second level of unpacking revolves around teachers selecting activities and curriculum models based on their beliefs and philosophy, and determining how the conceptual learning will be implemented. In other words, what activities and curriculum models will facilitate student learning most effectively? Using an analogy, the activities and curriculum are the vehicle used to get you to the final destination (meeting the standards). The type of car selected to make the trip is based upon personal preference. Some teachers prefer a sports car, whereas others want a Jeep. Some teachers will choose to use the Teaching Games for Understanding model (Mitchell & Oslin, Chapter 10), whereas others will select Outdoor Education (Stiehl & Parker, Chapter 9). Just as options on each type of car can vary (automatic transmission vs. stick shift; bucket seats vs. bench seat; convertible vs. hard-top), activities within the curriculum model vary according to the resources

Level 1: Conceptually	Level 2: Delivery and Content
• What are their intent? • How did they evolve? • How might they be interpreted?	• What curriculum model? • What activities? • How will conceptual learning be implemented?

FIGURE 2.1 Unpacking the standards on two levels.

unpack the standards   Define the standards to clarify what they mean, what skills students should be able to demonstrate, how they might best be achieved, and how to measure student success.

available and the personal preferences of the people doing the driving (teachers), or riding as a passenger (students).

Unpacking the standards requires that teachers examine their beliefs about teaching and learning in physical education. It requires defining what each standard means at each grade level, and how students might demonstrate achievement. Unpacking the standards asks several major questions: what do they mean, what skills should students be able to demonstrate, which concepts are essential for students to apply? After the standards are unpacked and interpreted, teachers will determine what content is best suited for the students in their particular setting, and select curriculum models that best match their philosophy and beliefs.

What Would It Look Like to Unpack the Standards?

As we unpack the standards it is important for us to clarify that we, the authors, believe the standards are integrated and interrelated; in fact, it is difficult to view them in isolation. The standards can be viewed differently depending on the activity or movement form for which they are applied and the curriculum model chosen for their delivery. This will become clear as you review our unpacking examples.

Standard 1: For some, developing competency in motor skills and movement patterns (Standard 1) is the focus of physical education; however, most would argue that this important component does not stand alone. Developing basic motor skills and movement patterns is essential for children as they learn to move in a physical activity setting. The Skill Themes curriculum model (Holt/Hale, Chapter 7) outlines the progression of skill development as progressing from mastery of basic skills to combinations of skills to more complex and specialized movements/skills, and finally to application of these skills in authentic and realistic settings. Human nature suggests that we tend to enjoy and seek to participate in activities in which we are successful. Helping young people develop skills (throw, hop, kick, leap) and then ultimately apply these skills to specific activity/sport techniques in which they experience success is the main focus of Standard 1. However, successful participation in dance, aquatics, sport, or outdoor activities requires not only mastery of these skills and movement concepts, but also integration of concepts and principles from the other standards.

Standard 2: Success with the more complex skills and activities mastered in Standard 1 requires understanding of movement concepts, principles, strategies, and tactics as they apply to the learning and performance of physical activities (Standard 2). The acquisition of sufficient skill in a sport does not necessarily allow young people to use those skills effectively in game play. A major focus of Teaching Games for Understanding (Mitchell & Oslin, Chapter 10) is to help participants understand when and why to use a particular skill and anticipating what the outcome is likely to be. This notion of encouraging young people to be more competent and knowledgeable games players and decision makers is the crux of Standard 2. Another view of this standard can be seen through the mechanical principles related to balance (lower center of gravity, widen base of support, weight balanced over base), which are critical for developing competent performers in various activities from dance to gymnastics to low-level initiatives to diving. Another example is making the connection between sport psychology and exercise physiology and understanding the implications for a young person's selection of and participation in a fitness program (McConnell, Chapter 13). The importance of linking these areas is seen with girls and young women who are plagued with concern about how they look. The resulting poor body image can have implications for their feelings of self-worth. Drawing on principles from sport psychology will assist these students in accepting who they are while concepts from exercise physiology will assist them to develop their own activity regimes through application of the FITT (frequency, intensity, time, type) principle.

Standard 3: What would it look like for students to participate regularly in physical activity (Standard 3)? Having students physically active during a sport experience on a daily basis, accumulating a set number of steps while completing an in-class hike, or taking part in a round of golf would all fit the standard. However, keep in mind that the activity selected is not the outcome but the means to achieving an outcome. In this case, the outcome is learners choosing to be physically active through an activity of their choice. Teachers might identify the following as skills, knowledge, or behaviors they would expect to see their students develop:

- Participate in physically active play outside of school
- Begin to recognize the connection between physical activity and good health (feeling good)
- Choose moderate to vigorous types of activities in which to take part
- Begin to use technical skills learned in physical education in self-selected forms of activity
- Monitor physical activity
- Set and monitor personal physical activity goals
- Knowingly select physical activities in the community that meet their interests
- Apply appropriate principles and concepts to their physical activity choices
- Demonstrate effective movement skills to be successful in chosen activities
- Apply behavior change principles to their own physical activity habits

Choice of curricular model will be based on programmatic philosophy and what the teachers identify as the goods of physical education. Then, decisions will be made on choice of content (activities) to match the model, to meet the needs of learners, and for which there are facilities and equipment.

Standard 4: Unpacking Standard 4, which is for students to achieve and maintain a health-enhancing level of physical fitness, might start with what we want them to achieve when they exit high school. For example, one district might begin with the expectation that students will design a fitness program with a monitoring system to log progress and keep a reflective journal focusing on their feelings about the experience. In this case, unpacking the standards would unfold in a progressive way, identifying the necessary skills and knowledge, including such components as a basic understanding of fitness concepts and terminology; taking responsibility for personal fitness; developing skill in planning, performing, and monitoring fitness activities; demonstrating an understanding of components of health-related fitness; applying appropriate training principles for developing fitness; and ultimately designing an appropriate personal fitness program that enables students to achieve desired levels of fitness.

Standard 5: How about students exhibiting responsible personal and social behavior that respects self and others in physical activity settings (Standard 5)? Students following classroom routines for using equipment safely, demonstrating fair play during competition, calling personal infractions when they occur in game play, or inviting a less-skilled peer to be a warm-up partner before class begins would demonstrate progressive achievement of this standard. Unpacking would require teachers breaking down specific and progressive outcomes that they would want to see their students demonstrate across K–12. This might include overarching topics such as employing safe physical activity behaviors; complying with rules, routines, and procedures; demonstrating appropriate etiquette; building a community of learners; participating ethically; demonstrating fair play; working independently or in groups; positively interacting in physical activity settings; resolving conflicts when they occur; and initiating responsible behavior. It is important to keep in mind that social responsibility can be taught through physical activity and curricula designed to focus on these components.

Standard 6: Students valuing physical activity for health, enjoyment, challenge, self-expression, and/or social interaction is the focus of Standard 6. Opportunities for participation in physical activity vary by such factors as community, age and ability of participant, and venues available. Helping young people to identify their interests, assess their ability levels, and access locations in the community where they might seek to participate and improve skills is an important role for physical education. In some ways, Standard 6 might be considered a by-product of the other standards. For instance, if children and youth are able to develop competent skill and movement patterns, use appropriate concepts and strategies to implement these developing abilities, have exciting and challenging opportunities to be physically active, and possess a level of fitness to participate and succeed in a fair and socially responsible way, then it is likely they will develop a value for their choice of activity. Achieving success will enhance self-esteem, enjoyment, and the desire to continue to pursue physical activity. It might be that the Cultural Studies curriculum (O'Sullivan & Kinchin, Chapter 12) is one way for young people to come to understand the place of physical activity in their own lives, school, and community and to ultimately make a difference in what teachers offer to meet their needs and interests.

Each of these examples demonstrates how the standards might be unpacked and interpreted for program design. It will be up to each teacher and each school district to interpret the standards based on values, beliefs, philosophy, and what is ultimately deemed important for students to know and be able to do as a result of their physical education programs. We need to continually remind ourselves that we will not be able to do everything, teach every activity, provide each student with exposure to all that is available in our field—this suggests that we make good choices about the activities we choose after unpacking the standards rather than trying to cover everything. In addition, we need to continually remember that the activities we select are not the outcomes but the means to achieving an outcome.

In reading the scenario presented in Figure 2.2, note how these middle school teachers chose to focus on NASPE Standards 3, 5, and 6. Their interpretation of the standards was based on their desire for students to appreciate and enjoy nature, the out-of-doors, and participate cooperatively and respectfully in outdoor activities. It is also apparent that there is at least one other standard that goes beyond physical education that is a major focus: environmental goals that are drawn from the health standards. This lends support to the notion that the standards are not isolated, but might be viewed and taught interactively both within physical education and across other content areas.

A Philosophy

What is a **philosophy**, and how is it developed? A philosophy is made up of the beliefs and values of those responsible for delivering the program, the students the program serves, and the community within which the program is housed. As a teacher, it is critical that you come to terms with what you believe about physical education and how those beliefs play out in practice. What a teacher believes to be of most value to students, and how they should experience learning and be assessed on it, will have an impact on what happens in the name of physical education. These philosophical viewpoints will help determine what is

philosophy   What a person believes and values.

As the teachers at Truman Middle School set out to plan the year, they decide that they want to offer students choices within their physical education requirement. One option was influenced by the district being located in a part of the country that has access to rivers, lakes, and Puget Sound, in addition to large mountain ranges that offer an abundance of outdoor activities. The teachers would like to provide their students with the opportunity to come to appreciate and enjoy nature, the out-of-doors, and participating in outdoor activities (NASPE Standards 3 and 6). In addition, they are concerned with the negative and sometimes abusive behaviors that they have been witnessing among their students, and would like to help them learn to interact more cooperatively and respectfully with one another (NASPE Standard 5). When considering these two "big picture" goals, the teachers decide that combining two main theme curriculum models, adventure education with outdoor education, is the direction to move for one of their course options.

Mrs. Charboneau is going to deliver the outdoor adventure program to the students across the entire semester. She has determined that while Standards 3, 5, and 6 are the major emphasis, she will indeed be able to provide opportunities for her students to achieve aspects of Standards 1, 2, and 4, as well. Here is the plan. Four end-of-semester goals are set for the students to achieve. Learners will successfully and cooperatively participate as a group on a 3-day camping trip, safely set up and maintain the campsite, participate skillfully in outdoor and adventure activities such as hiking, fishing, kayaking, and a 7- to 15-mile hike, and problem solve any situations that arise. Physical education will become the arena in which this content is taught and practiced throughout the semester.

Part of the standards-based curriculum are formative and summative assessments that demonstrate not only whether learning is taking place, but that, in fact, it does occur. A series of weekly student journal entries reflecting cooperative efforts, combined with teacher observation, will reveal how the class is doing at becoming a camping community and respecting one another. In addition, the teacher is going to keep a log of the number of conflicts that arise during class in an attempt to see if students are becoming better able to avoid conflicts, or resolve them when they do occur. Tasks such as setting up a campsite on the sports field and demonstrating how they will store perishables and other food sources, will provide evidence of readiness in the camping area. Developing sound bites to share with the class on topics and concepts such as leave no trace, hiking with a buddy, or steps to avoid hypothermia will become part of the preparation, and also serve as assessments. On Tuesdays and Thursdays, cardiovascular fitness days to prepare for the long hike, the students will wear heart rate monitors and keep a log of the time they spend in their training zones. Ultimately, whether or not they successfully participate in and achieve their 3-day camping trip goals will be the true test of success.

This is an actual semester-long course taught at Truman Middle School in Tacoma, Washington.

FIGURE 2.2 An example of how teachers might implement a curriculum.

worth students' learning, what it will look like in the overall program, what is emphasized, and how it is delivered. Although a teacher's beliefs cannot be the sole determinant of what a program will include or how it will be delivered, it is crucial that teachers know what they believe is important, and how that might mesh with teaching colleagues and translate into a programmatic philosophy that will guide decisions based on the standards (Figure 2.3). How will the program philosophy be translated into practice, into choices for student learning, into what the program will stand for, into reality?

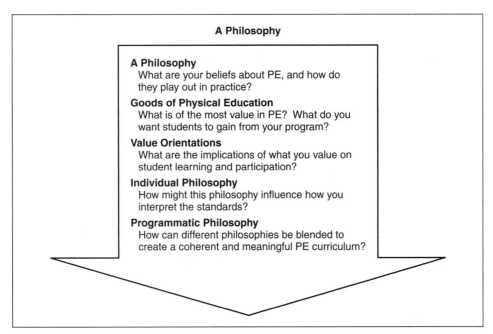

A Philosophy

A Philosophy
What are your beliefs about PE, and how do they play out in practice?

Goods of Physical Education
What is of the most value in PE? What do you want students to gain from your program?

Value Orientations
What are the implications of what you value on student learning and participation?

Individual Philosophy
How might this philosophy influence how you interpret the standards?

Programmatic Philosophy
How can different philosophies be blended to create a coherent and meaningful PE curriculum?

FIGURE 2.3 Developing a philosophy.

Goods of Physical Education

To develop a philosophy toward physical education and its role in the education process, Siedentop and Tannehill (2000) suggest that teachers begin by asking, "What goods do students acquire from a physical education program?" In other words, what do we consider to be of most importance in physical education? What skills, knowledge, and behaviors do we want students to achieve before they leave our programs? Some would say the primary good is students having the skills and knowledge to design and participate in a lifetime fitness program; others would suggest the ability to participate successfully in a variety of games and sports. Participating in an ongoing physical activity program might be another response, whereas having the "know how" to camp and recreate in the out-of-doors will be most important to someone else. Cooperating with others in problem solving and group challenges that could carry over into all aspects of life might be the response of one physical educator, whereas students taking responsibility for their own physical activity experiences might be what is most important to a colleague. Obviously, our answers will be varied and based on our own experiences and passions, the characteristics and needs of the students in our programs, nuances of the communities in which we teach, and what is currently valued by society.

When attempting to identify what you consider to be the **"goods" of physical education**, think about what it is that you really want students to gain from your program. What do you want them to be able to do that will help them lead healthy and physically active lives? Although one of the goals of education is to transmit our culture from one generation to the next, we need to be cautious that we don't merely transmit traditions of the past without considering what could be in the future. This suggests that we identify "goods" that have implications for the future and a changing society. You can't know the frustration of observing a physical education program today that looks exactly like the one I experienced when in primary and secondary school. Forty years ago, the program met my needs, was enjoyable, and gave me the skills and knowledge to make physical activity choices. However, this is a different era, society has changed, physical activity opportunities have changed and expanded, what we know about motivating youth to be physically active has grown, and the needs of youth due to lifestyle choices are markedly different. With this and more in mind, the "goods" of physical education are hopefully different as well. Develop your list of the "goods" of physical education for primary, intermediate, middle school, and high school.

What a teacher considers the "goods" of physical education, as well as his or her philosophy towards physical education, is based upon participation in movement experiences and many years as a student in physical education classes. As you will see in the next section, Ennis (2003) extends the notion of what a teacher values, to the decisions made in the development of curriculum.

Value Orientations

Ennis refers to a teacher's beliefs about education and learning as the teacher's **value orientation** (Ennis, 1992; Jewett, Bain, & Ennis, 1995), which reflects his or her views on "what students should learn, how they should engage in the learning process, and how learning should be assessed" (Ennis, 2003, p. 111). Typically, a teacher's value profile reflects a blend of these value orientations (Ennis & Chen, 1993). The contextual factors discussed later in this chapter will influence whether teachers are able to teach all that they consider important, and in ways that are consistent with their philosophy and values. As you read through a description of the five value orientations, note where the emphasis is placed, on physical education content, the needs and interests of individual

---

"goods" of physical education   What a teacher believes to be of the most importance in physical education.

value orientation   Teachers' beliefs on what students should learn, how they should learn it, and how it should be assessed.

learners, and/or the goals of society. Attempt to determine how your own values fit in to each of the orientations described and what a program would look like to meet these teacher values.

DISCIPLINARY MASTERY. Mastery of the subject matter is the major focus of this perspective, and defines a body of knowledge as what students should know and be able to do in physical education. Disciplinary mastery is the predominant value orientation in physical education, and is reflected by students who are able to first demonstrate basic movements, skills, and concepts, and then successfully use them in more complex and realistic applications. The current thrust toward standards and accountability supports the disciplinary mastery perspective. Disciplinary mastery is most effective when teachers have access to adequate facilities and equipment, time for students to gain proficiency, class size that allows high rates of practice and frequent teacher feedback, and students who are interested in learning the content.

LEARNING PROCESS. When viewed from a learning process perspective, providing students with process skills to continue learning is as important as the content itself. With the knowledge explosion that we are experiencing in all content areas, and a lack of time for students to learn all that is important, the need for students to learn process skills has become critical. These skills include technology, communication, problem solving, self-assessment, conceptual abilities, and application of new skills and knowledge. Teachers who focus on learning process deliver content in systematic and progressive ways that require learners to grapple with what they are learning, use their knowledge and skills to problem solve, and develop their own solutions to situations in physical activity settings. Students are most successful with this type of learning environment when they are already independent learners, and are able to work cooperatively with their peers.

SELF-ACTUALIZATION. Focus on the student is the cornerstone of the self-actualization perspective. The focal point becomes individual growth, development of self-esteem, and the setting and meeting of personal goals. This learning environment would emphasize individual achievement and excellence over subject matter content. When moving toward a self-actualization curriculum, the movement, sport, and fitness tasks and activities are designed to match the needs and interests of students. All students feel valued in this type of program as their voices and interests are sought and incorporated into programmatic decisions. Students are most successful when they are willing to persevere, even in difficult situations. The self-actualization teacher is most successful when given the flexibility to design programs with individual students as the focus.

SOCIAL RESPONSIBILITY AND JUSTICE. Equity, social justice, and developing interpersonal skills and relationships in a physical activity setting that emphasizes race, gender, and class equity, are highlighted within this orientation. Students learn to cooperate; examine issues related to fair play, gender roles, and equal opportunity; and make decisions about ways to overcome injustices they identify. Students are encouraged to and are given opportunities for developing positive personal behaviors to respond to injustice. They learn to take responsibility for their own behavior in equity situations through thoughtfully developed, applied, and progressive lessons. Teachers are able to reach these types of outcomes when given license to offer a flexible physical education that has equity and social justice as its focus.

ECOLOGICAL INTEGRATION. The ecological integration perspective views the individual holistically within the larger natural environment. This suggests a balance among subject matter content, the needs and interests of the individual, and the social setting—matching the content to the learning in selected settings so that students learn meaningful "real-life" applications. Individual students and groups of students learn to work together toward common goals, and come to understand when compromise is necessary to address individual and/or group concerns. The final outcome is students who are able to apply what they learn in one setting to situations that occur in another, while keeping the best interests of all participants at the forefront. Having adequate time to effectively design instruction and learning experiences that allow students to gain knowledge, as well as social responsibility within personally meaningful situations, is a challenge.

Articulating an Individual Philosophy

As individual teachers reflect on what they see as the goods of physical education and identify what they value about the learning process, they need to intentionally develop their own philosophy. This personal philosophy of physical education might serve as a lens through which to view the standards, and guide interactions with teaching colleagues about programmatic and curricular decisions.

Developing a Programmatic Philosophy

At this point teachers are ready to work with their colleagues to link their beliefs to the standards, and begin to develop a programmatic philosophy to guide teaching and learning in physical education. Where possible, we strongly encourage involving all physical educators in the process of selecting "goods," identifying what they value, and reflecting on how the standards might be emphasized across the curriculum. As suggested above, accepting ownership in a curriculum is a key factor in teachers using it; involvement in the process is critical.

Blending the philosophies of a number of different teachers can be a stressful and challenging task, yet one that is necessary if we are to offer a meaningful and congruent physical education program to children and youth. One example of a philosophy of physical education (Lambert, 2001) suggests that Standard 3 is the ultimate goal for youth to achieve by the time they graduate from high school (Figure 2.4). In order for students to reach this goal of demonstrating, practicing, and persisting in a physically active lifestyle, they must achieve the other standards as well. In other words, it is a holistic process of learning. To choose to be physically active requires students to value physical activity for any one of a number of reasons (Standard 6). Valuing is typically the result of having reached a level of competence in motor skills (Standard 1), and sufficient knowledge about how and when to employ those skills (Standard 2). Being able to participate cooperatively with others in physical activity (Standard 5) is also necessary for valuing and enjoyment. Reaching a level of fitness (Standard 4) that allows you to participate in physical activities of your own choosing becomes a by-product of your physically active lifestyle. Now, this is just one perspective. Another colleague might have a strong bias for teaching skill (Standard 1) and knowledge (Standard 2) as the major focus of physical education. Becoming knowledgeable and competent movers would be considered a precursor for achieving the other standards. This perspective might be based on the belief that the primary contribution to the overall curriculum is psychomotor, and that the cognitive aspects are necessary to carry out the psychomotor.

Neither of these two viewpoints is correct or incorrect, just different. Both philosophies will allow students to meet the standards; they merely approach the standards from different perspectives. However, in order for us to design a coherent and meaningful curriculum to meet the needs of our students, we need to be able to form some consensus on a programmatic philosophy that reflects each of our beliefs in such a way that we can each take ownership in its design and delivery. In the preceding example, if these teachers were to discuss what they think are the most important goals at the different age levels across K–12, they might find that they share similar perspectives on a number of standards to

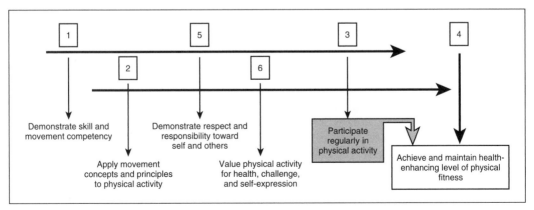

FIGURE 2.4 An example of Standard 3 as the ultimate goal of physical education.

emphasize at different points. For instance, they both might agree that students gaining competency in basic skills and movement concepts is the "key" for the primary grades, while learning to work cooperatively within a group is critical during the middle school years, and that being capable of designing a personal physical activity plan is necessary before graduating from high school.

A task that we have found useful during this collaborative process to help teachers identify which standards they believe should receive the most emphasis at each level is displayed in Table 2.1. Emphasis does not suggest that other standards will not receive attention, just that the main focus will be on the standard deemed most appropriate for a particular age level. Keep in mind that the standards can be distributed across the curriculum in different ways based on teachers' values and beliefs about what is most important. The NASPE

TABLE 2.1

Standards Emphasis at Each Level

Determine what you believe should be the major emphasis at each level by ranking the standards for each grade level range.

Standards	K–2	3–5	6–8	9–12
Standard 1 Demonstrates competency in motor skills and movement patterns needed to perform a variety of physical activities				
Standard 2 Demonstrates understanding of movement concepts, principles, strategies, and tactics as they apply to the learning and performance of physical activities				
Standard 3 Participates regularly in physical activity				
Standard 4 Achieves and maintains a health-enhancing level of physical fitness				
Standard 5 Exhibits responsible personal and social behavior that respects self and others in physical activity settings				
Standard 6 Values physical activity for health, enjoyment, challenge, self-expression, and/or social interaction				

standards document (1995, 2004) identifies student expectations and sample performance outcomes across grade level designations. Although it might be interpreted to mean that all standards receive equal emphasis at each grade level, this need not be the case because there are numerous ways the standards can be distributed to guide program development.

Building the Curriculum

Once a programmatic philosophy has been developed, it will guide all curricular decisions, of which there will be many. How does a teacher, a department, or a school district go about designing a physical education curriculum that has its focus on learners and learning? Ideally, this process should be an inclusive K–12 collaboration with all physical educators playing a role so that ownership might ultimately guide implementation of a sound and progressive curriculum. Unfortunately, and realistically, this is often not the case. Typically, committees are assigned the task of visiting or revisiting the K–12 curriculum, and individual teachers and departments are consulted as the process evolves. The result is often a curriculum that focuses on activities rather than learning, and programs that are not sequentially developed across K–12, which frequently are not meaningful to the children and youth for whom they are intended. Often we see a **curriculum guide** compiled that is intended to direct what is delivered in the name of physical education, yet it includes specific objectives for every conceivable activity, and as a result becomes unmanageable and impossible to deliver within the time available. One of the problems that results from this practice is what many have noted as teachers setting out to **"cover the curriculum"** (Lambert, 2003; Siedentop & Tannehill, 2000). Rather than focusing on student learning, the focus is on covering the content that has been outlined in the curriculum guide.

How do we move from the standards themselves to developing a meaningful curriculum to be delivered to children and youth? Perhaps the most crucial response to this is the idea of instructionally aligning 1) what we intend for students to learn, 2) how we assess to determine their success, and 3) what and how we teach and students practice. Figure 2.5 outlines steps for building the

curriculum guide   A formal document that identifies the objectives that students are to achieve in a subject area and the activities that will make up the content of the program.
"cover the curriculum"   When teachers focus on teaching everything outlined in the curriculum guide rather than focusing on student learning.

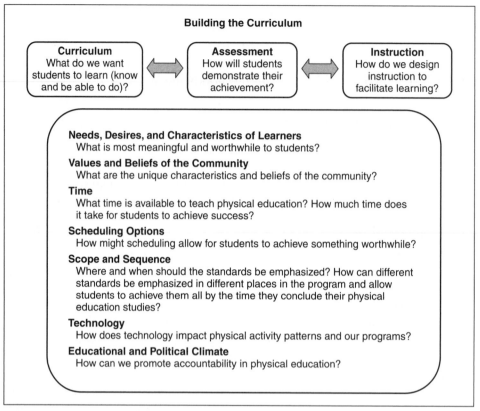

Building the Curriculum

| **Curriculum** What do we want students to learn (know and be able to do)? | | **Assessment** How will students demonstrate their achievement? | | **Instruction** How do we design instruction to facilitate learning? |

Needs, Desires, and Characteristics of Learners
What is most meaningful and worthwhile to students?

Values and Beliefs of the Community
What are the unique characteristics and beliefs of the community?

Time
What time is available to teach physical education? How much time does it take for students to achieve success?

Scheduling Options
How might scheduling allow for students to achieve something worthwhile?

Scope and Sequence
Where and when should the standards be emphasized? How can different standards be emphasized in different places in the program and allow students to achieve them all by the time they conclude their physical education studies?

Technology
How does technology impact physical activity patterns and our programs?

Educational and Political Climate
How can we promote accountability in physical education?

FIGURE 2.5 Steps in building the curriculum.

curriculum and highlights the notion of instructional alignment. **Instructional alignment** is equally as important at the district curriculum level as it is at the individual lesson level, because we know that the closer the alignment, the stronger the learning (Cohen, 1987; Walker, 1998).

Goals

The first piece of the instructional alignment triad is reflected in our goals for student achievement. Our programmatic values, beliefs, and philosophy guide us as we unpack the standards in an effort to identify what it is that students will learn in physical education. In a sense, our philosophy becomes the lens by which we develop our goals to reach the standards. We must keep in mind that

instructional alignment   Alignment of what we intend for students to learn (goals), how we determine student success (assessment), how we teach, and how students practice (instructional strategies).

standards reflect minimal expectations. Teachers can always go beyond the standards and expect more from students—usually resulting with students stepping up to the plate and being successful. Problems occur when teachers expect less from all students. Our programmatic philosophy will help shape what these expectations will look like and how we might challenge students to achieve above the minimum.

Assessment

The second piece of the triad is assessment. Designing assessments that match the learning goal is critical. What do we want students to achieve, and how might they demonstrate success? Does all learning have to be demonstrated in the same way? No. Just as all students learn differently, so do they demonstrate learning in varying ways. It is up to the teacher to provide opportunities for students to demonstrate their success, their mastery, their competence, and their level of achievement. Success is measured by student achievement, and what better way than to allow learners to select the way they can most effectively and authentically demonstrate that achievement.

Instruction

The final piece of the triad is instruction. How do we design instruction to facilitate learning? It must be done intentionally, thoughtfully, creatively, and in an inviting and individually motivating way. As Parker and Stiehl (Chapter 6) note, "What is taught is inextricably linked to how it is taught." Instruction is designed through a set of learning experiences that are facilitated through various instructional strategies and methods. These learning experiences must move learners through tasks that progress from less to more difficult, add complexity and diversity, and eventually lead to the meaningful performances that represent what you want students to learn. These tasks might involve skills/movements that are performed statically or dynamically, have increased numbers of movements, cause learners to move alone or with others, or require modified equipment to change complexity.

Curricular Considerations

Teachers will need to collectively make curricular decisions about the type of physical education their program will deliver to their students, to allow them to meet the standards and become physically educated individuals. Will the curriculum and instruction decisions teachers make always be the same? No. Not all children and youth must learn the same things, through the same learning experiences, nor should they be required to demonstrate what they know and are able to do in the same way. Teachers might better ask, "What are the important outcomes that I want these students to gain from this physical education program that will lead to achieving the standards set for physical education?" In order to reach these outcomes, teachers must discover the needs, desires, and characteristics of their learners, recognize what they value about teaching and learning, come to understand factors such as the values and beliefs of the community, consider how time constraints and scheduling options bind their decisions, recognize how technology has impacted education, and be informed about educational and political forces that influence students, teachers, and curricular decisions.

Needs, Desires, and Characteristics of Learners

From our perspective, the primary stakeholders in the curriculum process are the students and the physical education teachers. This view is based on the fact that teachers are the content experts, and the students are those for whom the curriculum is designed. The two together are those who actually "live" the curriculum. However, as teachers, we must be cautious in determining what we think learners need in order to reach the standards without consulting them about their interests, identifying their learning styles, understanding the life issues with which they must contend on a daily basis, and a host of other factors that will impact their learning.

How do we go about identifying the needs of our learners and using the information we garner to inform our decisions? Peters (1988) suggests we listen: listen frequently, carefully, and systematically, listen for facts, feelings, and perceptions. What are we listening for, and how will we recognize it when we hear it? Often adults—including teachers—don't listen to children and youth as much as we could, and miss some of what might inform us about their needs. Beyond listening, observing student performance, and identifying where they struggle, discovering how they spend their time away from school, talking with parents to gain a different perspective on a young person's life, conducting surveys and needs assessments, and assessing performance in classes are all ways to identify learner needs. Providing learners the opportunity to delve into their own physical activity experiences and those of their family, school, and community might be fostered through the Cultural Studies curriculum (O'Sullivan & Kinchin, Chapter 12). As we plan for learning, we might think of students' needs as the gap between the skills and knowledge they currently have and can apply, and those we wish them to possess. The "key" is to fill that gap through meaningful and worthwhile content that is engaging to learners.

During her student teaching, one of my preservice teachers was frustrated that her pupils were not cooperative, seemed disinterested in taking part in activity, and were basically ruining her lesson. When asked if the lesson was exciting, challenging, or relevant to the students' needs and interests, her response was, "probably not." When asked if the lesson was designed for students to be actively involved in making their own decisions or choices, her response was, "no." When asked if she would want to take part in the lesson if she were a student, she responded, "not really." So, why was she surprised that her students chose mutiny?

We are not suggesting that a curriculum be based solely on what students want to do. What we are suggesting is that teachers find out what is most meaningful and worthwhile to students. What is exciting to them? Which activities do they choose to take part in outside of school? Do they prefer to work alone or in groups? Are they competitors or recreational players? Are they interested in the out-of-doors, or do they prefer fitness or rhythmic type activities? Do they want to dance or play games? Do they have a desire to discover more about themselves and their family involvement in physical activity? Teachers need to intentionally design programs that allow students to participate in a preferred activity that will motivate them to persevere in their efforts to improve and develop skills, knowledge, and understanding. At the same time, it is important to introduce students to new activities that they might eventually come to enjoy and even prefer. Too often we see the same physical education being offered year after year, despite the changing needs and interests of students. Common sense tells us that a third grader enjoys different activities at different levels of participation than a tenth grade student. As Lambert (2003) states, "Although we certainly want students to enjoy what they are doing—why else would they be motivated to try or persist—our primary goal should be that they enjoy and engage in something worth learning" (p. 131).

Sagor (2002) suggests that we all possess five needs and the inherent desire to satisfy them. He goes on to explain that satisfying these needs will result in a full commitment to an activity or event:

- Need to feel competent
- Need to belong
- Need to feel useful
- Need to feel potent
- Need to feel optimistic

He describes how these needs were satisfied through activity by the skateboarders we talked about in Chapter 1 (Lund & Tannehill). As they achieved mastery of their skateboard skills their sense of *competence* developed, they recognized the link between their hard work and their success (*potency*), and acknowledged that to continue to be successful they must continue to "put in the time" (*optimism*). These skateboarders became affiliated with and members of a group who used a common language and wore distinctive clothing (*belonging*), and through sharing experiences and helping one another in learning new skills and achieving success, they developed a sense of *usefulness*. The message for us to draw from the experiences of these skateboarders is to design curricula that will meet students' needs in motivating and challenging ways.

Only then will they be willing to commit themselves to excelling at learning, and develop the desire to persist at trying.

Growth and developmental characteristics of learners are critical considerations for curricular design. When determining teaching practices that are developmentally appropriate for all children, we must consider each child individually. We must examine their changing needs and abilities, their body composition and size, their physical activity patterns and fitness levels, their previous experiences, and levels of skillful movement. Resources to guide us have been developed by NASPE, and are thoroughly outlined in a series on appropriate instructional practices for elementary, middle, and high school levels (2004, 2009a, 2009b, 2009c).

Diversity among our student population in American schools is growing annually. We see this diversity in racial and ethnic backgrounds, religious beliefs, economic and social class distinctions, skill and fitness levels, students for whom English is their second language, differences in learning styles, sexual orientation, motor and cognitive disabilities, and body size and composition, to name a few. In recent years, teachers have become more conscious of and more concerned with providing learning opportunities for all children and youth who attend our schools. With this growing awareness and need to reduce the achievement gap among American youth, we have chosen to include a chapter focused on providing meaningful and inclusive learning experiences for all students (Timken & Watson, Chapter 5).

Values and Beliefs of the Community

Although the learners are the primary benefactors of a curriculum, it is crucial that we recognize that others can inform our decisions and provide us with a broader, and perhaps clearer perspective of life in a given school district, and the implications this has for curriculum development. For example, understanding the unique characteristics of a community will help us recognize the beliefs and values of those who directly influence the school district and its programs. Do they support health and physical education? Do they believe our content is an integral part of a child's total education? Are there ethnic, religious, or cultural beliefs that will impact our curricular decisions? Are there recreation programs within the community that might support programmatic efforts? Is the community located in a region that has access to specific venues (e.g., lakes and rivers, walking or hiking trails, bikeways, bowling lanes, tennis courts, swimming pools)? Are there neighborhoods that require bus transportation, and therefore limit student access to after-school activity designed to support physical education program options? Conducting a systematic analysis of the community and identifying factors such as economic and physical resources; the ethnic, religious, and educational backgrounds of the residents; social and recreational opportunities available; and political forces that impact schools will provide pertinent information to consider when designing the curriculum. O'Sullivan, Tannehill, and Hinchion (in press) describe a school ethnography assignment based on an in-depth analysis of the school and community and interpretation of the implications for their teaching practice.

Not only should physical educators consult the community about the beliefs and values they want youth to acquire, but we must also educate them about "best practice" in physical education. Many in the community did not like physical education when they were growing up, and continue to believe it is not worthwhile. Others believe physical education should be exactly what it was in the past: tradition built on exercise and restricted to sport. It is our responsibility to help the community understand what we are attempting to do in physical education, the goals and standards that guide our programs, how we intend to facilitate students achieving those standards, and how this links to what is important and relevant to children and youth. For example, one middle school teacher introduced disk activities (ultimate, freestyle, field events, golf), and was told by the administration and parents that this was not appropriate content for physical education. "These are activities that are done in parks on weekends and aren't educating students," they said. It was up to the teacher to help them understand that disk is appropriate, focuses on learning motor skills, and will in fact enable students to achieve one or more of the NASPE standards (Standards 1, 3, and 5). Using the games classification system (Almond, 1986), Ultimate is an invasion game, while disk golf is a target game. If we build on the teaching games for understanding philosophy (Mitchell & Oslin, Chapter 10) our focus would be on students being able to transfer knowledge of what to do and when to do it across similar game forms. Instead of teaching Ultimate, soccer, hockey, and basketball as isolated games with specific skills, we would help learners determine how to solve tactical problems that are common to all invasion games, which on-the-ball skills to use (specific to each invasion game), and the off-the-ball movements to support them. It would also be appropriate to point out to parents, administrators, and others in the community that if kids are playing disk activities on weekends, it would be terrific if *all* kids knew how, could be successful, and wanted to participate.

Time

As we consider the extent of what we have identified as significant for student learning in physical education, and the knowledge, skills, concepts, and attitudes it would take for students to achieve success and mastery, we might ask, "How will we have time?" In the state of Washington it has been suggested that it would take 24 years of daily interaction with every content area for a student to reach all of the Essential Academic Learning Requirements–EALRs (state standards). We know that our children and youth do not have this kind of time with our content. In physical education we often have 30 minutes once a week at the elementary level, which of course equates to two hours per month, or 18 hours per year, hardly enough time for students to reach all of the standards. Similar time crunches exist for physical education at the middle school and high school, as well. So, teachers must make choices on which standards to emphasize at different grade levels, and consider which expectations their students can conceivably reach in the time available, keeping in mind that our focus is on student learning as opposed to covering the content.

Teachers must calculate the amount of available time they have to deliver content, provide students practice of the content, and assess student performance and achievement. Across the district and at each level, the amount of time available will be quite different as requirements for physical education, class length, and loss of time due to circumstances outside of our control all vary. Using the simple formula of multiplying the number of class sessions offered per week, times the number of weeks in the school year, times the length of each class session, gives you an estimate of the time available for instruction, learning experiences and practice, and assessment of learning.

    Number of class sessions per week
$\times$ Number of weeks in school year
$\times$ Length of each class session
= Estimate of time available

However, this is just the first estimate; we also must take into consideration those times when we lose physical education due to such uncontrollable events as assemblies, pep rallies, and teacher inservice days. Based on past experience, how much time might this be? It will vary, of course, yet we suggest that 8 to 10% of the available days will be lost. In addition, be sure that you don't count time allocated for dressing at the beginning and end of middle and high school physical education into the time available for student learning.

    Estimate of time available
$-$ 8–10% of available days for loss of time due to uncontrollable events
$-$ Minutes for dressing at middle and high school
= Available time for student learning in physical education

Once you have determined time estimates across the K–12 curriculum, it provides you a foundation upon which to base the program design, and the distribution of content into this time framework. The key is to limit the scope of the curriculum to those activities that you really have time to teach.

Another issue related to time asks the question, "How much time does it take for learning to occur?" You might consider how long it took you to become skilled in your chosen physical activity. As you identify goals you want your students to achieve, lay out how much time you will devote to teaching it and allowing students to practice through meaningful and challenging learning experiences. It is often quite a shock to realize that you don't have time to teach all that you believe is important for them to learn, and that you must make still further choices.

Scheduling Options

Typically, physical educators do not have control over or a voice in scheduling decisions for their content and classes. At the elementary level, we see classes ranging from 30 to 45 minutes one, two, or three days per week, often a 4-day rotating schedule, and generally with students from one class passing those from another at the door as they enter and leave the gymnasium. This schedule is most often determined by classroom teachers in conjunction with the administration, and takes classroom teachers' planning time into consideration. At the middle and high school levels we often see students grouped for other content areas (i.e., math, music, language), with physical education scheduled to accommodate these specific course needs. More and more frequently we see 6-period days giving way to 3- to 4-period days of 80- to 120-minute classes. This can be a blessing for our content area because it provides more time for student mastery, or it can be a disaster when teachers do not use the extra time wisely. Two hours to be actively involved in physical activity might be considered too much for students to handle, so some teachers are offering the more traditional 50-minute lesson, extending time in the locker room, and then having students come in to the gym and wait. What an unfortunate way to handle what others have found to be a boon for physical educators and their programs (Bryant & Claxton, 1996; Shortt & Thayer, 1998–99). We see courses being designed within courses as a possible way to effectively use the blocked time frame. For example, some schools might offer 30 minutes of fitness followed by adventure or cultural studies. This would allow students to work toward Standard 4, and then move on to other standards through various curriculum models. Other teachers are using the extra time during a sport education season to facilitate students becoming more literate games players who are better able to play the game successfully, rather than just perform isolated skills, or for building a sense of affiliation within teams.

The "key" is to select an organizational arrangement that allows sufficient time for students to achieve something worthwhile in physical education. This suggests that we become knowledgeable about how scheduling is done in our settings, know who the players are that impact these decisions, determine how much time we need to allow students to achieve standards, and make certain that we are invited to participate in these administrative discussions. Only then will our content be considered based on its needs relative to student learning.

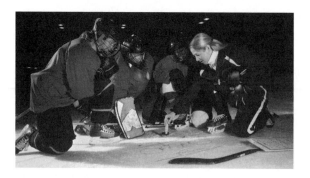

Scope and Sequence

What is a scope and sequence, and what might it look like in a standards-based curriculum? The **scope** of the curriculum traditionally refers to the content to be taught, its focus, and the activities selected within the content. **Sequence** refers to the order or progression in which learning activities are presented. As we select activities for our programs, we must consider those that will allow us to reach our goals, those that we have the facilities and equipment to deliver, and perhaps most importantly from our perspective, those that are meaningful, relevant, and worthwhile for our students. We must keep in mind that not all learners will have the same desires, passions, interests, or goals. When teaching toward standards, our task is to help each student find a physical activity outlet that he or she will enjoy, and have the skill to participate in over a lifetime. We must help students discover what it is they enjoy about physical activity: the competition, the group nature of activity, the individual pursuit of competence, or whatever else motivates them. This prompts two questions:

> *Should we deliver a **multiactivity program** where students experience short units of a variety of activities?*

No, by providing a coherent and meaningful curriculum, our programs should help students make informed and positive choices that might stay with

scope   Traditionally refers to the content being taught, its focus, and the activities selected within the content.

sequence   Refers to the order or progression in which learning activities are presented.

multiactivity program   A program characterized by a wide variety of activities intended to expose students to physical activity options. Units are short in nature, often as many as 10–12 per year, with little time for students to become proficient in any one activity. The focus tends to be on students being active rather than on learning.

them throughout their lives. The short units traditionally associated with a multiactivity curriculum do not allow students time to gain sufficient competence in any activity. We believe that competence will lead to success and that this success is critical for developing lifelong participation habits. As you move through this book, you will see how this can be done effectively by selecting from the main theme curriculum models to provide depth, coherence, and a specific focus.

Should we teach only content and activities that students will use as adults?

Some would suggest, yes. It is our belief that we should not get caught up in treating young people as miniature adults. Although we want them to be able to apply what they learn in physical education across their lives, we need to allow them to participate in, learn from, and enjoy activities they value as children and youth. For example, the likelihood of a young man skateboarding into adulthood is not strong, yet as a teenager, this might be an important outlet for him, and one at which he excels. Although some would argue that he has not gained a skill that he can carry over into adulthood, we would argue that he has gained a sense of accomplishment, has experienced success, as well as the knowledge that hard work and practice are necessary to achieve competence; all attributes which are surely worth learning. A young girl may not choose to play soccer when she leaves school, but during middle school this is an engaging activity during which she interacts with her peers and learns to be a supportive and enthusiastic team player. Teaching children and youth the process of learning through activities they find enjoyable and meaningful will be our best effort at helping them to choose to be physically active, and have the skill and knowledge to do so.

With a standards-based curriculum, scope and sequence can be viewed a bit differently. If the standards are what guide our design of the curriculum, then we might also view where and when the standards are emphasized as part of a program's scope and sequence. As you completed Table 2.1, you identified where you thought each standard should be emphasized, and hopefully as a group of district teachers you were able to discuss, negotiate, and come to agreement on a district perspective (see Table 2.2 for one district's effort). There is no correct or incorrect choice on where the emphasis is placed—it will look quite different from one district to another. The "key" is to link it to what you value for students at specific levels, while at the same time making sure that students will become competent on all standards by the time they finish with their physical education studies.

If our focus is on student learning and the specific needs of our learners, the activities and curriculum models chosen to reach the standards might vary among schools within a district as well. Although every child and young person might have the opportunity to reach the standards, they may be given different options and opportunities due to the school setting, the facilities and equipment

TABLE 2.2

One District's Effort at Prioritizing Standards to Be Emphasized Across K–12 (Ranked 1, 2, and 3)

Standards	K–2	3–5	6–8	9–12
Standard 1				
Demonstrates competency in motor skills and movement patterns needed to perform a variety of physical activities	1	2	2	
Standard 2				
Demonstrates understanding of movement concepts, principles, strategies, and tactics as they apply to the learning and performance of physical activities	2	3		
Standard 3				
Participates regularly in physical activity			1	3
Standard 4				
Achieves and maintains a health-enhancing level of physical fitness				1
Standard 5				
Exhibits responsible personal and social behavior that respects self and others in physical activity settings	3	1	3	
Standard 6				
Values physical activity for health, enjoyment, challenge, self-expression, and/or social interaction			3	2

available, the resources in the community to support different options, and student interests. This would suggest that the sequence of learning activities might vary markedly within a school district. Is this appropriate? If choices were based on these five points (setting, characteristics and needs of learners, facilities/equipment, community resources, personal interest of teachers and students), then we think so. As you will recall, students learn in different ways; have different interests; can learn and reach the standards through a variety of activities, learning experiences, and curriculum models; and can demonstrate their achievement in a variety of ways.

The *Moving into the Future* document (NASPE, 2004) provides guidance to physical educators through a description of student expectations based on what a student should know and be able to do at the end of grade level ranges. In addition, it identifies sample performance outcomes in the form of behaviors we might see students demonstrate as they progress toward achievement of the standard. We would like to emphasize that the sample performance outcomes are just that, samples. They do not represent a comprehensive list of what students should know and be able to do. They merely represent a "starter kit," and it is up to the curriculum committee to decide the performance outcomes that will be appropriate for students in that community to meet the content standards. How you use these materials will depend on what you have learned about yourself, the students, and the community, and what you have available in your own setting. You and your colleagues will outline what your own students will be able to do at different points along their journey through your physical education program.

Technology

Technological advances have had a huge impact on children and youth in our culture as we see them spending more time playing computer games or surfing the Internet, and less time being physically active. Our young people are generally more computer and technology savvy than their parents and, in many cases, their teachers. The advancement of technology into our public schools has grown rapidly, yet applications in some educational settings are limited by a lack of teacher technology literacy, funding problems that prevent some school districts from taking full advantage of what is available, and issues with keeping up with such a rapidly changing field. In physical education, we have access to a variety of technology tools that can enhance teaching and the learning experiences of students, such as Palm Pilots, laptop computers, heart rate monitors, digital cameras, and pedometers, to name a few. We have connections to the Internet in schools, and an abundance of information that can be accessed there; software programs that allow teachers to track student progress, report grades to parents, and develop newsletters using desktop publishing; and electronic messaging systems that provide teachers with opportunities to interact with colleagues, parents, and students. As we make curricular decisions, we must consider the impact of technology on physical activity patterns and behaviors of the future, as well as how it impacts programs today. There is much discussion of late on the appropriateness of using video games and activities as part of the physical education curriculum. Hayes and Silberman (2007) challenge us to think differently about the use of these resources as a means to motivate, increase understanding, and improve performance. Leight (2008) describes a blog as being similar to an online journal. She provides ideas on their use in physical education by sharing four types of blogs that can be employed: teacher communication, dialogue generator, student, and teacher. In a recent article, Banville and Polifko (2009) share ideas on how to use digital video technology to record pupil performance with a system that allows them to immediately view and critique that performance. An example of a webquest activity that can be incorporated into the physical education program and motivate interaction by young people is included on the website to accompany this text.

Educational and Political Climate

Curricular reform is on the agenda in all states with the focus on standards and accountability. Several states have used the NASPE standards as the framework to design their own standards, which in turn have been directly linked to curricular reform efforts (e.g., New York, South Carolina) and state assessment systems. How standards, accountability, and curricular reform initiatives are playing out varies from state to state, which is consistent with our decentralized system of education in this country. Most states are developing state assessment systems of student learning in all content areas. Physical education is still on the periphery in some states, and not among the content areas assessing student achievement of the standards. In still other states, physical educators are being required to teach a period of reading to students who failed this portion of the state assessment. A few states are requiring schools to design and implement classroom-based assessments in physical education as a precursor to becoming part of a state assessment system. If physical education is not able to move into the accountability arena with other content areas, this could ultimately have an impact on its status, and whether it is retained as a requirement. It behooves every physical educator and curriculum development committee to be informed about what is taking place within his or her state, to advocate for accountability, and to take an active role in influencing decisions that impact programs.

Implications for Instruction

As we suggested previously, it is difficult to separate instruction from curriculum. If instruction is not done well and has not been intentionally designed to facilitate students reaching specified learning goals, then we have not been successful in developing students who can meet the standards we have identified as most worth their achieving. Designing a curriculum to meet standards carries with it several instructional implications of which we should be familiar, including teaching the process of learning and backward design.

Teaching the Process of Learning

When we teach students the **process of learning,** they are actively involved; they pose questions and grapple with how to answer them; they move from a problem to be solved to gaining the knowledge, skills, and principles they need to

> **process of learning** Involves active learners posing questions, problem solving possible answers using their knowledge and skills, and transferring the new knowledge to other content and settings.

solve it; and they realize how this new learning might be transferred to another situation (Lambert, 2003). As Lambert suggests, "content and facts follow concepts and principles" (p. 139) through an experiential process of learning.

Frequently, learning in schools is achieved through the teaching and practice of isolated skills and knowledge, which is not characteristic of how we live, and not as rich as it could be. We don't live with different aspects of our lives separated into boxes, but rather in a holistic way as a complete person. The standards may be viewed in just such a way. Although the standards are written individually they must be viewed as overlapping, interlocking, integrating, and holistic. We may emphasize one or another at different times, yet they must be pulled together and likened to an individual as a whole and complete person. The outdoor adventure scenario (Figure 2.2) provides an instructionally aligned example of planning and teaching to the standards, and represents teaching the process of learning rather than isolated skills and knowledge.

To intentionally plan for this depth of learning requires us to know where we are headed, what our intentions are for student learning, and what it will look like when they finish our program. This is best achieved through curriculum design that is based on the principles of **backward design** (Wiggins & McTighe, 1998), because it "emphasizes what students should know and be able to do with what they know when they exit high school" (Lambert, 2003, p. 140).

Backward Design of the Curriculum

Backward design (Wiggins & McTighe, 1998), the outcomes approach (Spady & Marshall, 1991), or design down curriculum process (Lambert, 2003) suggests designing from exit goals back toward the beginning, from where you want to go to where you start, from high school down to elementary school. And, of course then the "key" is to deliver back up, to teach forward toward the outcomes you have selected as the worthwhile knowledge and skills for students to achieve when they exit high school (Figure 2.6).

Three questions to guide our work through the backward design process are:

What do we want students to know and be able to do as a result of participating in our programs?

Answering this requires us to identify our intended outcomes that emerge as we unpack the standards. This is the important "stuff" of our content area,

---

backward design   Intentional planning in which the teacher begins with the exit goals and designs the curriculum toward those goals; from high school down to elementary school.

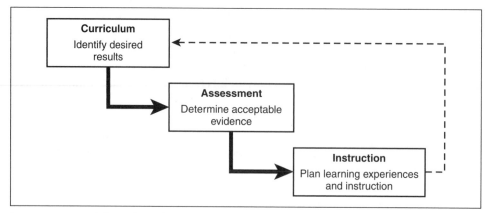

FIGURE 2.6 Bacward design (down) and delivery forward (up).

and the focus of student learning. Due to there being more content than students can realistically achieve, we must make choices on what we think is most important for students to achieve in physical education. These might be considered what Wiggins and McTighe (1998) call "enduring understandings" (p. 70), and represent what we want students to retain as they progress through our programs. Similarly, Erickson (2002) encourages us to teach the key concepts that will help students understand the relationships between significant learning experiences.

How will we know when they have been successful?

This is where assessment comes in. What evidence will demonstrate that students have learned and have achieved the standards? Identifying what will serve as acceptable evidence should be determined up front, and the assessments themselves designed prior to beginning instruction. This will ensure that there is alignment between what we want and what we measure.

How can we get them there in the most challenging and engaging ways possible?

Instruction is the means for achieving the goals we identify as worth students' knowing and being able to do (learning). Instruction must be intentional and purposeful, yet does not happen until after the learning goals and assessment are determined. Aligning instruction with goals and assessments is necessary if learning is to occur.

Lambert (2007) uses a three-legged stool as a metaphor to emphasize the importance of these three steps: curriculum, assessment, and instruction. If all three legs of the stool are given equal weight, the stool is solid. If any of the legs is removed or not attended to equally, the stability is removed.

Questions to Guide the Design of a Standards-Based Curriculum

Now that you have been introduced to the pieces of curriculum design, let's put it all together. When standards are used effectively to guide development of curriculum, the result is a program that reflects continuity and coherence across the K–12 program. As we suggested early on, the ideal situation would be to have all physical educators involved in the process with input from students and others. However, realistically, curriculum development or redesign usually takes place by committee. The committee must be intentional about seeking input throughout the process so that it results in a shared endeavor. Questions to guide curricular design that have been discussed in-depth previously in this chapter are identified below. Grappling with them and coming up with answers that all teachers can live with is necessary if the program is to achieve its intent.

1. What will the standards "look like" when unpacked at each level?
2. What do we view as the "goods" of physical education?
3. What are our shared values/beliefs?
4. What is our programmatic philosophy for physical education?
5. Which standards should be emphasized at each level?
6. Which of the main theme curriculum models can facilitate student learning and achievement of the standard(s) at each level?
7. What worthwhile and meaningful learning goals will meet the standard(s)?
8. How much time will it require to teach these goals at the respective grade levels?
9. How can students demonstrate success, mastery, or achievement of the learning goals, and ultimately, the standard(s)? What assessment evidence will be acceptable?
10. What is the most effective way to facilitate students meeting these goals/standards?
11. How can learning be achieved in interactive and holistic ways by teaching kids the process of learning?

As noted previously, instructional alignment is as important at the curricular level as at the instructional level. When making your curricular decisions, make sure that there is alignment between what you believe is of most value and the instructional strategies and learning experiences you develop. Alignment of goals, assessment, and instruction will strengthen and reinforce student learning.

Summary

Quality programs stand for something important and worthwhile. They are based on a clearly articulated philosophy of physical education that develops as teachers come to terms with what they believe is most important for students to learn. Quality programs reflect an alignment between learning goals that evolve from the philosophy, the assessments that determine if students reach the intended goals, and the instructional practices that provide students the opportunity to achieve success.

As we move through the curriculum development process, our decisions must be influenced by factors related to our beliefs about physical education, the needs of our learners, opinions and perceptions of the community, and contextual issues related to time, facilities, and scheduling. We must keep in mind that curriculum development is about change. It is about improving what is and what has been. It is about moving into the future with learning experiences and assessments that are designed to move students toward filling the gap between what they now possess and what we have identified as worthwhile for them to know and be able to do in physical education. It is about making choices on how to best facilitate learning for our students in a coherent and cohesive way.

References

Almond, L. (1986). Reflecting on themes: a games classification. In R. Thorpe, D. Bunker, & L. Almond (Eds.), *Rethinking games teaching*. Loughborough, UK: University of Technology.

Banville, D., & Polifko, M. F. (2009). Using digital video recordings in physical education. *Journal of Physical Education, Recreation, and Dance, 80*(2), 17–21.

Bryant, J., & Claxton, D. (1996). Physical education and the four-by-four schedule. *The Physical Educator, 53*, 203–209.

Cohen, S. (1987). Instructional alignment: searching for a magic bullet. *Educational Researcher,* November, 16–20.

Ennis, C. A. (2003). Using curriculum to enhance student learning. In S. J. Silverman & C. A. Ennis (Eds.), *Student learning in physical education: applying research to enhance instruction* (pp. 109–127). Champaign, IL: Human Kinetics.

Ennis, C. D. (1992). Curriculum theory as practiced: case studies of operationalized value orientations. *Journal of Teaching in Physical Education, 11*, 358–375.

Ennis, C. D., & Chen, A. (1993). Domain specifications and content representativeness of the revised value orientation inventory. *Research Quarterly for Exercise & Sport, 64*, 436–446.

Erickson, H. L. (2002). *Concept-based curriculum and instruction: teaching beyond the facts.* Thousand Oaks, CA: Corwin Press.

Hayes, E., & Silberman, L. (2007). Incorporating video games into physical education. *Journal of Physical Education, Recreation, and Dance, 78*(3), 18–24.

Jewett, A. E., Bain, L. L., & Ennis, C. D. (1995). *The curriculum process in physical education* (2nd ed.). Boston: WCB/McGraw Hill.

Lambert, L. T. (2001). A presentation delivered at the request of the Washington state Office of Public Instruction.

Lambert, L. T. (2003). Standards-based program design: creating a congruent guide for student learning. In S. J. Silverman & C. A. Ennis (Eds.), *Student learning in physical education: applying research to enhance instruction* (pp. 129–146). Champaign, IL: Human Kinetics.

Lambert, L. T. (2007). *Standards-based assessment of student learning: a comprehensive approach* (2nd ed.). Reston, VA: National Association for Sport and Physical Education.

Leight, J. (2008). Technology tips: lifting the fog on instructional blogs. *Journal of Physical Education, Recreation, and Dance, 79*(2), 52–56.

National Association for Sport and Physical Education. (1995). *Moving into the future: national standards for physical education.* Boston: McGraw-Hill.

National Association for Sport and Physical Education. (2004). *Moving into the future: national standards for physical education* (2nd ed.). Boston: McGraw-Hill.

National Association for Sport and Physical Education. (2009a). *Appropriate practices for elementary school physical education.* Reston, VA: AAHPERD.

National Association for Sport and Physical Education. (2009b). *Appropriate practices for high school physical education.* Reston, VA: AAHPERD.

National Association for Sport and Physical Education (2009c). *Appropriate practices for middle school education.* Reston, VA: AAHPERD.

O'Sullivan, M., Tannehill, D., & Hinchion, C. (in press). Teaching as professional inquiry. In R. Bailey (Ed.), *Physical education for learning: a guide for secondary schools,* New York: Routledge.

Peters, T. J. (1988). *Thriving in chaos.* New York: Knopf.

Sagor, R. (2002). Lessons learned from skateboarders. *Educational Leadership, 60*(1), 34–38.

Shortt, T., & Thayer, Y. (1998–99). Block scheduling can enhance school climate. *Educational Leadership, 56*(4), 76–81.

Siedentop, D., & Tannehill, D. (2000). *Developing teaching skills in physical education* (4th ed.). Mountain View, CA: Mayfield.

Spady, W. G., & Marshall, K. (1991). Beyond traditional outcome-based education. *Educational Leadership, 49*(2), 67–72.

Walker, M. H. (1998). The fundamentals of quality design. *Streamlined Seminar: A Newsletter, 16*(3), 1–4.

Wiggins, G., & McTighe, J. (1998). *Understanding by design.* Alexandria, VA: Association of Supervision and Curriculum Development.

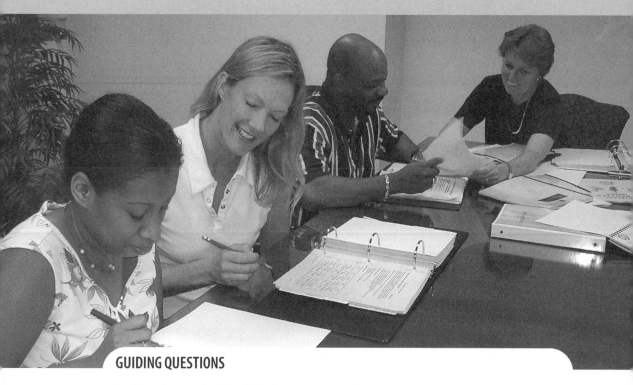

GUIDING QUESTIONS

1. How does evaluation differ from assessment?
2. What components/elements does good evaluation include?
3. Why should you do an evaluation?
4. When would you use a preformative evaluation? Summative?
5. What information does each of the various stakeholders have for the evaluation process?
6. What are some ways to obtain data from direct sources for a curricular evaluation?
7. What types of indirect information might be important data for an evaluation?
8. What would your curriculum evaluation plan look like?

Evaluating Your Physical Education Curriculum

Jacalyn Lund, Georgia State University
Deborah Tannehill, University of Limerick

Introduction

It is exciting to develop a new curriculum or implement change to an existing one. Unfortunately, too often curriculum development or curricular changes are based on the whims of teachers within a department rather than a result of informed decisions based on key pieces of data. As stated previously in this book, curricula should be designed to allow students to meet the district, state, or national standards that both guide and govern the program. The success of those curricula should be measured systematically to determine which changes, if any, need to be made to keep the curriculum dynamic and meet the needs of the program. The purpose of this chapter is to explain the role of evaluation in curriculum design, and offer strategies for gaining information necessary to make an informed decision about the existing curriculum or to implement change. At the conclusion of this chapter, the reader will know what a thorough evaluation entails, and will have a process for evaluating physical education curricula.

What Is Evaluation?

Although some people use the terms *evaluation* and *assessment* interchangeably, the two are not the same. Assessment is the process of gathering information from multiple sources to make educational decisions about students. Chapter 4 provides several different strategies for assessing the three domains: psychomotor, cognitive, and affective. **Evaluation** differs from assessment in that it involves interpreting merit or worth, using information gathered to make that decision (Guskey, 2000). Whereas assessment involves the gathering of information, evaluation is the judgment or decision based on specific criteria that results when the evaluator examines the data. As Guskey points out while explaining his definition, we make several evaluations informally on an almost daily basis. We decide what to wear based on evaluating the temperature or weather. We evaluate our latest haircut and decide whether to return to that same stylist. When we buy a new car, the decision is based upon evaluation of current needs, dependability of the previous model owned, and so on. The evaluation process used to make decisions about curricula is much more formal than those described previously. It involves informed decisions about the merit or worth of the curriculum of a school or district based on information gathered systematically.

Several models of evaluation have been used in education. The model that this book will propose is built on the work of Ralph Tyler, who developed an evaluation model based on comparing intended outcomes with actual outcomes (Madaus, Stufflebeam, & Scriven, 1998). Additionally, we will draw on the work of Hammond, who felt that it was equally important to look at why goals are not being met in an attempt to make change for the future (Guskey, 2000).

What Is Good Evaluation?

Before looking at the various steps of curricular evaluation, it is important to recognize what makes an evaluation good. This section will discuss several characteristics of good evaluation. If a district is going to undertake an evaluation of its curriculum (which should be done on a regular/ongoing basis), the evaluation should have the following characteristics.

Systematic

Basing a decision on limited knowledge is risky. When good evaluation is done, the information should be collected systematically to ensure that all viable sources of information are examined. By planning data sources to use prior to beginning an evaluation, omissions are less likely. Data sources for curriculum evaluation will be direct (e.g., surveys of students and teachers in the program; a self-study of program features) and indirect (e.g., number of students participating in after-school or non-school activities; enrollment in elective classes).

> **evaluation**   The systematic appraisal of worth based on a thorough and detailed examination of data.

An outline of the evaluation procedure should be developed to ensure that all necessary data sources are considered. Timing may also be a factor when gathering data for an evaluation, as some information may be needed before moving to a second phase, whereas other information can be collected simultaneously. By planning what the evaluation will encompass, along with when data collection will occur, the process will be orderly, deliberate, and thorough. Information gathered should be sufficient to measure the intended outcome.

Objective

Good evaluations should be unbiased, be fair, and avoid being self-serving. Conducting an evaluation with the intent of proving a point or showing that a product is good negates the purpose of the evaluation. An honest effort to obtain unbiased information should be the goal of an evaluation. Ignoring certain information, or failing to obtain it because it would not support a given way of thinking, will not produce a quality evaluation.

Involve All Stakeholders

When planning an evaluation, the **stakeholders**, or those who have an interest in the process, should have input. When doing a curricular evaluation, stakeholders might include students, alumni of the program, parents of current and past students, physical education teachers in the department, non-physical education teachers in the building or district, administrators (principals, assistant principals, and superintendents), support staff (counselors, guidance office personnel), school board members, and members of the community who do not have children in school. These individuals will provide a variety of perspectives, and give multiple lenses through which to view the program. Information from these stakeholders should be solicited in a variety of ways. Focused interviews and surveys are the most common methods used for gathering data from the stakeholders. When obtaining information from stakeholders, it is important to ask them questions that they have knowledge about. For example, a parent might have an opinion about whether his/her child is active beyond the school day, and whether the child enjoys participating in activities, but may have little knowledge about current trends in physical education, and therefore could provide little information about ideas and/or new activities. Likewise, an administrator knows how the program contributes to the mission of the school, and can provide insight about how the program fits into his or her "big picture" vision of education.

stakeholders   Those who have an interest in the evaluation process.

Be Thorough

When planning an evaluation, it is important to identify all the data necessary to make an informed decision. Although some data sources might be easier to access than others, it is important to get the information needed to judge the merits of the program. For example, although a survey might be the most convenient way to obtain information from a parent or student, it may not allow the respondent to adequately express concerns or positive feelings about topics not addressed on the survey. Focus groups provide an alternative method for gathering information from different people. Often, additional issues will emerge while discussing a point among several people. Obtaining information about student participation in non-school activities might reveal new trends and areas that students would find interesting to learn. For example, one private school had a team sport-dominated curriculum. A survey of parents would have indicated the need to add golf and tennis to the program, because many of the graduates go on to pursue business and professional degrees, and need these skills for success in their adult worlds. A good evaluation must not only explore information from a variety of sources, but also gather this information in the best possible manner. The type of data sought should determine how the information is obtained.

Use Defensible Data Sources

Validity and **reliability** are two important factors to consider when doing an evaluation. Regarding validity, one must look at appropriate items to obtain valid data. For example, measuring a student's success on the standards cannot be done by only using data from a fitness test. Physical education encompasses much more than fitness. There are many other factors to consider when evaluating the "goodness" of a program. Information obtained during an evaluation must be from viable sources, and the conclusions drawn from it must be valid as well. Making poor judgments about good data will not produce a good evaluation. In addition to being valid, information gathered in an evaluation should be collected in a way so that the data sources are reliable. If a study is reliable, it should not matter who is collecting the data, nor should the time of day or the day of the week when the information was obtained. Information must be obtained in such a way that results could be replicated.

validity   The degree to which a test measures what it is designed to measure.
reliability   The degree of consistency with which a test measures what it is designed to measure.

Include an Evaluation of Context

Sometimes the context in which an evaluation is being conducted impacts the findings. For example, students living near a national forest have greater opportunity to engage in outdoor activities than do students in the middle of a large urban city. Context would also be considered when deciding to use after school participation as an indicator of program quality when students are bussed in from miles away. When choosing content for a curriculum, several factors regarding context can affect that curriculum. Factors typically addressed in the statement of context include weather and/or climate, possible religious influences, local activities derived from the national origins of community settlers, economic wealth of the community, community facilities available, and miscellaneous regional factors (mountains, lakes, forests). Contextual factors will also have an impact on activities included in a curriculum because of available facilities and interests of community residents.

Justifiable Conclusions

Data alone do not make an evaluation. A good evaluation looks at the information and lets the professional judgment of the person or team writing the evaluation guide the final decision. Although data should inform the decision, they should not determine the decision. Evaluators should remember that some of those involved in the evaluation might not be as "informed" as others. Physical education has changed over the years, and some parents, teachers, and administrators could be judging the program that they participated in rather than the one currently being evaluated. Physical education teachers who read professional journals and attend conferences are more likely to know current trends than people from the community. As stated earlier, the stakeholders should provide input, but the team preparing the final report must carefully weigh the results when making a judgment about the quality of the program. Collecting pertinent information and then making an incorrect decision based on this data is of little use. To prevent this from happening, multiple people should examine the data to determine the results. If discrepancies between the evaluators occur, these should be discussed and resolved. The conclusions derived in an evaluation should be appropriate.

What Are the Purposes of Evaluation?

There are several reasons for conducting an evaluation. An evaluation can measure the effectiveness of current programs, or look at trends to determine whether new programs should be added. Evaluations can also be used to justify the existence of a program. The purpose of the evaluation will determine the data sources used for the process. This section will explore several reasons for doing curricular evaluations.

Are You Doing What You Intend to Do, and How Well Are You Doing This?

The first reason for doing an evaluation is to determine whether your goals for the program are being met. Assuming the programmatic goals align with the standards, the following questions might begin the process of looking at how well the curriculum is meeting the intent of those standards:

- Are graduates of the program able to perform basic, as well as sport and activity-related skills, to be successful participants after graduation from high school?
- Do graduates of the program have sufficient skill to learn new sports and/or physical activities (i.e., those not covered in the program)?
- Do graduates of the program have sufficient content knowledge to participate in a variety of activities?
- Do graduates have sufficient content knowledge to learn new activities that may or may not be related to those taught in the program?
- As adults, do graduates of the program have sufficient skill to participate in activities that they enjoy and were introduced to in physical education?
- Are graduates physically active?
- Have graduates reached an appropriate level of fitness?
- Do graduates of the program have sufficient knowledge about fitness that they could develop a health-related fitness program?
- Are graduates of the program able to participate in physical activity safely?
- Do graduates of the program enjoy participating in physical activity?

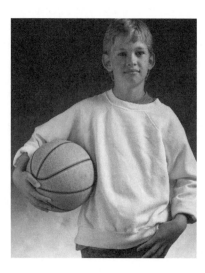

- Do students feel successful when engaged in physical activity?
- Do students play fairly when participating in physical activity without being reminded by an adult or supervisor?

Answers to these questions and others can be found in a variety of ways. The examples provided in this chapter are designed to give those developing curriculum the means for determining the answers to questions about the effectiveness of the physical education curriculum.

To Judge the Satisfaction of the Students

Not only should physical education curricula be meeting programmatic goals, the students who are participants should also have some degree of satisfaction. When creating physical education curricula, it is important to realize that not everyone will enjoy everything that is offered. However, the physical education curriculum should strive to meet the needs of everyone at some point in the curriculum. It could be that some students do not feel that course offerings are adequate. On the other hand, some activities suggested by students may not be popular enough to offer every semester. These students could possibly have their needs satisfied by offering less popular courses on an annual or biannual cycle. Lack of facilities or cost may make the activity difficult or impossible to offer. All of these factors must be taken into consideration when attempting to meet the needs of students.

Program Improvement

Many physical education programs have a variety of features that make them effective. However, curriculum planners should always be seeking ways to make programs better. When obtaining information from program stakeholders, questions should address not only things that are currently being done well, but also things that could be improved in the future. New activities might need to be added, or facilities upgraded or additional ones built. Certain procedures and policies might need revamping to make things run more smoothly. Scheduling, class size, and frequency of class sessions might need revisiting to meet the needs of the learners. All these ideas are critical to meeting the needs of those involved, both directly and indirectly, with the physical education curriculum.

Accountability: Are You Doing the Things That You Intend?

We live in an era of accountability. School districts are held accountable for everything that they do, and the physical education curriculum is no exception. In these days of tight budgets, administrators must determine whether the money allocated to physical education is worth the results. Some curriculum evaluation questions that address accountability are: Is the money in your program spent wisely? Is there a way to deliver the program more effectively and efficiently? Is the program meeting its intended goals? The bottom line on evaluation is that it should be designed to meet the instructional goals for the program. Clearly identifying the purposes and goals of the physical education curriculum, and measuring the degree to which the goals are met for accountability purposes, is a vital step in curriculum evaluation.

When Should You Evaluate?

In the past, much curriculum revision occurred during the summer months when teachers were not involved with teaching and coaching responsibilities. School districts have discovered that curriculum revision is a worthwhile inservice activity because of the discussions about philosophy, whether the curriculum is meeting the needs of the students and community, scope and sequence within a level (elementary, middle, high), and K–12 alignment. Many school districts that have contract days allocated during the school year for teacher inservice activity have chosen to use some of these days to examine and revise the existing curriculum.

A curriculum can be evaluated at various times, depending on the purpose of the evaluation and the needs of the program. A **preformative evaluation** or planning evaluation is done prior to beginning an activity, program, or project. For example, several physical education curricula are now adding climbing walls to their facilities. A preformative evaluation would look at the impact of having a climbing wall prior to investing a lot of money in the project. A preformative evaluation would begin by identifying what is to be accomplished, developed, or built, and then determining the goals for the project (Worthen & Sanders, 1987). Before the wall is considered, teachers must think about whether it will be a vital part of the total physical education program (e.g., what standards will it help students achieve?), or if it is merely an expensive toy that will have too many students waiting in line to participate. The next step would be to examine the process used to execute the plan. The evaluation would include a thorough analysis of the steps necessary to complete the project. An appraisal of the needs for the project, resources available (people, equipment, existing facilities, safety/security issues) for both building and implementation once it is built (what instructional strategies and skills will teachers need in order to allow them to deliver it successfully?), and any other pertinent information would be included in the evaluation. The last step of a preformative evaluation would be to determine how success will be measured. By carefully planning prior to implementation, expensive mistakes (in terms of people and resources) can be avoided.

preformative evaluation   An evaluation that is done prior to beginning a project or process.

A **formative evaluation** takes place during the activity. It can help redirect time, money, personnel, and other resources (Worthen & Sanders, 1987) as the project is in progress. Formative evaluations are used to evaluate where the curriculum currently is, and where it is headed. They can be done multiple times on a reoccurring basis, and ask, "Are we achieving success?" In a sense, formative evaluations are proactive, as they seek information that will help make change while there is still time to redirect efforts. After implementing a curricular change, school districts should do a mid-year evaluation to determine whether the changes have been positive and if further adjustments to the curriculum are necessary.

When most people think of evaluation, they think of a **summative evaluation** that is done at the conclusion of a project. Summative evaluations are ways to measure the success of a project or a plan, and determine what has been accomplished. Used mainly for accountability purposes, an external evaluator would use the information in a summative evaluation to determine whether the project was worth doing. Schools that are governed by an accrediting agency, such as the North Central Association, use summative evaluations. In this instance, data gathered are used by the evaluation team as they make their decision about the quality of the program. Summative evaluations ask questions to determine, "Were we successful?" as they make judgments about the results. Frequently, quantitative data is used in a summative evaluation (e.g., fitness scores, results of skill assessments or portfolios, interview and survey results).

Most evaluations could function as any one of the three types identified above, depending on the nature of the information gathered; the emphasis of the evaluation changes depending on the stage of the project (Guskey, 2000). In some instances, formative evaluations could be considered an early version of the summative evaluation. For instance, parent surveys could provide information to make changes to a curriculum during the year, and could be used as a measure of satisfaction while doing a summative evaluation. The purpose of the evaluation will be stated in the goals for the evaluation, and those will guide evaluators as they determine the types of questions that should be asked and the information necessary to answer those questions.

Guskey (2000) warns evaluators to avoid "evaluations" that merely provide information about what occurred. Although it is interesting to gather information about things such as the number of years of teaching experience, level of education, or number of workshops or college classes attended, these

formative evaluation An evaluation that occurs while a project is in progress.
summative evaluation An evaluation done at the conclusion of a project to measure the success of the project and to determine what has been accomplished.

demographics are documentation of what occurred rather than a measure of results. As such, these data contain insufficient information on which to make a judgment of value or worth. The information is interesting, but is not an evaluation.

How Should You Evaluate?

An evaluation should begin by looking at the goals of the curriculum and determining the degree to which they are being met. To do this, various data sources must be identified, as well as the instruments used to gather information from these sources. One part of the evaluation will probably look at some measure of whether students are meeting the performance standards set by the district or state. Some states are working to develop, or have developed, statewide assessments. Student performance on these would be excellent indicators of whether students are meeting the standards. If the curriculum to be evaluated does not have state assessments that measure how well students are meeting the physical education standards, then these should be developed for the program. Chapter 4 of this book talks about assessments that can be used to measure student achievement. The ultimate goal of a physical education program should be to develop students who are physically educated when they graduate. Assessment data on student performance should be included in the program evaluation. Although this information should be at the core of the curriculum evaluation to determine the program's worth, it is not the only information to consider while doing the evaluation.

As previously discussed, the second part of the curricular evaluation will include a direct measure of the opinions of stakeholders. Surveys (written or phone) and focus groups are the most common formats for collecting data from stakeholders. Surveys composed of checklists or Likert scales (see Figures 3.1 and 3.2) have answers that are easier to code than open-response questions, and are easier for respondents to complete (Salant & Dillman, 1994). However, if a survey with checklist or Likert responses fails to have the appropriate questions or response choices for respondents, it will not provide useful information. Figure 3.3 is an example of several questions that could be used for data collection with administrators during a focus group.

A program is only as good as its teachers. Although we feel very strongly that a quality program should have a teacher certified to teach physical education, we also recognize that having a degree in physical education does not automatically mean that the person is a good teacher. An evaluation should not only list the qualifications, degrees, and/or certifications of faculty members, but also have a method for measuring teacher effectiveness. Most districts have administrative teacher evaluations. These may be useful for looking at the quality of instruction. Time on task is another way to look at teaching

Physical Education Survey

Date _____ Class Period _____

Gender (circle one)   Male   Female

1. I love physical education class.

    Strongly Agree   Agree   Disagree   Strongly Disagree

2. My teacher cares about me.

    Strongly Agree   Agree   Disagree   Strongly Disagree

3. My teacher makes physical education class fun.

    Strongly Agree   Agree   Disagree   Strongly Disagree

4. I feel physical education is an important subject.

    Strongly Agree   Agree   Disagree   Strongly Disagree

5. My friends influence the way I behave in physical education class.

    Strongly Agree   Agree   Disagree   Strongly Disagree

6. I will continue to take physical education classes when they are no longer required.

          Yes   No   Undecided

7. I know what I'm getting graded on in physical education class.

    Strongly Agree   Agree   Disagree   Strongly Disagree

8. Physical education grades should be partially based on a student's level of fitness.

    Strongly Agree   Agree   Disagree   Strongly Disagree

9. Physical education grades should be partially based on how hard you try.

    Strongly Agree   Agree   Disagree   Strongly Disagree

10. Physical education grades should be partially based on whether you dress for class and participate.

    Strongly Agree   Agree   Disagree   Strongly Disagree

11. Physical education grades should be partially based on your level of skill for the sport/activity done in class.

    Strongly Agree   Agree   Disagree   Strongly Disagree

12. Physical education grades should be based on written tests about strategies, rules, etc.

    Strongly Agree   Agree   Disagree   Strongly Disagree

13. I think that written exams are appropriate in physical education.

    Strongly Agree   Agree   Disagree   Strongly Disagree

14. I think that my physical education grade is important.

    Strongly Agree   Agree   Disagree   Strongly Disagree

15. My parents think that my physical education grade is important.

    Strongly Agree   Agree   Disagree   Strongly Disagree

16. I try very hard in physical education.

    Strongly Agree   Agree   Disagree   Strongly Disagree

Figure 3.1 Example of a student survey on attitude toward physical education.

Adapted from Carlson, T. (1995). "We hate gym": student alienation from physical education. *Journal of Teaching Physical Education, 14*, 467–477.

Continued

17. My friends consider me physically fit.

    Strongly Agree   Agree   Disagree   Strongly Disagree

18. How do you rate your skill level compared to that of your friends?

    Much Better   A Little Better   A Little Worse   Much Worse

19. How do you rate your fitness level compared to that of your friends?

    Much Better   A Little Better   A Little Worse   Much Worse

20. Participating with friends makes physical education enjoyable for me.

    Strongly Agree   Agree   Disagree   Strongly Disagree

21. How do you rate your psychomotor skills?

    Very Good   Average   Not So Good   Never Play

22. I am afraid of making mistakes in front of others in my physical education class.

    Strongly Agree   Agree   Disagree   Strongly Disagree

23. I know how to develop a fitness program.

    Strongly Agree   Agree   Disagree   Strongly Disagree

24. I enjoy doing physical education activities outside of class (e.g., team sports, individual sports, etc.).

    Strongly Agree   Agree   Disagree   Strongly Disagree

25. In physical education, I prefer to work in a group rather than by myself.

    Strongly Agree   Agree   Disagree   Strongly Disagree

26. Other students like having me on their team.

    Strongly Agree   Agree   Disagree   Strongly Disagree

27. I don't mind getting hot and sweaty during physical education class.

    Strongly Agree   Agree   Disagree   Strongly Disagree

28. I am reluctant to participate in physical education because of the way I look in shorts and a t-shirt.

    Strongly Agree   Agree   Disagree   Strongly Disagree

29. I have faked injury/illness to get out of physical education class.

    Strongly Agree   Agree   Disagree   Strongly Disagree

30. I try harder when I enjoy the activity we are learning.

    Strongly Agree   Agree   Disagree   Strongly Disagree

31. I often make fun of the unskilled students in my physical education class.

    Strongly Agree   Agree   Disagree   Strongly Disagree

32. When I am good at a sport/game, I try harder.

    Strongly Agree   Agree   Disagree   Strongly Disagree

33. I like sports/games better when I am good/successful at playing them.

    Strongly Agree   Agree   Disagree   Strongly Disagree

34. Compared to other subjects, physical education is easy for me.

    Strongly Agree   Agree   Disagree   Strongly Disagree

FIGURE 3.1—CONT'D   *Continued*

35. I enjoy trying games/sports that I have never played before.

      Strongly Agree   Agree   Disagree   Strongly Disagree

36. I suit up for physical education.

         Always   Most of the Time   Some of the time   Never

37. I am reluctant to participate in physical education because I am required to change clothes in the locker room.

      Strongly Agree   Agree   Disagree   Strongly Disagree

38. Our locker room is a pleasant setting to change clothes (smells good, well-lit, clean, etc.).

      Strongly Agree   Agree   Disagree   Strongly Disagree

39. How do you feel about the number of different activities offered in physical education?

        Too Many   Right Amount   Too Few

40. Would you like to have a choice in activities that are offered?

        Always   Most of the Time   Some of the Time   Never

41. I prefer competitive activities rather than/instead of non-competitive (i.e., no winner or loser).

      Strongly Agree   Agree   Disagree   Strongly Disagree

42. When I participate in my physical education class, I often try to avoid being seen by the teacher. In other words, I become an "invisible player."

      Strongly Agree   Agree   Disagree   Strongly Disagree

43. I prefer team activities to individual activities.

      Strongly Agree   Agree   Disagree   Strongly Disagree

44. Are you a member of a school-sponsored athletic team(s)?

    I presently am on one   I was on one, but not now   I never was on one

45. Are you a member of a non-school athletic sport or club team?

    I presently am on one   I was on one, but not now   I never was on one

46. I participate in a physical activity outside of school where I have to get hot and sweaty, and/or breathe hard.

        Every Day   Once or Twice a Week   Occasionally   Rarely

47. Physical education class is a positive experience for me.

      Strongly Agree   Agree   Disagree   Strongly Disagree

48. I know the importance of physical activity.

      Strongly Agree   Agree   Disagree   Strongly Disagree

49. My three favorite physical activities are . . .

50. Overall, I enjoy physical education class.

    _____ Yes   _____ No

    If yes, please list three things you like most about physical education.

    If no, please list three things you like least about physical education.

FIGURE 3.1—CONT'D

Parent Survey

Please use the following scale when responding to the questions that follow:

1 = Never   2 = Sometimes   3 = Usually   4 = Always

1. Does your child enjoy his/her physical education class?	1	2	3	4
2. Does your child feel safe in physical education?	1	2	3	4
3. Does your child use skills learned outside of the class?	1	2	3	4
4. Does your child express frustration because he/she is not successful in physical education?	1	2	3	4
5. Do you receive feedback about your child's progress from his/her teacher?	1	2	3	4
6. Do you feel welcome to visit your child's physical education class?	1	2	3	4
7. Would you feel comfortable talking with your child's physical education teacher about his/her progress in the class?	1	2	3	4
8. Does your child share with you the content of (lessons taught/activities covered) physical education?	1	2	3	4
9. Do you feel that the content covered in physical education is preparing your child to be active as an adult?	1	2	3	4
10. Does your child ask you to participate with him/her in activities learned in physical education?	1	2	3	4

11. Which additional activities would you like to see covered in physical education?

FIGURE 3.2 Sample of a parent survey.

effectiveness. Computerized programs for teacher observation (e.g., ALT-PE) have been developed to facilitate that process. Reports provide data charts and time logs that show useful information for an evaluation. Figure 3.4 contains a self-appraisal of teaching skills that may also provide useful information. If a discrepancy between this self-appraisal and the administrator evaluation of teaching performance exists, part of the evaluation process might include a meeting between the teacher and administrator to look at and possibly resolve the differences. Because one of the purposes of evaluation is to improve the quality of a program, this may be an important step in that process.

Facilities, both indoor and outdoor, should be included in program evaluation. Questions about facilities might include: Is there adequate space to accommodate the number of students scheduled into the area? Are locker

Administrator Evaluation

Questions for a focused interview.

1. Is this program your idea of a quality physical education program? Please explain your answer.

2. Do you feel that students leaving the physical education program have the skills they need to be successful at the next level? Why or why not.

3. Are there activities that you feel should be added to the existing physical education program? If any, please explain.

4. Are there activities that you feel should be deleted from the existing physical education program? If any, please explain.

5. Do you believe that physical education is an important part of the curriculum?

6. What could the teachers in this program do to improve its quality?

7. Do you feel adequate time is allocated to physical education?

8. How would you rather use the physical education facilities at your school?

9. What facilities would you consider adding in the future?

10. Do students graduating from your program meet the national physical education content standards?

FIGURE 3.3 Example of questions used for a focused interview administrator evaluation.

rooms safe? Are locker rooms clean? Do they offer privacy for students while changing and showering? Are locker rooms supervised when students are present? Are fields in good repair? Other factors included in the delivery of a physical education program include having adequate time and ensuring that the teacher-to-student ratio will provide a quality learning environment (see Figure 3.5).

Indirect Measure of Program Effectiveness

In addition to direct measures about various aspects of the curriculum, there are several indirect indicators of the quality of the physical education program. Which of these indicators to include will be based on a variety of factors. Those conducting the evaluation should consider all of these indirect measures as possible data sources, and then use only those that are most appropriate for their program.

Teacher's Name _____

Teacher Evaluation

Is the physical education program meaningful in your school? Rate the following questions based on the scale below.

    1 = Never   2 = Sometimes   3 = Most of the time   4 = Always

_____ Is the atmosphere set so that students can be successful?

_____ Are the students evaluated during each activity unit?

_____ There is negative peer pressure when students are working in groups.

_____ Are skills taught in a safe, sequential progression?

_____ Are all students given the opportunity to be leaders?

_____ Positive change is evident in the program from one year to the next.

_____ Students have the chance to be creative in the classroom.

_____ Positive skill-related feedback is seldom given.

_____ The lessons have a learning goal as the focus.

_____ Opportunities for boys and girls are not equal in the classroom.

_____ Activity time in class is above 50% on the majority of the days.

_____ Excitement in class is low because students don't enjoy participating.

_____ Students show improvement from one week to the next.

_____ Activities are so challenging that students cannot be successful on them.

_____ There is positive behavioral feedback occurring on a daily basis.

_____ There are a variety of activities presented to the class.

_____ The teacher's enthusiasm is low.

FIGURE 3.4 Sample teacher lesson evaluation form.
Adapted from the work of Elizabeth Gramelspacher, Noah Mangus, and Shaun Roberts. Reprinted with permission.

Participation in After-School Programs

As stated in Chapter 1, we consider after-school programs to be an extension of the physical education curriculum. After-school programs, such as sport or activity clubs, intramurals, or interschool competitions, allow students to participate in activities learned during physical education class. Although the level of participation in interscholastic competition is beyond the scope of physical education, in some smaller schools, students might actually begin participating in an activity in physical education, and continue participation at the interscholastic

Program Evaluation Questionnaire

Date: _____

Directions: Rate your answers from 1 to 4, 1 meaning not established and 4 meaning well established. Circle the number you feel fits best. At the end of each section, add the circled numbers together and write the total. After the questionnaire is complete, add the totals of each section and then write that number in the blank where it says "OVERALL TOTAL."

CURRICULUM

1. There is a written, planned, sequential curriculum available and used.	1	2	3	4
2. Instructional activities are selected to help each student to achieve established program goals.	1	2	3	4
3. The curriculum involves appropriate activities, goals, and instruction meeting each student's needs.	1	2	3	4
4. The curriculum illustrates an appropriate scope and sequence.	1	2	3	4
5. The students are introduced to many activities that are developmentally appropriate.	1	2	3	4
6. Opportunities are created for students to create and consistently improve their solving skills and character development.	1	2	3	4
7. Objectives and exit requirements are stated and implemented into teaching.	1	2	3	4

TOTAL _____

INSTRUCTION

1. Daily instruction is provided to all students.	1	2	3	4
2. The instructional program creates the opportunity for student involvement and success.	1	2	3	4
3. Technology is incorporated into lessons on a consistent basis.	1	2	3	4
4. The teacher acts as a positive role model for the students by illustrating healthy living choices.	1	2	3	4
5. The teacher demonstrates professional commitment through involvement in professional organizations.	1	2	3	4
6. The teacher applies and uses various teaching methods and instructional strategies and personalizes classes so students may grow and succeed.	1	2	3	4
7. The teacher creates and implements lessons with high time on task.	1	2	3	4
8. The teacher stresses and implements lessons that create sportsmanship.	1	2	3	4
9. Appropriate instruction is given to those students with special needs.	1	2	3	4
10. The teacher provides frequent, specific, individual feedback to all students.	1	2	3	4
11. The daily instruction hits at least one state standard.	1	2	3	4
12. Character development is addressed on a daily basis.	1	2	3	4

TOTAL _____

FIGURE 3.5 Example of a physical education program evaluation.
Work created by Jessica Weller. Reprinted with permission.   *Continued*

level because of an interest piqued in class. This movement into higher levels of competition can be seen as an indicator of the quality of the physical education program. Participation in clubs and intramurals are also good indicators of student success and interest in the activities covered in class. Although gymnasium space may be limited, whenever possible, physical education curricula should be

ASSESSMENT
1. Curriculum, instruction, and assessments are related to one another.   1   2   3   4
2. The teacher uses multiple methods to evaluate each student on the   1   2   3   4
   psychomotor, cognitive, and affective domains.
3. Assessments are appropriate and objective.   1   2   3   4
4. Evaluations serve a guide for instructional planning.   1   2   3   4
5. The assessment criteria are explained to the students at the beginning   1   2   3   4
   and throughout the unit.
6. Program evaluation serves as an indicator of effective teaching   1   2   3   4
   strategies.
7. Summative evaluation of students identifies whether or not students   1   2   3   4
   have met the course goals and objectives.
8. The teacher consistently assesses each student on character   1   2   3   4
   development.
9. Assessment results are shared with each student.   1   2   3   4

                                        TOTAL _____

STUDENT
1. Students participate in a safe environment.   1   2   3   4
2. Students wear appropriate clothing for all activities.   1   2   3   4
3. Students are self-directed in conducting their own physical fitness   1   2   3   4
   programs.
4. Change of clothing is encouraged after participation in vigorous   1   2   3   4
   physical activity.
5. Students take responsibility for their actions, the equipment, and   1   2   3   4
   the facilities.

                                        TOTAL _____

FACILITIES, EQUIPMENT, AND SUPPLIES
1. There is enough equipment for each student to actively participate   1   2   3   4
   thoughout a lesson.
2. The facilities and equipment are examined on a daily basis.   1   2   3   4
3. Repairs to facilities and equipment are made in a timely manner.   1   2   3   4
4. The school provides adequate locker rooms, towels, and   1   2   3   4
   individual showers.
5. Locker rooms are clean and secure.   1   2   3   4
6. The teacher makes use of all available facilities and space.   1   2   3   4

                                        TOTAL _____

LEARNING ENVIRONMENT
1. An emphasis is placed on cooperative activities rather than   1   2   3   4
   competitive tasks.
2. Individualized improvement opportunities with personalized   1   2   3   4
   student feedback are provided in many forms.
3. The teacher and students demonstrate respect for one another.   1   2   3   4
4. A safe and comfortable learning environment is provided for   1   2   3   4
   every student.
5. The environment encourages students to succeed.   1   2   3   4
6. The learning environment stresses individual character   1   2   3   4
   development.

                                        TOTAL _____

OVERALL TOTAL _____   **/180**

Figure 3.5—Cont'd

supported with after-school opportunities for students. At the elementary level, rope jumping teams, dance clubs, or competitions involving small-sided invasion games might be found. At the middle school level, these same activities could be offered along with gymnastics, net games, and outdoor adventure activity field trips (camping, high ropes courses, cycling). High school intramurals could offer a chance for participation at a lower level of commitment and competition for any varsity sport offered. In addition, weight lifting clubs, martial arts (e.g., judo, jujitsu, tai chi), bowling, inline skating hockey, and other opportunities might be included. Enrollment in these activities should be tracked over time to see if there is a relationship between participation after school and activities offered through physical education.

Participation in Non-School Programs

These data may not be as readily available for program evaluation as information on school programs, but they still represent a possible data source. Some advanced physical education classes might use portfolio evaluation as part of the course requirements. Allowing or encouraging students to use portfolio entries from non-school programs could indicate student participation in them. Giving clubs permission to distribute promotional literature through the physical education program, and then making a follow-up call to program organizers may be another way to access the information. Because participation in non-school programs is one way to determine whether the physical education curriculum is meeting Standard 3 (participates regularly in physical activity), strategies for obtaining this information should be developed.

Preparation of Students: Do They Have the Necessary Skills to Move to the Next Level?

In the past few years, we have heard middle school teachers lament that students are not coming to them with basic motor skills. Students may know how to play basketball, yet they do not know what a skip or gallop is, cannot differentiate between a hop and a jump, and do not know what a level or a zigzag is. Other students know how to juggle and ride a unicycle, but they do not know what a backhand or forehand is, or what it means to invade space. It is important to ask middle and high school teachers whether students coming into their programs have the necessary skills to be successful in the activities offered. This is not meant to imply that every curriculum is identical, only that students should learn the essential skills that they will need to be successful at the next level of schooling. Student readiness might be determined with a survey or, if teachers of the district have the opportunity to meet during a district-wide inservice, this is a good question to have on the agenda. Too often when planning curricula, the elementary school teachers meet together, the middle school teachers meet collectively, and the high school teachers meet as a group. Interaction between the three levels is critical in both planning and evaluation of program effectiveness. By approaching curriculum development from a K–12 perspective, rather than a school-level perspective, the sequencing between levels becomes more seamless.

Enrollment in Elective Classes

Enrollment in elective classes can signify that students have had a quality experience in required physical education classes, and that they are motivated to spend time in additional physical education pursuits. It is important to note that in some instances failure to enroll in elective classes is not always an indicator of program quality. Some schools have so many courses required for graduation that it is difficult, if not impossible, for students to take elective classes. In some cases, funding limits the number of courses and/or teachers necessary to offer elective physical education courses. However, if it is possible for students to enroll in elective classes, this could be used as an indicator of success for a physical education curriculum.

Attendance, Dressing for Class, and Participation

Looking at attendance records is another way to determine whether the needs of students are being met. High attendance rates can be an indicator of whether students enjoy class activities and choose to attend class. Willingness to change clothes for class can be another indicator. Reluctance may indicate a dislike for the activity or lack of success. It also can indicate poor locker room facilities, or dress requirements that need to be updated. Some low-fit students' perceptions of body image may also be a barrier to changing clothes. In a similar fashion, students may come to class, but then decline participation. Some females or low-skilled males are reluctant to participate in popular activities, such as basketball, for which several members of the class have high levels of skill. This lack of participation should be taken into consideration when evaluating the curriculum. By expanding the curriculum, those students who are "turned off" by traditional activities can become engaged in class activities.

Grades

Grades can be a questionable item to use for program evaluation. If grades are truly based on learning (knowledge, skills, behavior), rather than attendance and dressing for class, and if this learning is evaluated in an objective (based on assessments) manner, grades can be an indicator of program success. If grades are based on whether the student showed up for class and exhibited minimal participation, they are not an indicator of program effectiveness.

Number of Students Who Have to Repeat the Class

The number of students who fail physical education could be another way to look at the program quality, assuming that the grade was based on achievement. The second part of this statistic is to look at the reason they failed. Tracking this statistic could be a simple process of developing a code that indicates why a student failed the class.

Curriculum evaluators might check to see that students understood expectations and requirements when they began the class. If several of those failing are unable to meet those expectations, other questions should be raised. Is adequate time allocated for physical education? Are standards of achievement set too high? Is the quality of the instruction sufficient to move students to the targeted level of achievement? Looking at the rate of failure for physical education, as well as the reasons for failure, could provide many insights about the curriculum.

Student Fitness Levels

Many schools mandate the administration of fitness testing twice a year, but fail to do anything with the results. Because fitness is one of the national outcomes of a physical education program, looking at fitness scores can be another way to evaluate the curriculum. Because fitness levels are linked to several health-related factors, a goal of having every graduate reach a given level of fitness is unrealistic. Programs should not be assessed on a fitness criterion, such as the number of students who can run a 6-minute mile. A health-enhancing level of fitness actually represents different things to different people. Many districts have a curricular goal that students will know how to become fit, rather than actually becoming fit. Fitness levels can be an interesting statistic to use in program evaluation. However, if fitness tests are administered, programs should look at the results as an indicator of the program content rather than for the levels of fitness. For example, Siedentop and Tannehill (2000) noted that many high school programs included only activities associated with older adults (i.e., golf, bowling, croquet), with no fitness activities included. Lack of availability of facilities both during and outside of class, or insufficient time, could be other factors limiting student fitness.

National Resources for Curriculum Evaluation

Planning curricular evaluations can seem to be a daunting task when first undertaken. If a curriculum evaluation has been done in the past, this report will provide useful information for planning the upcoming evaluation. If an evaluation has never been conducted, an outside professional evaluator, or a physical education coordinator from another district, might be contracted for the task. Although there are advantages to using an outside evaluator, that process can be very costly, especially in times of tight budgets.

Regardless of whether an outside person or agency is used to conduct an evaluation, an effective program will have an ongoing system for evaluation in place so that minor adjustments and changes can be made from year to year.

The National Association for Sport and Physical Education (NASPE) has several publications that cover many aspects of program evaluation. A series of publications for elementary, middle, and high school programs (NASPE, 1998a; 1998b; 2000) ask questions in a self-study format about areas of teacher qualifications and instruction, resources (e.g., time allocation, facilities, equipment), students, class size, use of assessments and technology, and curriculum.

NASPE STARS Program

NASPE has developed a means of recognizing quality physical education programs with its STARS Recognition Program. In this program, schools submit an application along with a portfolio of documentation about their school's physical education program. This program began in 2004, and includes criteria for the following areas:

- Time requirements
- Teacher qualification (licensed with a degree in physical education)
- Professional development of teachers
- Professional involvement of teachers
- Facility
- Equipment
- Teacher-to-student ratio
- Student health and safety
- Program mission statement
- Curriculum
- Instructional practices
- Student assessment
- Including students with disabilities
- Communication (intra-departmental and with parents)
- Program improvement/evaluation

There are five levels of recognition. Programs achieving the various levels of recognition are honored at the AAHPERD National Convention. Schools will receive a letter and certificate of recognition. For more information, contact NASPE at http://www.aahperd.org. Although this format is not comprehensive enough for use as a curriculum evaluation tool, it may provide ideas and categories for developing one for the district.

Physical Education Curriculum Analysis Tool (PECAT)

This instrument was developed by the Centers for Disease Control and Prevention (CDC), in partnership with physical education experts from around the country. It is designed to give educators a way to analyze the strengths and weaknesses of a physical education curriculum in terms of content, student assessment, and sequencing of activities. It is based on the six National Physical Education Content Standards, and provides rubrics for rating curriculum in those areas. The document includes scorecards, content rubrics, student assessment rubrics, and sequence rubrics. These are organized by grade level, and within the grade level are organized by standards. A curriculum improvement plan and resources section is provided to help analyze results of the curriculum assessment, identify strengths and weaknesses of the curriculum, and make decisions about the curriculum (to adopt, reject, or revise). Copies of PECAT can be downloaded from the CDC Web site, http://www.cdc.gov/HealthyYouth, or can be requested by email at HealthyYouth@cdc.gov.

What to Do with Results?

Once you have finished collecting data, it is time to look at results. Too frequently, reports are compiled and placed on a shelf, or filed away in a drawer. To spend the time and financial resources to do an evaluation and not use the results is a colossal waste. The report contains valuable information that will aid in creating a solid physical education program, or moving a good program to the next level, if this process is done with the objective of improving the curriculum rather than merely trying to affirm that everything is perfect. If you have interviewed or surveyed people, look at the results. Are they positive about your program? Do they think you have shortfalls that should be addressed? If you are getting the same message from several sources, this message needs attention.

The first step after data collection is to look at the curricular goals, and determine which of them have been met. A second part of this is to look at the degree to which students are meeting state or local standards to identify curricular strengths. After identifying program strengths, it is time to look at areas that did not meet programmatic goals, and therefore need improvement. A candid analysis of the current status of the program is a key step in making it better. After identifying the areas needing improvement, the evaluation must look at reasons for not meeting these goals.

After making a list of areas of concern, an action plan with a timeline should be developed. When creating a timeline, address the items of greatest need first. This involves prioritizing the list so that the most critical items get attention. After developing the timeline, a list of resources necessary to address the areas of concern should be developed. Some areas can be addressed relatively inexpensively, or may require more costly measures, depending on the depth with which they are addressed. Both of these solutions should be included on your list.

After completing this process, the list and timeline should be shared with school officials—building principals, school district administrators, and the school board or site-based management committee. To implement change, a meeting with those who have control over how resources are allocated to programs should be held. Start by reviewing the evaluation process, and sharing programmatic strengths and accomplishments prior to moving to areas needing improvement. By having a proposed action plan, you will let officials know that you have done your homework, and have identified which direction you wish to move for increasing program quality. Physical educators will convey a sense of knowing where they are going with the physical education program if they present an action plan. It is important to allow time to brainstorm with school officials to develop solutions to which they may have access and resources. If new facilities are needed, long-range plans for supporting these projects should be developed. If the possibilities are not presented to school officials, positive changes will be less likely to occur.

Improvement implies change (Guskey, 1996). A program cannot keep everything the same, and expect to get better. Those unwilling to make change will not be able to keep pace with the many innovations that are critical for developing a dynamic, viable physical education curriculum.

Summary

Evaluation is an important part of the curriculum writing process. We recognize that good evaluations cost money, and that many school districts are reluctant to spend resources on evaluating physical education when there is limited accountability for having a quality program. We feel strongly that evaluation is a necessary part of keeping a physical education program dynamic, while meeting the needs of the students and community. For that reason, evaluation, regardless of the scale on which it is done, should be conducted on a regular basis, and results of that study should be used to make any programmatic changes deemed necessary.

Good evaluation begins with the development of a plan for doing the assessment. Table 3.1 provides a framework for use in designing an evaluation plan for your school curriculum. Evaluation should be done as objectively as possible, using as many data sources as possible that will have the information necessary to make final decisions about the program. Preformative evaluations are done prior to implementing a new program or activity. Other evaluations are done to determine effectiveness, and to try to anticipate changes that will improve the existing curriculum. Good evaluations or judgments about merit or worth cannot be made with poor or limited information. When completing an evaluation, it is important to remember that the data should inform the decision rather than making it.

TABLE 3.1

Framework for Designing Your Curriculum Evaluation Plan
STEP 1

Initial Considerations	
Purpose of curricular evaluation	
(e.g., program effectiveness, to identify program omissions, program justification, program revision/ improvement, accountability)	
When will evaluation take place (depending on the purpose)?	
• Performative	
• Formative	
• Summative	
Resources available	
• NASPE publications	
• CDC analysis tool (PECAT)	
• District publications/documents	
STEP 2	
Outline of Evaluation Procedures: Action Plan	
• Stakeholders	
• Data necessary	
• Data sources (e.g., survey, interviews, pupil after-school involvement patterns)	
• Consider context	
• Evaluation team	
• Data analysis	
• Results and conclusions	
• Recommendations for change	
• Staff development opportunities	
• Timeline for change	

Continued

TABLE 3.1

Framework for Designing Your Curriculum Evaluation Plan—Cont'd

STEP 3

Steps in Evaluation	Data Source	Data Collection Instrument
• Review goals of curriculum; are they being met?		
• Opinions of stakeholders		
• Teacher effectiveness (including credentials)		
• Equipment and facilities		
• Scheduling (e.g., adequate time, teacher–pupil ratio)		
• Student involvement in after-school programs (e.g., clubs, intramurals, athletics)		
• Student involvement in non-school programs (e.g., clubs, recreation department, YMCA/YWCA)		
• Interaction across K–12 programs and teachers who deliver them		
• Student involvement in elective classes		
• Student attendance, participation, and suiting up in class		
• Student achievement as noted through grades (if based on learning)		
• Students who have repeated physical education		
• Student physical activity and fitness levels		

References

Carlson, T. (1995). We hate gym: student alienation from physical education. *Journal of Teaching Physical Education, 14,* 467–477.

Guskey, T. (1996). *Alternative ways to document and communicate student learning.* Read by author. Cassette recording no. 296211, Alexandria, VA: Association for Supervision and Curriculum Development.

Guskey, T. (2000). *Evaluating professional development.* Thousand Oaks, CA: Corwin Press.

Madaus, G., Stufflebeam, D., & Scriven, M. (1998). Program evaluation: a historical overview. In G. Madaus, M. Scriven, and D. Stufflebeam (Eds.), *Evaluation models: viewpoints of educational and human services evaluation* (12th ed., pp. 3–22). Boston: Kluwer-Nijhoff.

National Association for Sport and Physical Education (NASPE). (1998a). *Physical education: program improvement and self-study guide (high school).* Reston, VA: National Association for Sport and Physical Education, an association of the American Alliance for Health, Physical Education, Recreation, and Dance.

National Association for Sport and Physical Education (NASPE). (1998b). *Physical education: program improvement and self-study guide (middle school).* Reston, VA: National Association for Sport and Physical Education, an association of the American Alliance for Health, Physical Education, Recreation, and Dance.

National Association for Sport and Physical Education (NASPE). (2000). *Opportunity to learn: standards for elementary physical education.* Reston, VA: National Association for Sport and Physical Education, an association of the American Alliance for Health, Physical Education, Recreation, and Dance.

Salant, P., & Dillman, D. (1994). *How to conduct your own survey.* New York: John Wiley & Sons.

Siedentop, D., & Tannehill, D. (2000). *Developing teaching skills in physical education* (4th ed.). Mountain View, CA: Mayfield.

Worthen, B., & Sanders, J. (1987). *Educational evaluation: alternative approaches and practical guidelines.* White Plains, NY: Longman.

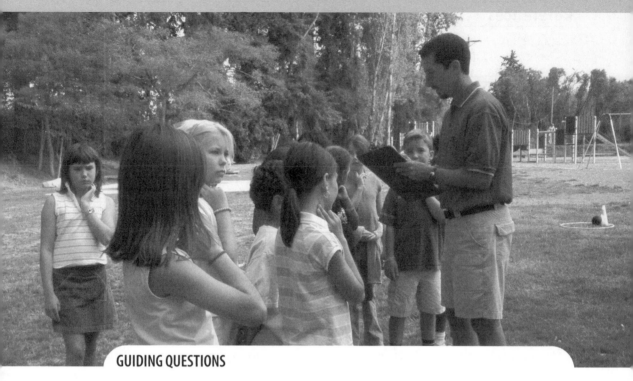

GUIDING QUESTIONS

1 How does formative assessment differ from summative assessment?
2 What questions might an assessor ask when trying to measure student learning?
3 How does performance-based assessment differ from traditional assessment formats?
4 Describe several ways to assess each of the physical education content standards.
5 For each of the performance assessments identified in Question 4, which type of rubric would be appropriate for that assessment?
6 How do curricular assessments differ from assessments that teachers use on a daily basis?
7 What process might be followed by teachers when developing curricular assessments?
8 What additional suggestions might teachers follow when developing curricular assessments?

Assessment in Curriculum Development

Jacalyn Lund, Georgia State University
Deborah Tannehill, University of Limerick

Assessment is an essential element in the movement toward using standards to determine what students should know and be able to do. Without assessment, teachers, programs, and districts have no way of knowing whether student learning did occur, and students have no sense of how they are doing with regard to their progress or achievement of the standards. Prior to the standards movement, much instruction operated under the notion of teach, test, hope for the best. This flippancy toward student learning becomes a thing of the past when there is accountability for student achievement. Some teachers resist using assessments while teaching physical education because the assessments decrease the time available for activity. Teachers must remember that physical education is about student learning and that time is needed to document that part of the instructional process so teaching can be more effective. Where possible, this chapter suggests types of assessments that can be integrated with student learning and, as such, are actually part of the instructional process.

After "unpacking" the standards to determine what students should know and be able to do, curriculum designers must decide what they are willing to accept as evidence that students have met these standards. The purpose of this chapter is to guide the development of assessments for those involved with the curriculum writing process.

Assessments can be viewed in two ways. First there is assessment *for* learning. These assessments are commonly associated with **formative assessments** where the intent of the assessment is to increase student learning.

> **formative assessment** Assessments that are on-going, largely informal, and appear throughout the instructional process.

Teachers can use formative assessments to see how much students have learned, and then plan future lessons based on this information. They also are an excellent means for letting students know teacher expectations, to inform them of their progress, and to let them self-assess their own development. The chapters on the various curriculum models provide some additional assessments that are specific to and appropriate for the model.

The second type of assessment is assessment of learning. These assessments are typically associated with giving a grade, and are considered **summative assessments**. They are given at the conclusion of student learning; students will have no chance to improve scores or learn from their feedback to improve performance.

Guskey (2000) uses the analogy of a cook making soup to illustrate the difference between formative and summative assessments. When the soup is being prepared, the cook tastes the soup to determine which additional ingredients to add. This is formative assessment. When the soup is served to the guests and they taste it, it is summative.

Some assessments could be used as either a formative or a summative assessment. The label of formative or summative is more an indication of when the assessment is given and how it is used rather than the type of assessment described.

Other books contain assessment ideas for physical education (Hopple, 2005; Lund & Kirk, 2010; National Association for Sport and Physical Education [NASPE], 1995; Schiemer, 2000). In fact, NASPE has developed an assessment series that contains many ideas for assessments for various curricular models and physical education activities. Additionally, NASPE is developing a new assessment program called P. E. Metrics that features several valid and reliable assessments for use in K–12 physical education (NASPE, 2008). Before describing some assessment formats appropriate for physical education, a discussion about designing assessments is necessary.

Thinking Like an Assessor

Too often, when teachers design assessments, they think like teachers. By thinking like teachers, they dwell on the problems associated with doing assessments rather than finding ways to measure learning. Many of the assessments that teachers describe during convention programs are actually good instructional activities, but are not assessments because they fail to specify criteria; they are developed with teaching rather than assessing in mind. Mere completion of a

summative assessments   Assessments given at the conclusion of the instructional process.

task does not guarantee a level of quality and does not ensure student learning. The addition of criteria to define the level of performance that students need to demonstrate to successfully complete the task is necessary if teachers are to use these tasks for assessment purposes. Wiggins and McTighe (1998) encourage teachers to think like an assessor when designing assessments, concentrating on finding the best way to measure learning. They pose several questions to promote the paradigm shift necessary to do this. The following is a discussion of those ideas as they pertain to physical education.

1. What would be sufficient and reveal evidence of understanding?

   Whereas teachers might be more interested in creating an activity that is interesting and engaging for students, assessors focus on creating activities designed to determine whether students have really grasped a concept or topic, or whether they have only superficial knowledge of the topic. Good assessments allow teachers to measure depth of understanding rather than just factual knowledge. An assessment that lets the teacher know if students have grasped a concept in an interesting, engaging, and challenging way would be the most effective type of assessment because it would also provide students with an incentive to achieve.

2. What misunderstandings are likely? How will I check for these?

   Sometimes students appear to have knowledge of a topic and can explain a certain phenomenon. However, further questioning reveals that the logic students are using to arrive at that conclusion is faulty, and that students don't understand the topic completely. For example, knowing about muscles and flexibility would be important for Standard 4. People frequently begin a warm-up for activity with stretching, because they think it will prevent injury. However, stretching cold muscles does little good and could potentially cause injury. A warm-up should begin with a cardiovascular activity that warms the muscle, followed by stretching. If trying to improve flexibility, stretching should be done at the completion of a workout during the cool down, rather than at the beginning. A good assessment will ask why students are doing something, in an attempt to uncover possible misunderstandings.

3. How will I distinguish between those who really understand and those who don't (although they may seem to)?

   Good assessments will differentiate between students who know the content and those who do not. At a surface level, students may appear to know content. However, as layers of knowledge are peeled away, it quickly becomes apparent who knows the materials and who does not. Good assessments peel the initial layers of knowledge back and reveal depth of understanding. A good written test will document knowledge of rules and strategies as they are applied to game play situations instead of merely having students reiterate or recognize the rule. Skill tests allow teachers to document whether students can perform the skill, and game play assessments provide a way for students to demonstrate that they know when to use the skill appropriately during the game.

4. What performance tasks must anchor the unit and focus the instructional work?

Although the assessment must measure the standard and various forms of student learning, the assessment must also be matched with an appropriate task. For example, if a developmental or skill theme approach was used to teach gymnastics, a required or compulsory routine would not be an appropriate assessment task; however, requiring students to create their own routines using concepts of weight transfer, using space effectively, and the like would assess the developmental concepts. The compulsory routine assessment might require students to do skills that were developmentally inappropriate for them whereas the created routine allows each student to select skills that are developmentally appropriate for the student's levels of achievement. If teachers wanted students to demonstrate the ability to show knowledge of a game by using skills at proper and strategic times, game play assessment completed during a class tournament would be an appropriate assessment.

5. Against what criteria will I distinguish work?

The question that good assessments try to measure is, "What is the gap between what a student knows and what he or she should know to reach the criteria?" When establishing performance criteria, teachers must set these at a level of difficulty sufficient for the students to meet the expected levels of learning and elements of the standards. Purposely setting the bar for performance at a low level to guarantee that all students will meet the criteria does a disservice to the program and the students. Additionally, teachers must realize that past levels of student performance may not be of sufficient rigor to satisfy the intent of the standard or expectation for learning.

Each of these items suggests that when teachers design assessments, they need to step away from items of concern as a teacher, and think like an assessor. In developing assessments for physical education, we encourage teachers to focus on how to engage students and evaluate learning rather than only the former.

Assessments Used to Measure Learning in Physical Education

The following are brief descriptions of the various types of assessments commonly used in physical education. Most types of assessments can be used for almost every curriculum model identified in Section II of this text. Some of the assessments are more commonly associated and used with some specific curriculum models than others. When this is the case, examples of use with the curriculum model are provided. At the same time, teachers are encouraged to use the various assessments with different curriculum models, even if we have not provided an example of such here.

Traditional Assessments in Physical Education

For many years, physical education teachers relied on three types of assessments to measure student learning; skill tests, written tests, and fitness tests have been the mainstays for assessing student learning in physical education. The following sections provide a brief overview of how some of these forms of assessment are used in physical education programs.

SKILL TESTS. **Skill tests** are typically used to measure a student's ability to perform a given skill, usually in a closed environment. They are useful for assessing some aspects of Standard 1, competency in motor skills and movement patterns. At the elementary level, an example of a skill test is the Test of Gross Motor Development, which has evaluations for several fundamental motor skills. In some programs, skill tests are used as proxies for the ability to play a given sport or skill. For example, if students passed skill tests on serving, the forearm pass, and the overhead pass, the assumption was made that they could play volleyball with a reasonable level of skill. Today, game play assessments are a nice complement for skill tests. The skill test assesses student ability to use the skill in a closed environment whereas a game play assessment assesses how well the student can apply the skills, using them at appropriate times and in appropriate situations. The Sport Education curriculum model (van der Mars & Tannehill, Chapter 11) might use skill assessments extensively.

Tests provide a way for students to practice skills in a closed environment. They serve as a good formative assessment, giving students feedback on their progress and indicating where they need to improve along with providing teachers with an idea about whether students have mastered the skill in a closed environment, and are ready to move on to more complex applications. If teachers set a criterion score (e.g., hitting a tennis forehand 10 consecutive times against a wall using correct form), skill tests can be used as a challenge to motivate student performance and learning. Sometimes it is difficult to assess a skill during game play because the student is never in the position to execute it (e.g., a spike in volleyball). Skill tests provide teachers with an opportunity to see how well the student can perform the skill. Skill tests should be seen as a milepost in skill

skill tests   Assessments of student psychomotor ability, usually done in a closed environment.

development with the ultimate goal being that students will have sufficient ability to use the skill correctly during game play. Skill tests provide students with a way to measure improvement. The best skill tests will simulate an authentic game play situation.

Many published skill tests were developed for use in research projects and/or studies. Because they have normative scores that give the researcher or test administrator an idea about the level of skill, they had to be conducted in exactly the same manner for each student. If normative scores were used as criteria, unless the testing protocol was exactly what the test designers had specified, the tests were invalid. Many skill tests are difficult to set up because nets must be set at a certain height, exact distances and exact equipment are required (type of ball, size of ball, etc.). French and her colleagues (French, Rink, Rikard, Mays, Lynn, & Werner, 1991) tested middle school students and found that most lacked sufficient strength to pass the overhead serve test in volleyball. Despite issues with published skill tests, many teachers find them useful for the reasons cited in the previous paragraph.

WRITTEN TESTS. Written tests are used primarily to assess Standard 2, understanding of movement concepts, principles, strategies, and tactics, although Standard 5 and parts of Standard 4 could be assessed using written tests. Because physical education teachers typically deal with a large number of students, written tests in physical education usually consist of selected response items (e.g., multiple choice, true/false, matching), fill in the blank, and possibly short answer essay.

Written tests give teachers an opportunity to assess cognitive knowledge for all students. Sometimes teachers try to informally assess cognitive learning during class time by asking questions. It is difficult to assess every student's knowledge with oral questions if the class is large, and written tests provide ways to measure individual student cognitive learning.

Too often written tests measure only factual information, such as the year when the game was first created, the height of the net or the dimensions of the court, or the number of players on a regulation team. Although there may be some value in knowing the history of a game, knowing tidbits of the game is probably not as important as knowing strategies for scoring points in the game or how to apply some of the rules. Although there is some value to testing basic knowledge, physical education content knowledge consists of much more than this level of learning (knowledge or comprehension). When writing questions for exams, teachers should limit questions to information that students will need to know for many years to come. To access student knowledge of higher levels of learning (analysis, synthesis, and evaluation), more complex questions need to be used on written exams. A multiple-choice question might offer different responses to the application of safety guidelines during a hiking trek. The possible responses would require students to take information learned in class and apply it to the question posed, thus measuring more complex levels of learning.

FITNESS TESTS. **Fitness tests** are used to evaluate the various components of fitness in Standard 4: cardiovascular endurance, muscular strength, muscular endurance, flexibility, and body composition. There are several different test batteries and variations for these tests. The Fitness Education curriculum model (McConnell, Chapter 13) would use fitness testing as an integral part of the model.

Fitness tests can provide teachers with important information about the fitness levels of students. If students score poorly in some areas, this indicates which types of activities are most beneficial for teachers to include in their programs. Fitnessgram has a software program available that explains to parents what the components are, what a normal range should be for a student of that age, the scores on various components of the tests administered, and remedial activities to address areas needing improvement. Given the recent attention to obesity, making parents aware of a student's level of fitness can be helpful and promote healthy habits in young people.

There has been much debate over the years about the usefulness of fitness tests. Some physical educators disagree with the choice of the tests (i.e., the sit and reach only measures flexibility in the hamstrings; what about flexibility in other areas of the body?). Another problem is that some teachers include tests of motor ability (e.g., 50-yard dash, shuttle run, softball throw, standing long jump) in the test battery. Another issue has been the debate between comparing students to normative data (Presidential Fitness Test) and using a criterion referenced score to evaluate student performance (Fitnessgram (2007). For a variety of reasons NASPE recommends that results of fitness tests not be used for determining student grades.

Performance-Based Assessments

In 1989, Wiggins called for a new type of assessment designed to measure learning in an authentic manner. **Performance-based assessments** are designed to measure student learning and understanding about a concept, rather than

fitness tests   Assessments used to measure the components of fitness, often including assessments of cardiovascular endurance, muscular endurance, muscular strength, flexibility, and body fat composition.

performance-based assessments   Assessments used to measure higher levels of student learning, such as a student's ability to apply knowledge while doing a meaningful or worthwhile task (one that is representative of work done in the field).

factual or superficial knowledge. Although some authors use the terms *authentic assessment, alternative assessment,* and *performance-based assessment* to define different types of assessment (Marzano, Pickering, & McTighe, 1993), in this book the three terms will be used interchangeably, which is in keeping with the way other authors use the terms (Herman, Aschbacher, & Winters, 1992; Lund & Kirk, 2010). Performance-based assessments have several characteristics that differentiate them from the traditional assessments described above. According to Lund and Kirk, performance-based assessments:

- Require the presentation of worthwhile or meaningful tasks that are designed to be representative of performance in the field
- Emphasize higher-level thinking and more complex learning
- Articulate criteria in advance so that students know how they will be evaluated
- Embed assessments so firmly in the curriculum that they are practically indistinguishable from instruction
- Expect students to present their work publicly when possible
- Involve the examination of the process, as well as the products of learning

Several different types of assessments are considered performance-based assessments. Many of them represent different ways to measure student learning than the traditional assessments explained in the previous section (i.e., open response questions or essays are an extension of written tests, game play is an extension of skill tests). The primary difference is that performance-based assessments move the testing format to a real-world setting. Because criteria are articulated to students prior to beginning the assessment, each of the examples of performance-based assessment would include a rubric or criteria by which the teacher would evaluate a product or student performance. The following sections contain a brief description of several types of performance-based assessments, suggestions for when they are used appropriately for assessment in physical education, and problems that can impact their use.

Assessments for Learning

As stated earlier, most assessments can be both formative (assessments used on a daily basis to help students learn) and summative (used for grading at the completion of a unit), depending on when they are used in the unit. The assessments described in the following sections are examples of assessments that inform teachers about whether their students have grasped the learning targeted for a lesson. They are excellent formative assessments, but would not by themselves provide sufficient evidence to verify student learning at the conclusion of a unit (e.g., a teacher would not want to make a judgment of student competence on a cultural studies unit based only on role play assessments) or as a measure of program success on a curricular assessment. Given the nature of these assessments, they are subject to what is called a value-laden paradigm and might be tainted by teacher bias caused by how students had performed in the past. That being said, they could be used as artifacts in a portfolio, thus becoming part of the evidence used to show student growth and learning over the course of study.

OBSERVATIONS (TEACHER, SELF, PEER). Given the performance-oriented nature of physical education, observation is an important component of assessing in physical education. Observations done when teachers give oral feedback to students about their performance are not considered assessments. If observation is used as an assessment, it must produce some type of written record of the performance. When doing observations, teachers should have a list of descriptors to use. Some examples of using teacher observation might include the teacher checking the components of a strategy to ensure that they are being demonstrated when a game play strategy is introduced (Standard 2). Students can do observations on themselves or other students using lists of the process components (critical elements) of a skill, while the teacher checks for the accuracy of the feedback provided by the observer. An example of a checklist is provided in Figure 4.1. Standard 5 might be assessed when teachers record incidences of when students willingly work with any partner assigned.

One advantage of using written observations is that teachers are more likely to look systematically at every student in class. When doing informal observations, teachers tend to scan the class to see what the majority of students

---

Checklist for Sportsmanship/Fair Play

The following is a checklist to evaluate positive sport behavior during contests. Check all behaviors observed for the player being observed.

Observed	Not observed	
_____	_____	Abides by the rules for the activity
_____	_____	Does not argue with others
_____	_____	Shares in group/team responsibilities
_____	_____	Gives others a chance to participate
_____	_____	Follows the directions of the coach/group leader
_____	_____	Respects the efforts of others
_____	_____	Offers encouragement to others
_____	_____	Volunteers to help others
_____	_____	Willingly participates in the activity

FIGURE 4.1 Example of a yes/no checklist rubric.

are doing. Sometimes students who are struggling or who are competent bystanders (those students who appear to be engaged in the activity but really are not) are missed. Self and peer observations ensure that all students in the class are watched and are held accountable for doing the specified task.

Peer and self observations should never be used to determine student grades unless the student doing the observation was simply given credit for completing the assignment (Standard 5). Students must understand that the purpose of the observation is purely to provide feedback to the performer, and not to evaluate the person for the purpose of giving that student a grade. If this knowledge is communicated to students, they will be more honest while doing their evaluations and provide better feedback. A second caution about using peer or self-assessment is that students do not naturally know how to observe the performance of others. Physical education teachers have spent many years perfecting observation skills. Students must be taught what to look for when doing the observation, and what an ideal performance should look like. Teaching students to observe and assess performance is like teaching any other skill; it involves explanation, demonstration, practice, and feedback. A written list of items to be observed is also crucial to the process and may be used as an aid when providing instruction on how to complete an effective peer assessment. Teachers should limit the list of traits to a number appropriate for the age of the students doing the observation.

ROLE PLAYS. The affective domain (Standards 5 and 6) is often very difficult to assess. **Role play** assessments present a scenario on a topic to students, and ask them to demonstrate how they would react to it. Many times the situation can be a problem that has arisen in class. An example of a role play assessment would be to assign two students the task of role playing the development of a strategy for working with two team members during a sport education unit who were very competitive with one another and both wanted to be the team's coach. In addition to assessing Standards 5 and 6, role plays could assess cognitive learning (Standard 2). A rubric is an appropriate way to share the criteria for assessments with the students. When assessing role plays, teachers must select traits that they wish to assess and develop appropriate levels of performance for each trait or descriptor.

Role plays provide many "teachable moments" as students present their solution to the problem from the scenario to their peers. Teachers can discuss the approach demonstrated and have class members react to the solutions pre-

role play An assessment in which students present a scenario and then demonstrate how they would react in that situation; role plays are useful as affective domain assessments.

sented. Role plays can make students aware of situations that are problematic to others in the class. The affective domain is difficult to assess, and role plays provide a platform for addressing and assessing it.

Students are typically asked to present their scenario and solution to the class, so role plays are very public events. Teachers must be careful when selecting topics, because students may easily be put into an uncomfortable situation. Also, if students are given an undesirable role, immature students may tease that student after class. Teachers also have to be careful not to typecast a student (e.g., having an obese student play someone who struggles with weight). Role plays are time-consuming to use for assessment, because they usually involve relatively few students. When too many students are involved in the scenario, it is difficult to determine whether students actually had input about how the problem was tackled. Reflections following the presentation of the scenario can be used to assess individual student involvement.

INTERVIEWS. When a teacher has students who do not express themselves well on written work, interviews can be an effective way to determine whether they know the desired information. Standards 2, 5, and 6 could be assessed with interviews. A teacher might ask each student to verbally explain his or her role in a defensive play, or to explain a strategy for defeating an opponent during a net game. The same is true with dispositions important to the affective domain. Much of the debriefing that occurs after adventure activities is actually a form of interview assessment. The Sport Education curriculum model also has good opportunities for using this form of assessment.

As previously stated, interviews are an excellent way to check for understanding with those who have limited writing skills. Using a combination of words and gestures, students can explain things that they are not able to communicate on paper. An interview might also be appropriate to ensure that students know content knowledge, such as the necessary steps for supporting partners (e.g., belaying) during outdoor activities. It may not be convenient to have a pencil and paper to administer a written assessment, but an interview could verify the knowledge, and thus ensure the safety of the person being supported. Teachers could use a checklist to record student knowledge and understanding of key points.

Time is an obvious disadvantage when using interview assessment. It would be difficult to use this form of assessment in a large physical education class. Also, privacy is an issue. Some students might be reluctant to share information about Standard 5 or 6 if they know that a classmate could hear the response. Privacy also becomes an issue when assessing cognitive knowledge. For example, one student might overhear the response of another without doing the work him- or herself, or students engaged in an orienteering lesson might benefit from hearing the response of another student identifying the coordinate for one of the control points of the course.

JOURNALS. **Journals** are an opportunity for students to reflect on their learning and progress, and the happenings of the class. The entries are excellent ways to assess Standards 5 and 6, providing teachers with a way to gain insight into student attitudes toward the class or toward a topic addressed in class. To improve the quality of journal entries, teachers provide a writing prompt to help focus student thoughts. Responses to writing prompts are typically more insightful than if a teacher allows students to simply write for a certain amount of time without specifying a topic. Teachers might also give students the option of doing a "free write," if something occurred during the class about which they wish to vent. It is recommended that teachers not assess journals for their content if evaluating the affective domain, but rather whether students made the entry. If students sense that they get credit only for certain types of entries, these are the types of responses that they will give teachers, and honesty will decrease.

Journals are a great way for a teacher to keep up with the feelings of members of a class. By having students respond to prompts, the teacher can determine how students are reacting to the lessons taught. Some teachers use journal writing to assess cognitive knowledge (Standard 2), and can detect student misinformation or misunderstanding on a topic covered. Journals would provide an excellent way to assess student learning in several of the curricular models including, but not limited to, Outdoor Education, Adventure Education, Cultural Studies, and Personal and Social Responsibility.

Once again, time is a factor for journal writing assessment; writing in journals can subtract minutes from class activity time. However, some teachers make this part of the daily routine, and students retrieve writing materials as class finishes and record their thoughts in a quick, efficient manner. Teachers also must spend time reading student entries. If students sense that teachers are not valuing the assignment enough to read their work, they will put little effort into the assessment.

Multi-Use Assessments

As stated earlier, assessments may be formative (used with lessons for improving student learning) or summative (used for a final evaluation of student performance as for a grade), depending on when and how they were used during the instructional process. The following sections of performance-based assessments, when used correctly, could be either type of assessment.

journals An assessment that provides students opportunities to reflect and write on events or topics in class.

Portfolios

Portfolios are collections of artifacts that, when considered collectively, demonstrate student competency or mastery of some subject area (Lund & Kirk, 2010). Portfolios are generally used to show growth or learning over time. For example, if a portfolio was used to evaluate an Outdoor Education bicycle unit, it might include a fitness pre-assessment, (to determine readiness to participate), a training proposal to eliminate any areas of low fitness, a webquest on bike safety, a project that allows students to document knowledge of how to properly adjust a bicycle or repair broken items on a bike, a log of miles completed during various training sessions, a reflection about participating in a culminating or competitive event, and a final reflective summary of progress that includes what the student learned through the experience. Portfolios are excellent ways to assess all of the content standards, depending on the requirements specified in the rubric and the artifacts included in them.

The advantage of using portfolio assessment is that students can have some choice in the artifacts used to demonstrate competence. Typically, the teacher specifies certain documents that the portfolio must contain (as in the example above), but also gives the student some choice about including additional artifacts. Students are required to write reflections about the artifacts, explaining why they were chosen and how they demonstrate student competence. Portfolios also provide an excellent opportunity to do cross-curricular assessments. Many schools have targeted improving writing skills for all students. Portfolios give physical education teachers an opportunity to measure learning in the content area, as well as contribute to overall school goals. Lastly, Standard 3 in physical education is difficult to assess. Portfolios can be a way to assess Standard 3 because logs of out-of-class activity can be included in the documentation.

One disadvantage to using portfolios is storage. Given the number of students that physical education teachers are responsible for, space to store these documents can be an issue. A second issue is that some teachers allow students to submit an unlimited number of artifacts, which turns the portfolio into a scrapbook. Artifacts for a portfolio must be carefully chosen from the working portfolio so they reflect the types of student learning that the experience provided. Another disadvantage is the time required to evaluate all this student work. It is suggested that students have a working portfolio in which they store possible artifacts, but turn in an evaluation portfolio containing selective pieces to document student learning.

portfolios   Collections of artifacts that typically are used to show students' competency or mastery of a subject area.

PROJECTS. **Projects** give students the opportunity to create something that demonstrates their knowledge of a topic. Typically a project demonstrates cognitive knowledge (Standard 2), but knowledge of fitness (Standard 4), as well as Standards 5 and 6, could also be evaluated with projects. Multimedia projects are very popular. Students might develop a PowerPoint presentation designed to teach officials the rules of volleyball that are commonly misinterpreted (Standard 2). A video showing safety practices when participating in outdoor activities (Standard 5) is another example of a project. Developing a rap about fitness is a project that demonstrates knowledge about fitness concepts and principles (Standard 4). Students might produce a puppet play depicting their enjoyment of physical activity (Standard 6).

Projects are an excellent way to allow students with multiple intelligences other than kinesthetic to use their talents, while demonstrating learning in physical education. Students are usually very motivated to complete these projects and will spend more time on them than they would to prepare for a written test. When projects are used, teachers may learn something about student talents or interests of which they were not previously aware. They also provide ESL students an opportunity to demonstrate learning in an alternative manner.

Sometimes teachers like to give students options or choices with projects, which results in students having a voice in the assessment and their own learning. Problems arise when the projects do not demonstrate the same type of learning or knowledge or are not of similar difficulty. Teachers need to make sure the project genuinely demonstrates learning rather than just being an activity that students will enjoy. If the project options demonstrate the same learning, a single rubric or several with minor variations would be appropriate. Additionally, if a project involves several students, teachers should include ways to evaluate individual effort to document that each member of the group has learned the desired information. If the assignment is completed out of class, teachers must make sure that all students have access to the resources they need (e.g., video cameras, computers) and that the project is truly the efforts of the student rather than ambitious parents.

GAME PLAY. Game play is usually part of a sport unit, and can easily be an assessment tool for teachers when an appropriate rubric is written to assess it. Psychomotor skills, cognitive knowledge (rules and strategies), cooperation and teamwork, and safety can all be assessed during game play. In short, depending on the rubric used, game play can be used to evaluate Standards 1, 2, 5, and 6. In Chapter 10, Mitchell and Oslin explain the Game Performance Assessment Instrument (GPAI), which is a game play assessment tool used to assess the use

projects Assessments that require students to create something that demonstrates their knowledge of a topic.

of tactical strategies during a game as well as skill execution. Sport Education and Teaching Games for Understanding are two curricular models that would make extensive use of game play assessments.

The advantage of using game play as an assessment tool in physical education is that it requires no additional time to assess because game play is an integral part of the instructional process. Students play a game as an instructional activity while the teacher evaluates student performance. Game play can be used as either a formative or a summative assessment.

Discrete skills are difficult to evaluate during game play. Sometimes students are out of position, and might use incorrect form to make a play. If a teacher were using game play to evaluate student form on a skill, the student would not receive a high score, despite making a spectacular play. Also, students might not have an opportunity to perform a skill during a regular game because the opportunity never arises. An assessment should not penalize students because of the lack of opportunity to demonstrate their skills.

With programmatic assessment, districts might elect to have outside individuals (not the teacher) evaluate student performance to ensure an unbiased evaluation. Because games can sometimes last a long time, it is undesirable to observe a regular competitive game. Instead, students are given a limited amount of time to demonstrate certain skills. The game is not a competitive game, but rather an opportunity to demonstrate certain skills as well as the knowledge of when these skills are appropriately used during the game. Students are told the components they must demonstrate, and are given the rubric used to evaluate these. In some respects, students must have greater skill to set up the appropriate game play situations than is the case if the situation occurred naturally during a game. By assessing game play in this scripted game, items that teachers wish to evaluate are more likely to be present than in a traditional competitive game.

EVENT TASKS. **Event tasks** are performance-based assessments that can be completed in a single class period (NASPE, 1995). Examples of event tasks include students being given a challenge or a problem to solve in their adventure unit, with the teacher assessing their cooperation and teamwork, students in a cultural studies curriculum developing an inclusive game, and students in a dance unit creating a dance that shows their knowledge of dance composition and choreography. An event task could be used to evaluate every standard, depending on the task and the accompanying rubric. Outdoor Education is another curriculum model that might use event tasks extensively.

event tasks   Performance tasks that can be completed within a single class period.

Event tasks have been used in statewide assessments. They are relatively simple to set up, and because they are completed in a single class period are efficient to administer. Some issues related to event tasks might include having sufficient equipment for every group in class to complete the task, or making sure that students have adequate prior knowledge to complete the task within the time frame. Teachers also should be sure that students do not find equipment too novel, and spend their time exploring the equipment rather than completing the task. As with all performance-based assessments, it is essential that students are given the rubric or criteria for evaluation when receiving the directions for the event task assessment.

ESSAYS. This type of performance-based assessment refers to a complex assessment that uses higher levels of thinking to evaluate student learning. **Essays** are representative of something that a person in the field might create or do. Some examples of essays might include writing a script for announcers at a tennis match (Standard 2), a publicist's report in a Sport Education unit, a brochure describing a new fitness program and how it addresses the various components of fitness (Standard 4), an article for the parents' newsletter about the new dance and rhythms program and its contribution to meeting the needs of all students (Standard 5), or following a cycling unit, an interview with "Lance Armstrong," talking about preparation for and the feelings experienced after winning the Tour de France (Standards 2 and 6). The Cultural Studies curriculum model contains several opportunities for using this type of assessment.

Essays provide a great opportunity for students to demonstrate content knowledge in creative ways. Students who might not appear to be "that interested" in physical education can really "get into" this type of asessment. Many schools are encouraging teachers to promote writing across the curriculum, so essay assessments provide an opportunity for physical education to contribute to that goal. Finished products are great for distribution during parents' night or an open house. In one elementary school, a student teacher did a heart obstacle course, giving her students facts about the heart and keeping it healthy. When students returned to their academic classroom, the classroom teacher had them record this knowledge, and use it to create a brochure. Parents visited the physical education class during an open house to have a personal tour of the obstacle course by their child and receive the brochure created by the class.

Students who struggle with writing may find this type of assessment challenging. Because some of these children are more verbal, they can work well with a group, and provide ideas that other students can capture in writing.

> **essays**   A performance assessment representative of what someone in the field would do, such as writing a dialogue, creating a brochure, or writing an article to demonstrate knowledge of a topic.

While working in groups it is important to share tasks across all students and avoid such practices as, females automatically being assigned as the writer. Additionally, if the teacher uses essays in class too frequently, taking time to write in physical education can subtract time available for physical activity. Block scheduling and "downtime" might alleviate this problem by providing extra minutes to use for writing activities.

OPEN RESPONSE QUESTIONS. **Open response questions** present a scenario that frames a problem for students, and then gives them an opportunity to solve it. Because there are multiple ways to approach the problem, there is no single correct answer. This is not to imply that every student response is appropriate. Students are expected to give a solution, and then provide a rationale explaining how they arrived at it. This gives students the opportunity to apply knowledge given in class to real-world scenarios. Different types of open response questions require different types of higher order thinking skills. Open response questions at first blush might resemble traditional essay questions. The major difference is that the answer to an open response question should begin with the words "it depends" (Lund & Kirk, 2010). A Cultural Studies or Fitness curriculum might make extensive use of open response questions. For example, a fitness unit might take one of the commonly advertised pieces of fitness equipment and through a series of scaffolded questions explore student knowledge of how to achieve fitness while exploring the value of the device.

Single dimension questions are fairly simple to write; it takes 10 to 15 minutes for students to respond to them. They usually require students to evaluate some information, and either draw a conclusion or take a stance. Students are required to justify that response with explanations, examples, or evidence. An example of a single dimension question that could be used to assess Standard 5 is the following:

> *You are the coach of a team participating in a sport education unit. A key game is being played today, and your best player has not been working very hard during practice. You must decide whether to allow the player to participate or punish the poor practice behavior by having him or her sit on the bench. Decide what you are going to do and give your reasoning for that decision.*

open response questions   Present problems and then require students to respond. The students' responses typically begins with "it depends."

single dimension questions   Open response questions that usually require students to evaluate information, draw conclusions, and then justify their responses.

Scaffolded questions contain a sequence of tasks or questions, each dependent upon a previous answer; questions are increasingly more difficult. **Multiple independent questions** have a series of questions that are not related to the previous question. **Student choice questions** allow students to select from a list of questions, each with similar content. An example of a student choice open response question for Standard 2 is the following:

> *Describe the importance of non-locomotor movements in one of the following activities: basketball, creative dance, pickleball, canoeing, or inline skating. Identify the non-locomotor movements in order of importance, giving your rationale for selecting that order.*

Response to provided information questions provide a prompt (e.g., some data, a picture, or a reading), and ask the students to respond in some way to the prompt. As with the other performance-based assessments, students will have the rubrics while writing responses. When writing rubrics, teachers must be sure that criteria are broad enough to allow for student creativity and for possible correct responses that were not anticipated. A narrow rubric that only allows very specific responses can turn a good open response question into an essay question.

Open response questions are excellent for measuring cognitive knowledge for Standards 2 and 4, or affective dispositions as in Standards 5 and 6. Because the questions require students to give reasons for the response, they can be used to verify understanding of important concepts. Although the single dimension questions may be appropriate for younger students, more complex questions would probably be used in elective classes with older students who have better writing skills and more depth of knowledge on a topic.

Time is a significant factor in using open response questions for assessment. Good open response questions require time and several revisions to develop. The accompanying rubric is also critical to the success of the question. Also, much teacher time is required to read and evaluate responses.

scaffolded questions   Open response questions that contain a sequence of questions, each dependent on a previous answer and each more difficult than the previous question.

multiple independent questions   Open response questions that ask a series of questions that are related, but are not dependent on the response given to the previous question of the series.

student choice questions   Open response questions in which students are presented with several questions that assess similar knowledge and are given the option of selecting which question to answer.

responses to provided information questions   Open response questions that provide information (e.g., data, picture, article) to which a student must respond.

STUDENT LOGS. Documenting outside participation in physical activity is difficult (Standard 3), but student logs provide a means for doing so. **Logs** are simply a list of activities or practice trials completed by the student. Sometimes Sport Education gives team points for practice outside of class. Logs used in class can measure improvement over time. Students might indicate success rates for various skills within a unit using a student log. Teachers would look at the logs to see whether these rates are improving. If not, remedial work is necessary. Some logs consist of blank spaces on which students can record their efforts, whereas others might indicate the type of activity desired, and students merely fill in the number of trials for that activity.

Logs can be motivational for students as they record activity or successes. Students might lose track of their output, and maintaining activity logs can help them see what they have accomplished. Logs also are useful artifacts for portfolios.

Unless teachers hold students accountable for their efforts, students might not be completely honest when completing their logs. A recent online fitness course offered in Florida was declared a failure, because students were dishonest in reporting their activities. Pre- and post-testing students might have decreased this problem, because students would have been required to show improvement that resulted from their efforts.

Establishing Criteria for Assessments

When students know teacher expectations for performance, learning is more focused and more effective (Shanklin, 2004). This section will explain ways and provide examples of ways, such as **rubrics**, to inform students about assessment criteria.

Checklists

Checklists, also referred to as performance lists (Arter & McTighe, 2001), can be used to identify the characteristics that should be included in the assessment. They are generally scored as either "yes" or "no," or simply have an area for the assessor to make a tick mark, thus indicating the presence of the trait. No judgment about the level of quality is made; the trait or characteristic is either present or not. See Figure 4.1 for an example of a checklist. Checklists are useful when evaluating simple performance, such as a peer or student/self-observation

---

logs   Lists of activities or practice trials completed by the students.
rubric   The criteria by which a performance, portfolio, or product is evaluated.
checklists   A list of elements or descriptors that are present or not present in the performance being evaluated.

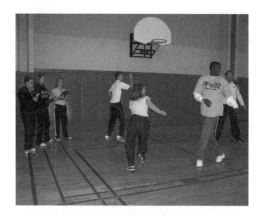

(Standard 1). They might also be used for evaluating journals because they require no teacher judgment of the quality of the content. Standard 2 could be assessed with a checklist if teachers showed students a video of skills and then required students to evaluate these skills for correct form using the checklist.

Checklists are relatively easy to construct and easy to administer. They can be very comprehensive (have several characteristics in them), and can still be completed in a timely manner. When using checklists for peer or self-assessments, it is suggested that the number of items listed be appropriate for students of that age. Checklists are very useful for evaluating the process, or the quality of the performance (e.g., critical elements).

All elements on a checklist are of equal importance; there is no way to indicate that one characteristic is more important than another. The second problem with checklists is that there is no way to indicate the beginning presence of a characteristic found in initial learning stages. Unless a trait is present as stated in the performance criteria, it should not be checked off. Lastly, checklists are difficult to use for grading. The only way for a teacher to determine competence is to have every item marked off.

Point Systems

The second type of performance list is a **point system**. It is very similar to a checklist, with one important distinction—the descriptors are assigned points, and the evaluator can indicate which of the items are more important by assigning more points to them. They could be used to evaluate assessments in Standards 1, 2, 4, and 5. Figure 4.2 shows an example of a point system rubric used for assessing a fitness portfolio.

point system   A list of characteristics to be evaluated that has an assigned point value for each characteristic; if the characteristic is present, then the designated number of points is awarded.

Scoring Guide for a Fitness Portfolio

____ Fitness Evaluation (15 points)

    ____ Abdominal strength (2 points)

    ____ Pacer or other test of aerobic endurance (4 points)

    ____ Flexed arm hang/pull-ups/push-ups (2 points)

    ____ Sit and reach (2 points)

    ____ Body fat (3 points)

        ____ triceps

        ____ calf

    ____ Resting heart rate (1 point)

    ____ Height (1 point)

    ____ Weight (1 point)

____ Fitness Plan (30 points)

    ____ Calculate target heart rate (2 points)

    ____ Calculate Body Mass Index (2 points)

    ____ Analysis of the current level of fitness (5 points)

    ____ Needs based on research (5 points)

    ____ Proposed workout plan (16 points)

        ____ Warm-up and recording chart (3 points + 1 point for chart)

        ____ Strength workout and recording chart (3 points + 1 point for chart)

        ____ Flexibility program and recording chart (3 points + 1 point for chart)

        ____ Aerobic program and recording chart (3 points + 1 point for chart)

____ Results (30 points)

    ____ Completed workout logs (10 points)

    ____ Weekly journal entries for exercise and nutrition (10 points)

    ____ Analysis of fitness improvements (10 points)

____ Future plans (15 points)

    ____ Strategy for continuing to exercise (5 points)

    ____ Analysis of barriers (5 points)

    ____ Goal for 6 months from now (5 points)

FIGURE 4.2 Example of a point system scoring guide.

As with checklists, point system performance lists are fairly easy to construct. Because points are assigned, they can be used for grading purposes. Descriptors that are most important can be given emphasis by being worth more points.

Problems arise with point system performance lists when teachers try to award partial credit for characteristics, without stating how students get partial credit. When the allocation of points for criteria is not clearly defined, teachers might award a different number of points to different students for equivalent work. A second problem arises when, in an attempt to make an assessment more clear, teachers might list several components to be included under a broader category, with points being assigned to the overall category. Problems arise here when some of the elements under that category are missing, and the teacher has failed to indicate the worth of those subelements. The sample point system in Figure 4.2 shows how to avoid that problem.

Analytic Rubrics

Analytic rubrics require the evaluator to make a judgment of quality about the various descriptors used, allowing acknowedgment of the rudimentary presence of a trait or characteristic. Because it takes more time to make a judgment about the degree to which a descriptor is present, fewer traits are generally used with analytic rubrics. There are two different types of analytic rubrics. **Quantitative analytic rubrics** use a number to indicate the degree to which the descriptor is present (see Figure 4.3). The number should be anchored by a word or short phrase so that the number has meaning and the person doing the evaluation has some indication about what the number represents. This practice also improves reliability. **Qualitative analytic rubrics** use verbal descriptions for the various levels. Because of the time involved to do the evaluation, qualitative rubrics typically have fewer traits or descriptors than do quantitative rubrics. Although any number of levels can be written, generally this is an even number so that the evaluator is forced to make a decision about level of quality and not simply award the middle score. See Table 4.1 for an example of a qualitative rubric.

Analytic rubrics are valuable for use with formative assessments. Students can see how their performance is rated with regard to each of the descriptors identified in the criteria. The descriptions associated with the qualitative rubric provide students with an opportunity to see what they must do to move to the

quantitative analytic rubrics   Rubrics that use numbers to indicate how each descriptor is evaluated against pre-determined criteria; the numbers are anchored with a word or phrase to indicate the level of performance that the number represents.
qualitative analytic rubrics   Rubrics that use verbal descriptions of the various levels for each descriptor being evaluated.

0 = Never 1 = Some of the time 2 = About half of the time 3 = Most of the time									
Changes levels to show variety									
Uses different pathways									
Uses space effectively									
Shows changes of force and energy									
Stays with the beat of the music									
Smooth transitions between balance and locomotor movements									
Shows contrasts (e.g., fast/slow, even/uneven, etc.)									
Dancers work in harmony with one another									
Uses various parts of the body to enhance aesthetics									
Creates focus by emphasizing the movement									

FIGURE 4.3 Example of a quantitative rubric.

TABLE 4.1

Example of a Qualitative Analytic Rubric

Assessment task: Student will send and receive an object with an implement or foot (10 trials for each) with a partner.

Games Activities: Level 2 Rubric

	1: Developing	*2: Acceptable*	*3: Target*
Control of object when moving	Student chases object when moving. Student avoids changing pathways; chooses only to manipulate object in a straight pathway. Student manipulates object slowly. Student loses control of object when looking up to pass or passes without looking. Object is maintained too close to the body and parts of the body get in the way or cause the student to lose control of the object.	Object is controlled at a moderate speed, keeping object at appropriate distance from the body or implement (e.g., hockey stick). Student attempts different pathways to manipulate object, temporarily losing control but regaining control quickly. Student slows forward progress in order to gain control of object before passing.	Object is controlled at an appropriate distance from the body or implement (e.g., hockey stick). Uses different pathways to move the object. Controls the object close to the body when changing speeds and when preparing to send the object. Student transitions from dribbling to passing smoothly.
Control of object when stationary	Object control is sporadic. Uses too little or too much force when manipulating object. Stance is shoulder width apart and not staggered.	Object is controlled at an appropriate distance from the body or implement but may need to shift stance regularly to maintain control/catch up with the object.	Object is controlled at an appropriate distance from the body or implement (e.g., hockey stick) using appropriate stance (e.g., staggered). Uses appropriate force when manipulating object (e.g., is able to send a "catchable" object to the receiver).

Continued

TABLE 4.1

Example of a Qualitative Analytic Rubric—Cont'd

	1: Developing	*2: Acceptable*	*3: Target*
Sending	Moving target is unable to gain control of sent object within a reasonable amount of time because object was sent to an inappropriate place or with inappropriate force. Sender does not step when passing.	Sends object with appropriate force to moving receiver most of the time (at times the receiver needs to stop and gain control rather than continuous motion). Uses good form.	Sends object with appropriate force to moving receiver (just in front of the receiver). Sends object to receiver using correct form (e.g., all critical elements). Sends object to receiver who does not have to stop and gain control of object (one continuous motion).
Receiving	Blocks the object rather than giving with the object to absorb force. Loses control of body balance while receiving the object.	Consistently (75%+) receives object with appropriate force when stationary. Usually (50%+) receives object with appropriate force when moving.	Provides for a target partner. Receives object with appropriate force (gives) when moving and when stationary.

next level. Because students are able to see the criteria, they can self-evaluate, and are usually motivated to work hard and move to the next level. When analytic rubrics are used for summative assessments, the various descriptors should be weighted so that more important items can receive greater emphasis.

Analytic rubrics are difficult to use for grading. In the example shown, there are 10 characteristics identified. If a student receives a 2 for two of the items, a 3 for four of the items, and a 1 for the remaining items, it is difficult to translate this into a grade. The grade should not be based upon the average of all the scores because every characteristic is not equally important. Also, provisions should be made that if a student receives an unsatisfactory score on one or more of the items they should not receive an overall satisfactory score on the assessment. A condition should be added that a student must score at least at an acceptable level of performance on all descriptors to have a satisfactory performance on the assessment.

Holistic Rubrics

Holistic rubrics are also verbal descriptions of the criteria for performance (see Figure 4.4). Instead of having each trait analyzed and scored separately, holistic rubrics look at the performance as a whole, and a single score for the performance or product is awarded. A paragraph containing descriptions of the various characteristics is developed for each level of the rubric. To receive the score at a given level, all of the characteristics indicated should be at that level of quality. If one or two items are at a lower level, then the lower score should be given. Exemplars, or examples of student work at a given level, are helpful to use while training a person to use holistic scoring.

Holistic rubrics are typically used for summative (final) assessments in which students have no chance to go back and improve performance. They are commonly used in statewide assessments, or for determining a grade because a single score is given. Also, because a single judgment is made, they tend to be much faster to use than analytic rubrics because analytic rubrics require the user to make a judgement of quality about each of the traits listed.

The disadvantage for using holistic scoring is that students are rarely at a single level for each of the traits or descriptors. It is hard for teachers to give the lower score when they know that part of the performance is actually at a higher level. Holistic rubrics are also more difficult for students to interpret. When they receive a score, they have no idea whether part of the performance was actually higher than the score given, which is why they are not usually used with formative assessments.

Using Curricular Assessments

If state-mandated assessments for physical education don't exist, teachers planning the curriculum will want to develop assessments that measure student learning at various intervals in a K–12 program. These assessments are directly tied to content standards, and are designed to determine whether students have attained the skills necessary to meet the specified goals. The process we used for developing physical education assessments for the Indiana Department of Education is similar to the one a writing team should follow when developing assessments for the curriculum. Figure 4.5 explains that project, as well as what teachers developing a curriculum need to do to develop a comprehensive assessment system.

holistic rubrics   Rubrics that look at the performance as a whole and make a single determination of worth; each level contains descriptions or criteria for the various traits or characteristics being evaluated in a single paragraph.

Rubric for a High School Dance Unit Assessment

Level 4: Can perform any dance step either facing one direction or turning. Can dance in any formation with a partner or others. Anticipates next step so as to facilitate transitions. Dance steps are automatic. Leads rather than following others when appropriate. Knows when additional steps or movements can be added to enhance the aesthetic quality of the dance. Student performs all steps in time with the music. No hesitation when changing tempos or rhythmic pattern. If a break in the music occurred, dancer would be able to get back on tempo with dance steps. "Hears" the tempo without having to count. Is able to move smoothly between steps while dancing with a partner, regardless of partner position. Movement flows from one movement pattern/step to the next. Uses eye contact and head movement to stylize dances. Smiles and demonstrates enjoyment while doing the movements. Uses body movements to emphasize/enhance dance moves. Dances with much confidence and style. Seeks diversity with dance partners and groups. Looks forward to dancing with others as an opportunity to get to know others in the class. Accepts errors from others (doesn't tease or belittle), and tries to help them with areas of difficulty. Demonstrates proper dance etiquette. Others enjoy dancing with this person.

Level 3: Dances performed include the following steps: polka, mazurka, waltz, two-step, Texas two-step, buzz turns, ball change (rock step, shuffle), and bleking. Dances can be performed in circles, two, or four couple formations. Can change direction and turn while dancing without partner(s). Can change directions and/or orientation in the room without difficulty while performing dance steps. Could explain steps to others if asked to do so. Student performs steps with the music. If errors do occur, the observer may not notice because the performer quickly gets back with the music. Student is able to adjust to changes in tempo, even with changes in the music tempo. May occasionally count to self to stay on tempo. Moves smoothly between different steps of movement patterns. Anticipates next step so there is no break between the steps. Can dance with a partner and move from one step to another. Incorporates head, arm, and leg movements when appropriate. Additional movements add to the aesthetic appeal of the dance. Moves with confidence. Willingly works with anyone in class either as a partner or group. Attempts to help those who experience difficulty. Demonstrates basic dance etiquette.

Level 2: Dances performed include the following steps: skipping, grapevine, schottische, slide, leap, gallop, and stamp. Most dances are done in circles (single, double, or broken). Performs simple/basic turns, and/or changes of direction. Knows the steps for the dances performed without watching others. May make occasional errors but can re-establish correct step pattern. Student performs steps and is usually with the music. If errors occur, can get back with dance's rhythm fairly quickly. May occasionally be on the wrong foot due to an error, but can correct this and re-establish rhythmic pattern. Can detect changes of tempo in the music. May count aloud to stay on the beat. Usually is able to move from one step to another without taking extra steps. When an error in the movement pattern is made, student is able to pick up new step. May hesitate or pause slightly between steps. Incorporates a few additional arm and/or head movements with dance steps. Additional movements may appear "stiff" or unnatural, but they are added. Works with a variety of students in class. Will dance with a partner.

Level 1: Can perform dances that include walking, running, and hopping movements. Most steps are done in lines or a single circle. May have difficulty turning. Can do dances, but shows some hesitancy. Watches others while performing to ensure correct steps. Student may perform steps correctly, but does not perform them with the beat. Student is slow to respond to changes in beat/tempo. Fails to hear changes in the music. Shows some hesitancy when changing between movement patterns or steps. May miss a beat or step. Performs basic dance steps with little or no style. Works with students similar to self. Rejects attempts by teacher when asked to work with those other than friends.

FIGURE 4.4 Example of a holistic rubric.

The process began by unpacking the state physical education content standards. Standards had been developed for every grade level, kindergarten through 9th grade. Assessments prior to those given at the exit standards are benchmarks that indicate student progress toward the exit outcome (Wood, 2003). We decided that we could group students and get adequate indication of student progress toward the exit outcomes, and thus not require teachers to administer yearly assessments. For this reason, assessments were written for K–1, 2–3, 4–5, 6–8, and 9. Teachers would be free to assess students at any time during that time frame to determine whether students had met the criteria specified for the assessment in the age grouping. By looking at the exit standards first, which in this state was grade 9, a determination was made about what graduates of the physical education program should know and be able to do. Starting with the exit requirements, a backward map for each standard was developed down to kindergarten, where students began their journey toward becoming physically educated. It was critical for members of the writing team to work through all the grade levels to get a smooth progression within each standard. At the elementary level, the writing team determined that the standards could be met with assessments for four categories of physical activity: dance, gymnastics/body control, net games, and goal games.[1] Within each category, assessments were developed that were progressively more complex in the upper grades and also required greater skill. At the K–1 level, the assessments were done in a relatively closed environment with the environment gradually becoming more open and more complex for grades 4–5. This allowed a gradual progression because at the 6–8 level students were expected to play small-sided games, do sophisticated dances, more complex gymnastics requirements, as well as other activities. The analytic rubric in Table 4.1 is actually an example of one of the rubrics developed for games at the 2–3 level.

At the middle school grades, teachers and students were given some choice about the types of activities in which they would demonstrate competence, because most programs do not have sufficient time to offer every sport and activity that would be developmentally appropriate for that age. A table was produced that grouped activities in much the same manner as found in Mitchell and Oslin's Chapter 10, Teaching Games for Understanding. Table 4.2 shows the chart that was developed for middle grades. It was decided that students would demonstrate competency (as defined by the rubric) in four activities and mastery in two others with no more than two activities coming from each category. This forced students to engage in a variety of activities, which is an important factor in meeting the standards.

[1]These areas are traditionally associated with the Developmental Model found in Chapter 7. When planning assessments at the district level, teachers will have the luxury of knowing resources available in the district. Assessments could be expanded to include activities from other curriculum models. We are not suggesting that this list of activities is suitable for all; it is an example of how a district might conceptualize its curricular assessments.

FIGURE 4.5 Developing a comprehensive assessment system.

If games and activities are grouped into categories with several common characteristics as was done in Table 4.2, then **generalized rubrics**, such as the one found in Figure 4.6, can be developed. The advantage of developing a generalized rubric is that fewer rubrics must be developed. Also, students and teachers become familiar with the descriptors and levels of performance, and

generalized rubrics   Universal rubrics that can be used to evaluate many different types of related performances.

TABLE 4.2

Chart of the Categories of Movement Forms for Middle School Assessments

Individual Activities	Fitness Activities	Rhythmics	Net Games	Goal	Target	Aquatics
Tumbling	Cycling Aerobic dance Weight training	Folk Square Line Social Aerobic	Badminton Pickleball Volleyball	Basketball Soccer Ultimate Floor hockey	Bowling Archery Golf	Swimming

they do not need to be taught, as would be the case with a task-specific (sport- or activity-specific) rubric. Looking closely at Figure 4.6, the psychomotor domain is not assessed directly. However, students must be able to demonstrate the psychomotor skills if they are to demonstrate the conceptual understandings indicated on this rubric. To ensure that students had these skills, teachers might use skill assessments while teaching these concepts. The skill assessments would not be included as the curricular assessment; they would be part of a teacher's instructional format.

High school assessments, although similar to those used at the middle school level, are more complex and demand increased levels of skill competence. Additional categories that encompass some of the other curriculum models and will meet the intent of the standards could be added to the table used for the middle school level, in order to accommodate the various curricular models. Also, some activities that are more developmentally appropriate for high school students are added to the existing categories.

The rubrics developed for this project are not perfect and will require pilot testing to "work out the bugs." The more any assessment is used and refined, the better the quality. Wood (2003) discusses the difficulty of creating a cut score for high stakes assessments. One of the methods of setting performance criteria described by Wood involves assessing skilled performers and unskilled performers (as defined by a panel of experts), and determining whether the assessment indicates the appropriate skill level. A detailed description of this critical process is contained in that publication. Six steps are suggested for the process:

1. Choose a review panel.
2. Choose a method or methods for setting cutoff scores.
3. Train panelists.
4. Set cutoff scores.
5. Compile evidence for validity and generalizability of cutoff scores.
6. Carefully document the process.

Along with developing assessments, a system to hold teachers accountable for administering the assessments and scoring them reliably must be developed.

Target Activities
Archery, Bowling, and Golf

Criteria for assessment
1. Demonstrates good form/technique and a slight stillness on the *ready position/ preparatory stance.*
2. Demonstrates good technique on movements of the *draw or backswing.*
3. Demonstrates a good *release/contact* and *follow-through.*
4. Demonstrates ability to *hit the target.*
5. Demonstrates knowledge of the rules or etiquette of the sport.
6. Demonstrates responsible personal and social behavior.

Scoring rubric for target activities (archery, bowling, and golf)
Proficient
1. Uses proper ready position; no more than 2 observable errors in 6 trials.
2. Uses good technique on draw and backswing; no more than 2 observable errors in 6 trials.
3. Demonstrates correct technique on release/contact and follow-through; no more than 2 observable errors in 6 trials.
4. Hits the target.
    Archery: at least 4 arrows stay fixed in target
    Bowling: knocks down a pin on at least 4 of 6 attempts.
    Golf: ball contacted and sent forward in air on at least 4 of 6 swings
5. Has thorough knowledge of rules in all situations and etiquette associated with the sport.
6. Can keep score accurately.
7. Is courteous to others, follows safety procedures at all times, and informs others when they do not follow these provisions.
Competent
1. Uses proper ready position; no more than 3 observable errors in 6 trials.
2. Usually uses good technique on draw and back swing; no more than 3 observable errors in 6 trials.
3. Usually demonstrates correct technique on release/contact and follow-through; no more than 3 observable errors in 6 trials.
4. Usually hits the target.
    Archery: at least 3 arrows stay fixed in target
    Bowling: knocks down a pin on at least 3 of 6 attempts.
    Golf: ball contacted and sent forward in air on at least 3 of 6 swings
5. Solid knowledge of the rules.
6. Is courteous to others and follows safe procedures at all times without being reminded by others.
Developing
1. Uses improper ready position; more than 3 observable errors in 6 trials.
2. Uses improper technique on draw and back swing; more than 3 observable errors in 6 trials.
3. Does not demonstrate correct technique on release/contact and follow-through; more than 3 observable errors in 6 trials.
4. Does not usually hit the target.
    Archery: fewer than 3 arrows stay fixed in target
    Bowling: knocks down fewer than 3 pins in 6 attempts
    Golf: ball not sent forward in air on at least 3 swings
5. Is unsure of rules and how to keep score; makes errors regularly about proper etiquette.
6. Is unaware of others during performance; violates safety procedures, creating an unsafe environment for self and others.

FIGURE 4.6 Example of a generalized rubric for target sports.

This is an important step to ensure that the assessments are administered correctly and that teachers are scoring student results accurately. Ideally an independent review team that makes a site visit to the school should score student performance. Most districts lack the resources to do this, so training teachers to use the assessments properly and accurately is seen as an alternative. Fay and Doolittle (2002) note that assessments would fail without teacher training on how to use them. South Carolina has implemented an accountability system with its state assessments where schools videotape the assessments and send 20% of their results to the state department every three years to be checked for accuracy in scoring. This process is very time consuming and expensive, but it has proven to be educational for physical educators in that state. Leaders in South Carolina are encouraged by the results, and feel that the quality of physical education programs is improving as a direct result of the state assessment system. Similar types of teacher development are possible for a school district that implements its own curricular assessment system.

In summary, when creating assessments for curriculums that are not governed by state assessments:

1. Begin by looking at the standards, and determine what students should know and be able to do to demonstrate that the standards are met.
2. Decide at which levels benchmark assessments will be administered to determine whether the standards have been met.
3. Develop assessments designed to measure the degree to which students are meeting standards, starting with the exit standards and moving backward through the grades.
4. Set levels of performance for the tasks.
5. Determine an accountability system to ensure the implementation and accuracy of the assessment process.

Many of the assessments explained in the previous section could be used to measure student attainment of the standards. To avoid overwhelming teachers by requiring multitudes of assessments, districts should use larger, more holistic assessments for assessing curriculum benchmarks, which can assess several standards in an authentic, realistic manner. These larger assessments will allow teachers and students to spend sufficient time to accurately assess student achievement of the standard(s). Portfolios, projects, or student performances are some examples of the "big picture" assessments that might be used for curricular assessment.

Suggestions for Developing Big Picture Assessments Appropriate for Curricular Evaluation

Developing curricular assessments is not an easy task to do alone. Working in a group gives many perspectives and opinions. The disagreements that arise can strengthen the resulting assessments when they are resolved through compromise. For example, the group working on middle school assessments in Indiana had over 150 years of teaching experience among them. Lengthy discussions ensued over seemingly minute points. The group talked for over an hour trying to decide whether to assess the serve in net games. A good serve on a net game will stop play (e.g., an ace). We needed to have a way to get the implement (ball or bird) into play so that students could demonstrate other aspects of game play. The result was that the serve was eliminated from the criteria despite its importance to game play. This is one example of numerous discussions that occurred during the assessment writing process. The following suggestions are offered to help when designing curricular assessments.

1. Develop generalized assessments that can be used for multiple activities.

   By using generalized assessments rather than task specific assessments, far fewer assessments will need to be written. This means that there are fewer rubrics to write, as well. Teachers could select any of the activities in the category to teach the important concepts, and avoid trying to teach every activity. Concepts are taught and emphasized as students focus on the key components of the game or activity. According to teachers in the field who tested the assessments, students were able to see the connections between games within the category, and learning was more effective.

2. Use assessments that address multiple standards.

   When developing curricular assessments, you don't need a different assessment for every standard. Develop assessment tasks and rubrics that include as many standards as possible. For example, while choreographing a dance, students could demonstrate competency in psychomotor skills, cognitive knowledge, relationships with others, and enjoyment of the activity. The portfolio assessment in Figure 4.2 covers many standards using a fitness lens. An outdoor culminating activity offers the opportunity to assess cognitive knowledge, psychomotor skills, awareness of safety, and relationships with others. Using fewer assessments with better depth means that teachers will have fewer assessments to administer and less paperwork to complete, but will still have the opportunity to document the degree to which their students are meeting the standards.

3. Develop assessments prior to beginning the teaching process.

   In the past, teachers waited until the completion of the activity to develop assessments. Assessments were based on the activities taught. With a standards-based curriculum, the assessments are designed based on the standards, and activities are then selected that will allow students to demonstrate competency on the standards rather than on the activity. This represents a huge paradigm shift for many physical educators, but when curricula are assessed in this manner, learning has much better alignment with the standards. When teachers know how they will assess students, instruction becomes more focused and they are able to emphasize learning that is important for student success.

4. Use assessments that can be used during the learning process so that assessment becomes an integral part of learning.

   With a standards-based curriculum, it is often difficult to separate learning from the assessment. Using an outdoor activity, students may be participating in a bicycle trip, but they also are demonstrating skills, various components of fitness, knowledge about cycling, and relationships with others. The assessment is a learning experience, and the learning experience becomes an assessment because of the accompanying rubric.

5. Assess the big picture rather than the detail.

   When designing curricular assessments, it is best to use more complex, larger assessments that measure concepts rather than activities. This will help focus on items that are really important in physical education. Ask yourself, "Twenty years from now, what do I want these students to know?" Assessments should be designed around these major ideas rather than details that students will soon forget.

6. Use simple assessments for elementary students and more complex assessments for older students.

   When designing assessments, keep them fairly simple for the younger students, and gradually make them more complex as students get older. Assessments can be made more complex when more students are involved, more equipment is used, the environment is more open, and so on. Simple assessments will be easier to set up and also easier for students to complete. Older students are better able to handle additional complexity.

7. Make sure students know how you will assess as well as knowing the criteria that will be used for the assessment.

   There is no reason to keep students in the dark about what you are assessing and the criteria that you will be using to do so. By giving students the assessments in advance, they can prepare for them. Many teachers fear that this becomes teaching to the test. Wiggins (1989) points out that if the test is worthwhile, that is not a problem. A recent study introduced skill tests early in a badminton unit (Shanklin, 2004). Students of all ability levels (more, average, and less skilled) in the treatment group had more responses with correct form than those target students in the control group. Many of the assessments used in physical education are by themselves worthwhile endeavors. By giving students criteria with the assessment, they can self-evaluate their ability and progress, and make the learning process more effective.

8. If you have several schools at various levels (elementary, middle, secondary), make sure that every school at each level uses the same curricular assessments.

In some large districts, students may transfer from one school to the next. Within these schools, contexts will be different, students will be different, and facilities will be different. Given all this variation, activities taught will also probably vary. Assessments must be designed that look at learning conceptually, and can still assess the standards despite justified variability. If the curriculum is aligned between schools and the same *curricular* assessments are used, moves within the district are easier for students. This also helps teachers, because they don't have to develop high stakes assessments by themselves. District in-services provide excellent opportunities for teachers to develop the assessments that they will use to evaluate whether students are meeting the standards. It is much easier to create quality assessments when working in a group than while working in isolation. Reliability is critical with these high stakes assessments, so training at professional development sessions is strongly encouraged.

9. When developing assessments, make sure there is alignment between levels; steps between levels should be gradual.

Curriculum and assessments cannot be developed by one level (elementary, middle, high) in isolation from other levels. Teachers must work together to ensure that assessments have a good flow from one school level to the next. An excellent approach is to start with the exit standards and assessments, and work backward from there. This backward design approach to developing assessments will help ensure alignment on a K–12 basis.

Many of the assessments explained earlier in this chapter could be used to measure student attainment of the standards. Table 4.3 is a summary of the differences between lesson and curricular assessments. To avoid overwhelming teachers by requiring multitudes of assessments, districts should use larger, more holistic assessments for assessing curriculum benchmarks, which can assess several standards in an authentic, realistic manner. These larger assessments will allow teachers and students to spend sufficient time to accurately assess student achievement of the standard(s). Portfolios, projects, and student performances are some examples of the big picture assessments that might be used for curricular assessment.

Summary

Assessment is a vital part of the curriculum process. If well written, assessments measure the degree to which students have demonstrated competency on the standards and inform students of their achievement. The important thing to remember when writing assessments is to start with the standards, and decide what you expect students to know and be able to do to meet them. From there, decide what you are willing to accept as evidence that they have achieved desired knowledge, skills, and behaviors. Assessments help measure the effectiveness of

---

TABLE 4.3

A Comparison Between Lesson Assessments and Curricular Assessments

Lesson Assessments	Curricular Assessments
Typically are developed by the teacher (teacher generated)	Developed by a district, state, or outside group
Varies according to lesson content	Based on curriculum standards
Purpose is to determine whether students have reached the objectives for the lesson	Purpose is to determine whether students have met the standards (i.e., is the student physically educated?)
Formative: Lead to improving student performance and/or learning	Summative: Measure whether students have mastered programmatic standards
Used to evaluate lesson effectiveness	Used to evaluate program effectiveness
Administered by peer, self, or teacher	Administered by the teacher or an outside review panel
Results are used to drive instruction; inform the teacher what needs to be taught on the next day of the lesson	Inform the school district or state whether adjustments need to be made to the curriculum
Provide feedback to the students and/or teacher about student success	Provide feedback to teachers and/or administrators about program success
Tell the students whether they have been successful for the day	Provide feedback to administrators about program strengths and areas needing improvement
Students are expected to demonstrate competency/mastery on a given day.	Students are expected to demonstrate competency within a range of time.
Become more complex as students move through the unit	Become more complex as students progress through the curriculum (are more complex and involve higher levels of learning at the upper grades)
Use content or face validity	Use other methods to determine validity
May not have reliability established	Reliability formally determined; evaluator has been trained to increase reliability

---

the curriculum. They play a vital role in physical education, and help to document to others that learning has occurred. In today's educational climate, physical education programs must have a solid assessment plan to document student learning.

References

Arter, J., & McTighe, J. (2001). *Scoring rubrics in the classroom*. Thousand Oaks, CA: Corwin Press.

Cooper Institute for Aerobics Research. (2007). *Fitnessgram/Activitygram test administration manual* (4th ed.). Champaign, IL: Human Kinetics.

Fay, T., & Doolittle, S. (2002). Agents for change: From standards to assessment to accountability in physical education. *Journal of Physical Education, Recreation, and Dance, 73*(3), 29–33.

French, K., Rink, J., Rikard, L., Mays, A., Lynn, S., & Werner, P. (1991). The effects of practice progressions on learning two volleyball skills. *Journal of Teaching Physical Education, 10*(3), 261–274.

Guskey, T. (2000). *Evaluating professional development.* Thousand Oaks, CA: Corwin Press.

Herman, J., Aschbacher, P., & Winters, L. (1992). *A practical guide to alternative assessment.* Alexandria, VA: Association for Supervision and Curriculum Development.

Hopple, C. (2005). *Teaching and assessment in elementary physical education* (2nd ed.). Champaign, IL: Human Kinetics.

Lund, J., & Kirk, M. (2010). *Performance-based assessment for middle and high school physical education.* Champaign, IL: Human Kinetics.

Marzano, R., Pickering, D., & McTighe, J. (1993). *Assessing student outcomes: performance assessment using the dimensions of learning model.* Alexandria, VA: Association for Supervision and Curriculum Development.

National Association for Sport and Physical Education. (1995). *Moving into the future: national standards for physical education.* Reston, VA: National Association for Sport and Physical Education, an association of the American Alliance for Health, Physical Education, Recreation, and Dance.

Schiemer, S. (2000). *Assessment strategies for elementary physical education.* Champaign, IL: Human Kinetics.

Shanklin, J. (2004). *The impact of accountability on student response rate in a secondary physical education badminton unit.* Unpublished master's thesis. Ball State University, Muncie, IN.

Wiggins, G. (1989). A true test: toward more authentic and equitable assessment. *Phi Delta Kappan, 69,* 703–713.

Wiggins, G., & McTighe, J. (1998). *Understanding by design.* Alexandria, VA: Association for Supervision and Curriculum Development.

Wood, T. (2003). Assessment in physical education: the future is now! In S. Silverman & C. Ennis (Eds.), *Student learning in physical education: applying research to enhance instruction* (pp. 187–203). Champaign, IL: Human Kinetics.

Additional Resources

Arter, J. (1996). Performance criteria: the heart of the matter. In R. E. Blum & J. A. Arter (Eds.), *A handbook for student performance assessment* (pp. 1–8). Alexandria, VA: Association for Supervision and Curriculum Development.

Black, P., & Wiliam, D. (1998). Inside the black box: raising standards through classroom assessment. *Phi Delta Kappan, 80*(2), 139–148.

Black, P., & Wiliam, D. (2004). Working inside the black box: assessment for learning in the classroom. *Phi Delta Kappan, 86*(1), 9–21.

Cohen, S. A. (1987). Instructional alignment: searching for a magic bullet. *Educational Researcher, 16*(8), 16–20.

Guskey, T., & Bailey, J. (2001). *Developing grading and reporting systems for student learning.* Thousand Oaks, CA: Corwin Press.

Hensley, L., Lambert, L., Baumgartner, T., & Stillwell, J. (1987). Is evaluation worth the effort? *Journal of Physical Education, Recreation and Dance, 58*(6), 59–62.

Jennings, J. (1995). School reform based on what is taught and learned. *Phi Delta Kappan, 76*(10), 765–769.

Kimeldorf, M. (1994). *A teacher's guide to creating portfolios.* Minneapolis, MN: Free Spirit.

Lambert, L. (2007). *Standards-based assessment of student learning: a comprehensive approach* (2nd ed.). Reston, VA: National Association for Sport and Physical Education.

Lazzaro, W. (1996). Empowering students with instructional rubrics. In R. E. Blum & J. A. Arter (Eds.), *A handbook for student performance assessment.* (pp. 1–9). Alexandria, VA: Association for Supervision and Curriculum Development.

Lieberman, L., & Houston-Wilson, C. (2002). *Strategies for inclusion: a handbook for physical educators.* Champaign, IL: Human Kinetics.

Marzano, R. (2006). *Classroom assessment and grading that work.* Alexandria, VA: Association for Supervision and Curriculum Development.

Mitchell, R. (1992). *Testing for learning: how new approaches to evaluation can improve American schools.* New York: The Free Press.

National Association for Sport and Physical Education. (2004). Moving into the future: national standards for physical education (2nd ed.). Reston, VA: National Association for Sport and Physical Education.

National Association for Sport and Physical Education. (2008). *P.E. metrics: assessments for elementary physical education* (p. 48). Reston, VA: National Association for Sport and Physical Education.

Popham, W. J. (1997). What's wrong—and what's right—with rubrics. *Educational Leadership, 55*(2), 72–75.

Popham, W. J. (2003). *Test better, teach better: the instructional role of assessment.* Alexandria, VA: Association for Supervision and Curriculum Development.

Popham, W. J. (2005). *Classroom assessment: What teachers need to know* (4th ed.). Boston, MA: Pearson Education.

Popham, W. J. (2008). *Transformative assessment.* Alexandria, VA: Association for Supervision and Curriculum Development.

Steffen, J., & Grosse, S. (2003). *Assessment in outdoor adventure physical education.* Reston, VA: National Association for Sport and Physical Education, an association of the American Alliance for Health, Physical Education, Recreation, and Dance.

Stiggins, R. (1997). *Student centered classroom assessment* (2nd ed.). Upper Saddle River, NJ: Prentice Hall.

Tomlinson, C. (1999). *The differentiated classroom: responding to the needs of all learners.* Alexandria, VA: Association for Supervision and Curriculum Development.

Westfall, S. (1998). Setting your sights on assessment: describing student performance in physical education. *Teaching Elementary Physical Education, 9*(6), 5–9.

Wiggins, G. (1989). A true test: toward more authentic and equitable assessment. *Phi Delta Kappan, 69,* 703–713.

Wiggins, G., & McTighe, J. (1998). *Understanding by design.* Alexandria, VA: Association for Supervision and Curriculum Development.

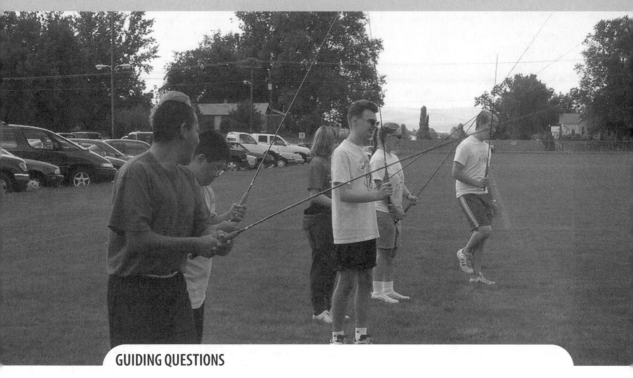

GUIDING QUESTIONS

1   What is curriculum? Is it *what* we teach, or is it *who* is teaching?
2   How and on what are an individual's beliefs and values developed?
3   How might some beliefs and values impact the teaching and learning environment?
4   How might some beliefs and values impact individual students?
5   What are some examples of institutional bias in education and in physical education?
6   What is meant by the quote "A savior mentality uninformed by awareness of the stark inequities of American society and untempered with historical and political understanding is inappropriate and even undermining" (Cochran-Smith, 2003; p. 374)?
7   What is meant by inclusive and culturally responsive teaching?
8   Why is inclusive and culturally responsive teaching thought to be important?
9   What are the characteristics of inclusive and culturally responsive teachers, and what do they do in their classrooms?
10 How can a physical education teacher be an agent of change?
11 What are some examples of how an inclusive and culturally responsive teacher might utilize some of the curricular and instructional models presented in this text?
12 What is meant by the quote by Elliot Eisner (2003/2004), "we need a radically different conception of what matters in education" (p. 10)?

Teaching All Kids: Valuing Students Through Culturally Responsive and Inclusive Practice

Gay L. Timken, Western Oregon University
Doris Watson, University of Nevada at Las Vegas

To a great extent teachers are the curriculum: affect, attitude, and persona have a much more powerful impact on classes than do [the subject matter] or the pedagogical techniques they employ. (Rosetta Marantz Cohen, as cited by Hellison, 2003, p. 97)

Introduction and Overview

Meeting the needs of a diverse student population is one of the most significant challenges facing educators in the 21st century. Currently, there are approximately 5.3 million youth enrolled in U.S. elementary and secondary schools; of that, about 35% are from racial and ethnic minority groups (Futrell, Gomez, & Bedden, 2003). It is estimated that 82% to 84% of teachers and administrators are white, 75% of teachers are women, and roughly 56% of principals are men (National Center for Educational Statistics, 2003). At the same time, the number of schoolchildren of minority status continues to rise; up to 69% of students in high-poverty urban schools are of color (Johnson, 2002) and more than 33% of children are of limited English language proficiency (Futrell et al., 2003). It is estimated that by 2020 more than two thirds of the school population will be African American, Asian American, Hispanic, or Native American (Meece & Kurtz-Costes, 2001). Yet only 32% of teachers entering the profession feel they can adequately address the needs of children from diverse backgrounds and less than 15% are fluent in another language other than English (as cited in Sachs, 2004).

Each child carries to school a proverbial "backpack" stuffed full of their multiple identities, which come from their cultural backgrounds; heritages; socioeconomic backgrounds; racial and ethnic characteristics; religious and spiritual backgrounds; sexual orientations; language proficiency; and countless other qualities that result in the sum total of who they believe they are. These identities come in varying degrees of shapes and sizes and, as such, have differing impacts on how each child navigates the world. Moreover, these identities will impact how teachers will successfully teach their students. This chapter is about awareness—awareness of one's own struggle with **bias**; the historical, social, cultural, and political structures deeply rooted within us; and how these structures impact our teaching. The necessary steps of investigating our bias will assist us in providing responsive, inclusive, and meaningful educational experiences for all kids.

In the United States, people with disabilities, including over six million special education students (Olson, 2004), continue to fight for access. Many public buildings remain inaccessible to wheelchairs, and many of the disabled continue to battle public perception. Even today, disabled people, including K–12 public school students, must litigiously challenge structural and institutional inequities through the use of the Individuals with Disabilities Education Act (IDEA) and the Americans with Disabilities Act (ADA). This occurs even in the world of sports (i.e., Casey Martin, PGA golfer). Might teachers' expectations of disabled students be lower than for those who are able bodied, based on both the social and institutional construction of bias? Can we avoid **athletic privilege**?

In the United States, girls and women have equal access to participate in physical activity as a result of the passage of Title IX. However, girls and women remain the least active segment of the U.S. population (U.S. Department of Health and Human Services, 2000). Participation of girls in physical education is equally disappointing. It is estimated that only 33% of elementary school students and 27% of secondary school students are physically active during physical education class (Fairclough & Stratton, 2005, 2006). It is well estab-

bias   A predisposition or prejudice, such as holding inappropriate and/or incorrect assumptions about people who are different.
athletic privilege   A form of elitism whereby those who are more athletically inclined are accorded higher status and privilege, socially, economically, and politically. For example, the athletic achievements of schools often are more recognized (i.e., trophy case at the school entrance) than are achievements of debate teams, music ensembles, or foreign language clubs.

lished that as children age physical activity levels decrease, with girls demonstrating a more marked decrease than boys. In addition, during physical education class, girls' physical activity levels are below those of boys at all levels—elementary, middle, and high school. How might physical education teacher bias regarding gender impact the physical activity behavior of girls, both in and out of school?

In the United States, obesity is perceived as a personal weakness instead of a socioeconomic or political dilemma. Present day media help construct stereotypes and assumptions about people who are overweight and obese, in part by juxtaposing messages of over-consumption with images of ultra-thin (women) and "ripped" (men) bodies who are "dieting," taking supplements, or both. Might our own buy-in to media-configured images, and our insensitivity to the social construction of "body" as a culture contribute as much to the obesity "epidemic" as to disordered eating? How might personal and societal perceptions of obesity and related biases filter into teaching and learning in physical education?

In the United States, the political climate toward the lesbian, gay, bisexual, transgender, and queer (LGBTQ) community can be hostile. Although nearly every public school has a zero-tolerance race-based discrimination policy, nearly 20% of LGBTQ youth report experiencing hostility, violence, and rejection from teachers and administrators (D'Augelli & Hershberger, 1993; Human Rights Watch, 2001). In addition, it is estimated that approximately 20% of lesbians and 45% of gay males have experienced violence by peers in the school setting (Taylor, 2000). Physical education provides these students with an even more hostile and oppressive context as the confluence of homophobia and normative heterosexuality come together. For males, physical education and sport are viewed as the proving ground for masculinity, while for girls, the demonstration of characteristics typically attributed to male physical prowess (e.g., power, speed, agility) is cause for question of their sexuality (McCaughtry, Dillon, Jones, & Smigell, 2005). The threat of violence notwithstanding, many youth experience daily verbal derogatory remarks or name-calling during school and physical education class (as cited in McCaughtry et al., 2005; Sykes, 2004). How might a teacher's beliefs and bias toward homosexuality figure into discriminatory practices, particularly in physical education?

In the United States, because of economic disadvantage and one's race, not all children are provided a fair start, such as early and enriching educational opportunities, adequate pre- and post-natal health care, nutrition, quality housing and safe neighborhoods, day care, and after-school care (Anderson Moore & Redd, 2002; Kailin, 2002; Moore, 2002; Payne, 1996; Redd, Brooks, & McGarvey, 2002; Weinstein, 2002). Although it has been noted that upwards of 70% of youth who live in and attend schools in urban settings are children of color, high poverty, crime, drug use, and joblessness result in a teaching context that at best is described as challenging. Urban physical education teachers face demands associated with limited facilities, space, and equipment; lack of professional development opportunities; unsupportive administration; and unmotivated, disinterested, and disruptive students (McCaughtry, Bernard, Martin, Shen, & Kulinna, 2006). How might the cumulative effects of teachers' expectations throughout a student's education—year after year, and for both race and low income (Ferguson, 2003)—function to open doors, or to close them?

Teachers touch the lives of nearly every child, and have the opportunity to make a positive difference through **culturally responsive teaching** and **inclusive practices,** or perpetuate social, cultural, and political inequities in their teaching and in their curricular choices. For the many teachers who truly have good intentions and idealistic notions, Cochran-Smith (2003) reminds us that the naïve "change the world" sentiment is dangerous: "A savior mentality uninformed by awareness of the stark inequities of American society and untempered with historical and political understanding is inappropriate and even undermining" (p. 374). Essentially, the most noble of intents can still be harmful.

All individuals, teachers included, do harbor personal assumptions and opinions about others, but the notion of "other" or "different" is the **social construction of bias** and perpetuated within the rules, policies, and practices of our most esteemed institutions, one being education (Kailin, 2002; McIntosh, 1989). As teachers, we need to be aware of and move beyond socially constructed and individual bias, beyond our preconceived expectations of students and their potential, in order to teach *all* kids. So this is our point of departure as we begin to unveil and explore the inequities in education; and we cannot clearly envision our task of teaching *all* kids without some understanding of how we got here. As our students explore and begin to understand the contents of their "backpacks," so too must we.

culturally responsive teaching   Both a frame of mind and actual teaching practice in which teachers are responsive to the culture, needs, interests, learning preferences, and abilities of each student.

inclusive practices   A term adapted from physical education literature. For the purposes of this text, inclusive teaching is about providing physical education experiences for all children and youth in the regular classroom setting and access to rich curriculum and instruction as well as supporting each student's persistence toward excellence regardless of ability/disability, body size/type, or ethnicity/socioeconomic status.

social construction of bias   Prejudice that develops as a result of social networks or interchanges or that is learned from others. For example, we come to form opinions and make assumptions about other people from family, peers, friends, and media.

The Impact of Bias in Education

The greatest similarity among people is our common humanity and the greatest difference is how we are treated. (Kailin, 2002)

Stereotypes and assumptions are commonly associated with race, gender, and class, but also occur for those less proficient in English, individuals with differing religious affiliations (or none at all), and those who are less athletically inclined. Kailin (2002) suggests that all people, including teachers, administrators, and counselors, carry with them learned stereotypes and assumptions that ultimately inflict harm on children—*all* children. For example, children of color and children who live in poverty may feel the brutal effects of being **marginalized**, ignored, feared, and stereotyped. On the flip side, those children who bear witness to such discriminatory acts by authority figures who are predominantly white and from the **dominant culture** inevitably internalize such messages. This discriminatory cycle continues when people fail to question the messages and the consequences implicit in such treatment.

Inherent in any student–teacher exchange are messages—messages that are intended and unintended, messages that are implied and those that are inferred. Although some messages are overt or explicitly stated by teachers (i.e., treat each other with respect), other messages are subtle and/or require no overt statement at all (i.e., some student-athletes are allowed to dominate play without consequence). According to Dodds (1983), the subtle messages students receive or experience via the hidden curriculum can overpower much of what a teacher intends or enacts (as cited by Rink, 2002; see Figure 5.1).

Kailin (2002) provides examples of teachers who considered themselves open-minded and fair, yet unconsciously acted out their assumptions and bias during interactions with students, or in the form of curricular choices (i.e., hidden curriculum). The following are examples of the hidden curriculum. One teacher was unconscious of her low expectations of students of color, and frequently provided sharp warnings to black girls and boys, while allowing or ignoring the bossy and chauvinistic behavior of one white female student. Another teacher,

marginalized   Specific to those students who do not receive the full benefits (if any), those who are negatively impacted, and/or left out as a result of biased or indifferent teaching.

dominant culture   In the United States (and specifically in education), the dominant culture is the white culture. Those within the dominant culture create rules and policies that often privilege those within the dominant culture. For example, given that 82–84% of teachers and administrators are white, they can be considered the dominant culture of education.

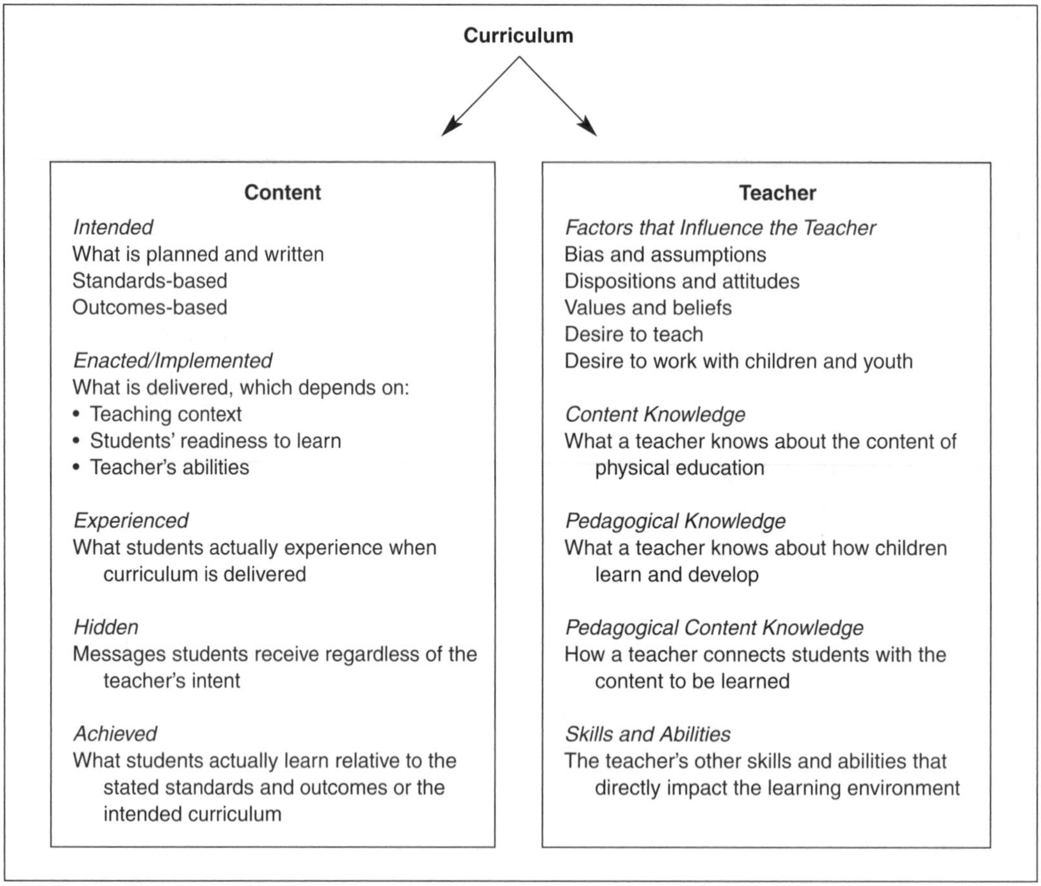

FIGURE 5.1 The intended and delivered curriculum.

without recognizing the teachable moment on stereotypes and racism, continued to read a story about a Native American character described as savage and a slow, simple-minded drunk. Students were likely internalizing these messages and images with the potential to project them onto Native Americans in general, as they sat mesmerized by the story. To further amplify this point, American Indian imagery continues to be reproduced as school mascots, perpetuating the distortion of and reducing a non-white culture to "little more than a singular stereotype of a mythical be-feathered fighting figure" (Staurowsky, 1999, p. 388).

Recently, the physical education department head from a nearby high school asked for a review of the curriculum. The intended curriculum, or selected activities for the year, were as follows: basketball, volleyball, rugby, soccer, field hockey, lacrosse, badminton, football, and softball. Such a curriculum is representative of the more traditional team-oriented activities, serving only a handful of students. Activities such as yoga, inline skating, adventure or outdoor education, fitness education, and dance were given little to no consideration, making implicit a statement about what *is* and *is not* deemed important (hidden curriculum). Fortunately, after some discussion, the department's teachers acknowledged how some students in physical education might feel marginalized and threatened, and consequently protect their identities by adopting a "plague-like avoidance" to anything remotely physical, or pretending it just doesn't matter (Evans, Davies, & Penney, 1996).

Stereotypes and assumptions cross the race, gender, and class lines to include religious beliefs, sexual orientation, intellectual and physical disability, skill level, fitness level, body size and composition, and learning style. Unfortunately, examples in physical education are numerous. All too often, physical education teachers are uncomfortable with students who are overweight or obese, and operate on the premise that such students never really work very hard in physical education. Heart rate monitors often tell a vastly different story, showing these students to be in or above their target heart range. Low-skilled students fail to learn or significantly improve their skill when their more skilled classmates (or sometimes the teacher) dominate play and practice. Some teachers fail to respond to critical incidents, choosing instead to ignore or demonstrate indifference to the situation and to the students. Other teachers disregard their responsibility to protect all students when the "different" student is bullied, and the target of verbal and sexual harassment, cruel teasing, and physical abuse.

These stories serve as a reality check and springboard into discussion about how to overcome educator bias. Though teachers are situated within the broader social context and cannot alone reproduce inequities, teachers can and should begin to assess how they come to practice the craft of teaching from a place of tacit assumption and bias that, unwittingly, contributes to such disparities (Kailin, 2002). So, culturally responsive and inclusive teachers ask how they can be transformed into agents and allies of progressive social change that impact the lives of youth they teach.

Teaching All Kids: Inclusive and Culturally Responsive Teaching

Treat people as if they are what they ought to be and you help them become what they are capable of being. (Goethe)

Teaching *all* kids is about more than asking simple, equal access, equal opportunity questions; all kids can come to school, right? No? To delve further is to ask the *right* questions, fundamentally different questions that focus on individual achievement, individual excellence, and maximizing potential. Tomlinson (2003) helps us ask different questions. Instead of asking about children

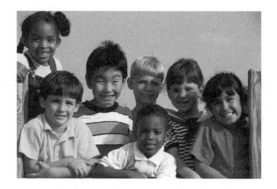

and their labels, in essence their deficits (e.g., obesity, low motor skilled, oppositional-defiant, low-income), a teacher should inquire into particular interests, needs, and strengths of students. Instead of asking, "How can I motivate these students?" ask "What releases the motivation born in all humans?" Ask "How might I adapt [my] agenda to work for the student?" instead of "What do I do if a student cannot accomplish my agenda?" (p. 9). A teacher's ultimate agenda is to support each student in his or her persistence toward excellence by maximizing access to rich curriculum and instruction.

Lest we forget, curriculum is as much about *what* we teach (Tomlinson, 2000) as is it about *who* is doing the teaching. Inherent to the caring approach comes the understanding that teaching is a moral activity, and as such, teachers have a moral obligation to care for every student and their individual capacities and interests (Noddings, 1992). This ethic of care should extend school-wide, as children should learn to care for (self, intimate, and global, others, animals, plants, environment, and ideas) as well as be cared for. Noddings' "challenge to care" was a reaction to school structures working against caring. Such structures—regimented standards-based, narrowly defined, single-minded goal, one-size-fits-all curricula and tests—contradict inclusive and responsive practice, and fail to recognize that students seldom come standard issue (Tomlinson, 2000).

It is useful to remember that teaching is "inevitably, inescapably value laden and never 'interest free'" (Evans & Penney, 2002, p. 5). As such, we must first recognize our own shortcomings as teachers, and muster both the desire and courage to be more introspective and insightful on matters of bias, power, privilege, and equity. If students are to have a chance at living in and contributing to a complex and equitable global society, it behooves teachers to be as culturally literate and sensitive as possible (Staurowsky, 1999). Being culturally literate and sensitive is far removed from the benevolent liberal and often undermining "celebrate diversity" approach (Kailin, 2002), and is in direct contrast to simplistic and superficial adaptations or modifications for learning.

Though adaptations are requisite to good teaching (i.e., all good physical education is adapted physical education), a more thoughtful, holistic, and comprehensive approach to teaching is essential to enable and empower the full spectrum of diverse learners teachers see on a daily basis.

Culturally responsive teaching is such an approach, a *frame of mind* (Weinstein, Curran, & Tomlinson-Clarke, 2003), implying that teachers are responsive to their students and their various cultures, needs, interests, abilities, and learning preferences (Irvine & Armento, 2001). In other words, the job of a teacher is to support and provide the best possible learning environment for all students regardless of their cultural and linguistic background (Richards, Brown, & Forde, 2007). Being culturally responsive means coming to understand and connect with the other 17 hours of a student's life outside of school—their jokes, music, dress, language, behavior, home life, role of family, community, and religion—and using that information when creating learning experiences (Kopkowski, 2006). Additionally, culturally responsive teachers are deeply committed to social change and not simply to a few multicultural strategies such as teaching an African dance for Martin Luther King holiday, playing soccer on Cinco de Mayo, or playing netball or cricket. We must ask questions that cut to the heart of biased educational experiences (Nieto, 2002/2003), but first we must be open to the idea that the educational system is plagued with bias and consider the students who are disadvantaged because of this. Questions such as those in the supplementary materials help teachers move past "ethnic tidbits" and "cultural sensitivity," and into the real issue of structural change, the real issue of teaching all children.

Villegas and Lucas (2002a, 2002b) share their vision of the cumulative and inseparable characteristics of a culturally responsive teacher. Their vision, and that of Irvine and Armento (2001), is used throughout this section, and has been extended to the context of physical education, and the models and approaches presented in this text.* We have taken license here to broaden their definition of "culturally responsive," and added the term "inclusive" to more specifically address the broad nature of physical education, and the broad range of students with whom teachers work daily; the range includes race, social class, gender, religious affiliation, ability, physical and/or intellectual disability, underweight, slight of build, anorexic, overweight and obese, sexual orientation, and limited English proficiency, for example. Villegas and Lucas (2002a) and Irvine and Armento (2001) provide examples of practices to guide teachers through the process of culturally responsive teaching (see Table 5.1). Their examples and others are provided in the following sections.

---

*Villegas and Lucas (2002a) provide citations for many of their suggestions for culturally responsive teaching. For the purpose of brevity of this chapter, the citations from various works are not included. The reader is encouraged to consult the Villegas and Lucas book for more detail.

TABLE 5.1

Cultually Responsive Teachers

Culturally Responsive Teachers Are . . .	Teaching Characteristics and Behaviors
Socioculturally conscious	Has cultural content knowledge • Recognizes cultural influences on student behavior Is aware of their own sociocultural history and identity • Recognizes and analyzes personal beliefs and values for the potential impact on students Demonstrates empathy, not pity, for students • Holds high expectations for students regardless of situation Works to build community within each class • Creates a safe and supportive learning environment • Employs some form of social responsibility model (e.g., Hellison, 2003) and/or full value contract (Henton, 1996) • Utilizes various curriculum models to build trust, cooperation, and communication among students • Creates social, psychological, and emotional safety nets for students • Creates and maintains a task-oriented climate for learning • Empowers learners by creating a climate of social justice and equity • Plans for and teaches to capitalize on the strengths of students • Diffuses the power differential between teacher and student, and among students
Holds affirming attitudes toward students	Is aware of personal beliefs and values relative to student cultures and characteristics • Recognizes beliefs about children, their culture, education, teaching, and learning that are inappropriate and harmful • Believes in the inherent value of all cultures • Values what each student brings to the classroom Embraces multiple approaches to learning, and different methods of thinking and interacting • Provides multiple ways to learn and demonstrate learning Builds on individual and cultural resources of students • Considerate of English language learners and allows students to learn in their first and second language • Attempts to learn a second language

Continued

TABLE 5.1

Cultually Responsive Teachers—Cont'd

Culturally Responsive Teachers Are . . .	Teaching Characteristics and Behaviors
	Thoughtfully considers student interests and varying abilities when planning curriculum • Conducts a student survey of their interests in physical activities • Includes a range of physical activities in the curriculum beyond the "typical" team-oriented sport-centered activities • Creates a student-centered curriculum Constructs learning experiences to accommodate for various learner needs • Alters field and equipment size/type • Modifies rules from the adult version to more child centered • Creates small-sided teams (3 vs. 3; 4 vs. 4) to increase opportunities to participate
Embraces a constructivist view of learning	Focuses on learner capabilities, not deficits • Works to help students capitalize on what they *can* do, instead of focusing on what they *can't* Believes that learners construct knowledge instead of absorbing it • Helps learners use preexisting knowledge and skills to learn new material (e.g., uses a student's soccer experience to learn basketball) Uses real-life situations and applications instead of contrived situations • Uses the Games for Understanding approach to learning, such that students are not practicing in a decontextualized manner Finds ways to make learning more problem-based whereby critical thinking skills are honed • Asks more questions of students • Creates situations in which students must work their way through a problem Utilizes assessment tools to propel student learning instead of simply evaluating it • Uses alternative and authentic forms of assessment to determine student learning • Uses multiple assessment tools to accommodate various student learning needs • Allows students to demonstrate learning in a variety of ways

Continued

TABLE 5.1

Cultually Responsive Teachers—Cont'd

Culturally Responsive Teachers Are . . .	Teaching Characteristics and Behaviors
Learns about students and their communities	Works to connect with all students
	Develops positive and enduring relationships with students
	Makes an effort to engage in the various cultures and communities represented in the classroom
Is committed to and develops the skills for being an agent of change	Is aware of institutional inequities
	Works to ameliorate those inequities by being involved at multiple levels (class, school, educational institution, community)
	Connects and collaborates with other teachers who also want to focus on social change

An Inclusive and Culturally Responsive Teacher Is Socioculturally Conscious

These teachers have **cultural content knowledge,** and recognize how student behavior is influenced by culture (group responses, remaining silent during teacher-led discussion, avoiding eye contact with adults; Weinstein et al., 2003, p. 270). Classroom management practices embody the value of all students, as teachers recognize how some disciplinary policies and practices are inconsistent and inequitable within and among groups (see Weinstein et al.). Thus, fair and consistent application of disciplinary and accountability policies across students is crucial.

A heightened sense of awareness of one's own sociocultural identity (introspective to race, class, and gender, for example) helps in comprehending the effects of historical and present-day forces on personal beliefs and values. Socioculturally conscious physical educators recognize their K–12 physical education experiences as vastly different than those of the majority of their childhood K–12 peers, as well as those of their current students. The faculty notion of "physical education was great for me, so it must be great for everyone" is offset by the realization that not all students love physical education. Having been "athletically privileged" and provided "elite status" (for many of us) was

cultural content knowledge   Having an in-depth appreciation and understanding of multiple cultures and how individuals' cultures influence their perspectives and behaviors.

as confirming as it was empowering. Might this have prompted teaching, specifically teaching physical education, as a career choice? Recognition of differential power structures helps create an understanding of false assumptions and inequities in education. Responsive teachers readily identify how athletic prowess is as overvalued in schools as it is in society, and respond equitably to such power differentials within and among students.

Empathy, not pity, is foundational to working with all students. For example, expectations of future potential are often based on a student's current performance, and current performance may limit a teacher's (and student's) expectations of future potential. Socioculturally conscious teachers, then, set high standards of achievement for all their students, and adjust their teaching such that a student's future potential is not limited by biased and assumptive practice. For example, students with disabilities or those from poverty-stricken homes should not be pitied but should be expected to achieve high standards in physical education.

All too often teachers unconsciously lower their expectations, which can result in fewer interactions with and less meaningful feedback to a student. The end result—students who are pitied can become marginalized, disaffected, and eventually dropouts. Empathy means varying the tasks and learning situations, providing more opportunities for practice, finding new ways to present material, altering/modifying task progressions, and using peer tutors, but always with the mindset of high expectations. It is important to note here that National Association for Sport and Physical Education (NASPE) standards can and should be broadly defined, and benchmarks created to meet the individual needs of each student; that said, the benchmarks for future potential should not be set too low based on assumptions of current performance.

Socioculturally conscious teachers recognize the importance of, and work to build communities within, each class. Classes as communities have complex, unique, and dynamic cultures (ways of being; Villegas & Lucas, 2002a), and teachers must help students understand and navigate school and classroom culture. Students need help learning how to develop and self-regulate behavior to maximize social participation (i.e., when and how to interact with teachers and other students appropriately), but it would be inappropriate for a teacher to expect each student to conform to the dominant culture at the sacrifice of their own (e.g., some students may continue to dress according to cultural practices while still engaging in physical education; Weinstein et al., 2003). Hellison's (2003) Social Responsibility model helps teachers shift responsibility to students so they not only learn to monitor and regulate their behavior, but also learn to take responsibility (Parker & Stiehl, Chapter 6). First, however, students must be able to define and recognize both appropriate and inappropriate behavior, and reflect on the personal and social effects of such behaviors (Standard 5). Helping students define appropriate personal and social behavior through awareness talks and individual counseling time, in a group, and one-on-one, are all useful methods. Equally important here is the teacher's awareness of the process of their own personal and social responsibility—that is, the teacher models appropriate behavior of respect, being a good listener, and demonstrating caring, for example.

Cooperative learning activities embedded in Adventure Education (Dyson & Brown, Chapter 8) experiences can help initiate the process of building learning communities that are safe, respectful, and caring. Appropriately sequencing activities is critical to building a learning atmosphere based on trust, cooperation, and communication. As students are ready, they take on more demanding tasks that require higher levels of cooperation and trust. Inherent in cooperative and adventure activities is the need for teachers to learn the art of facilitation, which is vastly different than what we now call teaching. Meeting Noddings's (1992) call for caring is also imbued in Outdoor Education (Stiehl & Parker, Chapter 9), as caring for others (Standard 5) and for the environment becomes as much a focus as does physical activity (Standard 3). Being mindful of the intent of the standards, the curriculum models, and the need for carefully constructed and systematic progressive activities is requisite in achieving safe and respectful learning environments. In essence, just doing a couple of cooperative activities or hiking, for example, will not bring about the desired classroom environment and student achievement. To meet the needs of every child, a teacher must deliberately plan the curriculum with this in mind and then deliver the curriculum with appropriate instructional practices.

It takes a great deal of desire and skill on the part of the teacher to create a learning environment that is safe, promotes mutual respect and caring (of cultures, abilities, religions, and other differences), and is supportive of students' academic, social, and physical activity goals. Henton (1996) offers the Full Value Contract as a method for increasing the value and safety of self and peers by creating a classroom that: 1) is physically and emotionally safe for students to take personal risks and meet challenges, 2) helps students assume responsibility and be more accountable for their own learning, and 3) encourages both academic and personal growth of students. For example, students can create a list of characteristics and actions requisite to creating a safe learning environment, and then commit in writing to supporting that environment through their actions and words. Another activity teachers can lead students through is the Helping Hand activity described in Table 5.2. To "play hard, play safe, play fair" (p. 73) is to fully participate physically, emotionally, socially, behaviorally, and cognitively. A note of caution: these activity ideas alone do not work in isolation; strategically coupling and consistently reinforcing (not enforcing) Henton's and Hellison's (2003) ideas can help build a safe learning environment.

TABLE 5.2

Understanding the Full Value Contract: The Helping Hand Activity

Give students a piece of standard-size white paper.

Have them outline their hand.

Each finger has a meaning; have students write on the sheet their response.

- Thumb: How do you like to be helpful to others in class?
- Pointer: What strengths do you bring to class?
- Middle: What bothers you while in class?
- Ring: What excites you about class?
- Pinky: What is a weakness of yours in class?

Have students respond to the questions, and then group the students in small clusters and have them share their answers.

Bring the whole group back together and have the class outline a class-wide hand and synthesize findings from the group.

This creates a helping hand the whole class has contributed to!

Socioculturally conscious physical educators recognize the public nature of physical education, and create **psychological and emotional safety nets** for students (Griffey, 2003; personal communication). Knowing the physical education classroom (and locker room) is a safe place to learn, a place free of ridicule, harassment, and social ostracism despite ability, interest, or body type provides some students a sense of relief. That is likely not enough for others, so a teacher's work is not done with the hanging of the proverbial rules and consequences sign, or with signs reading "integrity," "honesty," "play fair," or "respect." Problem situations will arise, and when they do, the "teachable moment," not the "teacher's moment" (i.e., soap box lecture opportunity), can help students find their way to responsible decision making and peaceful conflict resolution. Learning experiences and tasks with an element of risk should carry warning labels from the teacher, such as "This is a tough challenge and may require persistence, *and* I have faith you'll make it." Teachers should encourage students to take risks and meet challenges (Standard 6); however, it is not the teacher's definition of risk, but a student's that requires teachers to have a depth of awareness about each student. A macho and aggressive approach

psychological and emotional safety nets   Developed to help students psychologically and emotionally manage their way through the physical education environment. Analogous to how teachers create safe physical environments, teachers are ever mindful of each student's need to feel psychologically and emotionally safe.

here might serve to undermine a student's feelings, and diminish the very confidence it is intended to build.

A classroom that is more task than ego-oriented also serves to create a psychological and emotional safety net for students. Painful as they may be, teachers need to help students understand mistakes as a natural occurrence in the learning process; mistakes are not an indication of failure or personal worth, but instead provide the very opportunity by which to learn and develop. Some students may gauge their current and future ability, competence, and personal worth by social comparison—that is, by comparing personal performance against one's peers. This **ego- or ability-oriented** behavior can result in negative affect if that failure is perceived as incompetence instead of a natural process to learning. If performance is high, or perceived as such, ego-oriented students more likely remain motivated; if performance is low, or perceived as low, failure is attributed to lack of ability. In this case, effort and persistence, and thus performance in activity, deteriorates. Conversely, students who are **task- or mastery-oriented** focus more on the process rather than the outcome of an activity; that is, the central focus is on mastering a task, not social comparison. Task-oriented students view ability and intelligence as controllable factors, see failure as a temporary setback and make adjustments in effort and/or strategy to achieve desired results (Weiss & Chaumeton, 1992). Though personal dispositions can dictate one's proclivity to be ego or task-oriented, certain situational factors contribute, as well. For example, a teacher's own orientation may undergird his or her classroom, and predispose students, for better or worse, to one orientation or the other. Helping students focus on task processes (e.g., critical elements of skills) and self-referencing improvement over time would create more of a task-oriented learning environment, thereby increasing the possibility of sustainable effort and positive affect. This sustainable effort and positive affect could, in turn, lead students to meeting and/or exceeding each NASPE standard.

Clearly, creating a safe learning environment is critical to the success of students. However, socioculturally conscious teachers go beyond safe learning environments to create climates of social justice and equity—climates that empower learners to take part in a democratic process. Education beyond mere facts and simple knowledge is viewed as a vehicle for empowerment, and these teachers are acutely aware of the inequities in education, society, and even sport,

ego- or ability-oriented   A person (and learning environment) who references his or her skill or ability against his or her peers; the constant comparison to others instead of self-referencing improvement over time.

task- or mastery-oriented   Self-referencing improvement in skill and ability instead of peer comparison; focuses on the process of mastering the task.

and help students uncover and explore such inequities. For example, teachers of physical education might help students explore the social, economic, and political undercurrents to the obesity epidemic in the United States. Students could be encouraged to explore the social corruption of sport, even within their own school or physical education class. That said, teachers must be willing and able to "open up" or "unpack" to issues of inequity, even within their own classes. Allowing for student voice, choice, and decision making is also empowering, and with proper and non-authoritarian guidance, students can help determine appropriate units of instruction, or specific activities that fall in line with many of the models presented in this text. Such opportunities allow students to take part in their physical education experiences, thereby increasing relevance and meaningfulness. This decision-sharing process has less to do with student ability and more to do with a teacher's willingness to transfer power and control, or at least to share it.

Capitalizing on the multitude of student interests and abilities, and multiple ways of thinking and being, implies genuine respect, value, and caring. Acknowledging that some people enjoy physical activity about as much as they enjoy flossing their teeth can serve as a reminder of the various interests and abilities of students. Considering the many intelligences Howard Gardner has put forth, and utilizing (in both curriculum and instruction) the various strengths of students, for example, musical, logical, spatial, or linguistic, implies both respect and value of differences. Capitalizing on multiple intelligences comes easily in Sport Education (Siedentop, 1994; Siedentop, Hastie, & van der Mars, 2004; van der Mars & Tannehill, Chapter 10) when students take on roles consistent with their strengths (e.g., a highly linguistic student becomes a team publicist; the computer whiz becomes a statistician or videographer). Various roles and responsibilities within Sport Education can help students connect with their physical selves via various non-physical strengths. Transferring authority to students using roles and responsibilities within a Sport Education season helps diffuse, though never completely, the power differential between teachers and students. Power differentials between students must also be diffused as completely as possible, allowing for safety, mutual trust, respect, and care. That said, teachers must first be willing to identify the power structure and power differential, and then want to diffuse them.

These suggestions and models help teachers move past narrowly defined and otherwise traditionally based skill development and physical activity outcomes, to those that more fully encompass NASPE standards and the broader outcomes of education. With that in mind, care must be taken to preserve the very essence of these models, because teachers can quickly destroy what they have been carefully trying to build. A socioculturally conscious and caring teacher can employ any one of the curricular or instructional approaches to achieve a caring and equitable classroom, for it is less about the model and more about awareness: awareness of beliefs and values, awareness of both personal and curricular bias, awareness of respectful and equitable treatment of all learners, and awareness of and support for mutual respect between all learners.

An Inclusive and Culturally Responsive Teacher Holds Affirming Attitudes Toward Students from Diverse Backgrounds

Affirming classrooms are built on hope, optimism, and mutual and genuine respect. Affirming teachers are acutely aware of their own personal beliefs and values relative to other cultures and characteristics, and understand that although the dominant group has socially constructed **"normal,"** there is no greater inherent value for any one culture or characteristic. All students are viewed as capable learners who bring a wealth of experience and knowledge to the classroom. This is not to imply that all students come to school with the same knowledge base, language development, or physical ability. It is to simply state that every student has untapped potential, and affirming teachers, understanding the consequences of their attitudes and expectations on learning, work tirelessly to *support* each student's potential, instead of *overcoming* their deficiencies. Exposing all students to an intellectually rigorous curriculum, setting high expectations and performance standards, and consistently holding all students accountable for learning creates an environment for achieving excellence. That said, teachers must make explicit their expectations and high standards so students know precisely what they are expected to achieve. For example, students should know about the content standards for physical education and the expectations surrounding each standard. Posting the NASPE standards in "kid language" (e.g., elementary example, NASPE Standard 1: Be a good mover; NASPE Standard 2: Be a knowledgeable mover; NASPE Standard 3: Move each and every day), and then referencing each standard during units, individual lessons, and for assessment purposes helps connect learners with expectations.

An affirming response to a child's culture or community is to embrace multiple approaches to learning and different methods of thinking and interacting, all the while helping students learn to function effectively within society. This may mean providing three or four ways for students to both learn and demonstrate learning, which maximizes their strengths. For example, the "mover" or

"normal"   Typically defined by the dominant group. For example, the construction of "normal" in the United States is typically the following: white, heterosexual, male, middle class, able-bodied, Christian. Those that fail to conform to this social construction of "normal" are viewed as different and, possibly, deficient.

"kinesthetic" student may easily master and demonstrate skill and skillfulness (meeting Standard 1), but may struggle with written assignments or written exams (meeting Standard 2). Allowing students to demonstrate their cognitive understanding in a variety of media (i.e., written paper, poster board display, PowerPoint presentation, debate, oral presentation, portfolio, community project, or exhibition) is an affirmation of multiple ways of knowing and demonstrating knowing that runs counter to historical practices—the use of standardized assessment and evaluation procedures for students who seldom come standard issue. The demonstration of physical competence might also vary across students. For instance, a student with a physical disability may never display what we refer to as the "mature" action for a non-disabled individual; however, he or she may display appropriate physical performance for *him or her*. This implies the need for a good understanding of the student's capabilities (not deficiencies), the health restrictions due to the disability, and the appropriate use of the broad definition of each NASPE standard. A teacher may need to use specific adapted assessments (e.g., APEAS II; Bruiniks-Ozeretsky Test of Motor Proficiency) for students with disabilities and/or modify assessments for activities included in the curriculum. The assessment in Table 5.3 could be used with many students, as long as task modifications (e.g., shorter basket, different sized ball, position near basket) are embedded in both instruction and assessment.

Affirming educators build on individual and cultural resources of students. An example of an individual and cultural resource is language. Knowing that learning is connected to language development, for both first and second languages, and allowing bilingual students to use their native language to learn implies value for students and for their language. A physical educator could create a "word wall" to post common physical education terms, phrases, and instructions in both English and Spanish, for example. While taking written exams, students could have access to a bilingual dictionary, electronic translator, or even a second exam written in their native language. This has less to do with inappropriately enabling or disabling students, and more with helping them learn the content in ways that do not devalue specific cultural resources.

An affirming physical education curriculum would take into account all student interests (not just the dominant group or teacher interests) and varying abilities, and include a range of alternative forms of movement activities such as tai chi, rock climbing, or native dance. Connecting with and empowering disaffected and marginalized learners is the very essence of caring education—caring for students who care little for physical education or physical activity. Once again, allowing students to help determine the curriculum, and specific units of instruction and/or activities, is empowering and student-centered. Disaffected students may feel valued, and thus affirmed, when participating in a Sport Education unit. The unique contribution (i.e., team responsibilities; uniform designer, statistician, photo-journalist) to a team and a team's success helps

TABLE 5.3

Basketball Assessment

Names _____ Date _____ Class Period _____

Basketball Skills Checklist

Task 1: Goal Setting

Number of total shots you think you can make first attempt
while shooting around the key   _____

Number of shots actually made first attempt   _____

Challenge: set a new goal   _____

Number of total shots made with new goal   _____

After you have completed your second attempt, have your partner complete the following:

Criteria	Task Met	Needs Improvement
Shooting hand: fingers spread on ball, tips of finger pads resting on ball		
Non-shooting: fingers touching ball for support		
Shooting arm lined up with basket (throwing a dart)		
Focus eye on back of rim		
Body square to basket, knees bent		
Gooseneck finish: thumb points to shoes		

Set three goals for your partner.

1. _____

2. _____

3. _____

affirm a student's place on the team, in the class, as well as in the school community, and may serve to empower the student for future activity participation. Adventure Education can provide similar opportunities for unique contributions as students work together to achieve a common goal. One student's contribution may be more physical, while another's is more strategic or tactical; both are required to achieve success for the group, thus, both students are valued members. Moving from a traditional program and exposing students to

Outdoor Education activities such as hiking, orienteering, or mountain biking may not only provide affirmation of, but also truly connect with, student experiences and knowledge. In any case, within any curriculum, using a task-oriented instead of an ego-oriented learning environment, where progress is self-referenced and focused on improvement, effort, and mastery, would tend to serve students well (see Wallhead & Ntoumanis, 2004).

Affirming teachers construct learning experiences to accommodate learner needs and set learners up for success; for instance, changing movement requirements (kicking skills may be defined differently for a student in a wheelchair); altering field size (playing on a smaller field/court; long and narrow; short and wide); using modified equipment (volleyball trainer; racket with a shorter handle); adapting adult-form game rules (free throws taken from a point three steps in; no direct kicks); or playing small-sided games (four versus four, instead of a full-sided game; Block & Conatser, 2002; Kasser & Lieberman, 2003; Lieberman & Houston-Wilson, 2002). Such inclusive practices are indicative of an affirming attitude toward all students, and a belief that the original adult game form is not nearly as sacred as each individual student and opportunities to learn.

To be an affirming teacher is to value what students bring to the classroom, to hold high and affirming expectations, and to see all learners as capable of reaching their fullest potential. Genuine respect for and value of all learners, their culture, and community have less to do with any one curricular model and more to do with beliefs about children, teaching, and schools. Using Fitness Education or Skill Theme requires the same amount of respect for individual students and their diverse backgrounds as any other model.

An Inclusive and Culturally Responsive Teacher Embraces the Constructivist View of Learning

This is a challenge to the more traditional understanding of learning and teaching; teaching is telling, learning is absorbing. Villegas and Lucas (2002a) ground culturally responsive teaching in the constructivist orientation due to the inherent respect for each student's place of understanding. A less authoritarian and hierarchical approach, Villegas and Lucas see constructivism as focused on learner capabilities, not deficits. As teachers, we cannot overlook the vast array of resources (personal and cultural experiences, interests, capabilities) each child brings to school. A constructivist approach views knowledge as constructed by and embedded in each learner, not something "outside" a learner. Constructivist teachers help learners use preexisting knowledge, frameworks, and experiences to make sense of and connect with new ideas, concepts, and experiences. When teaching from the Games for Understanding perspective (Mitchell & Oslin, Chapter 10) and using the games classification system, students can apply preexisting knowledge of tactical problems from one game (Ultimate or pickleball) to another (soccer or tennis). Many of the game tactics in Ultimate are similar to the tactics in soccer, such as off-the-ball movements, or starting and restarting play. Once common tactics of one invasion game are learned, they can then be applied to other invasion games. This same principle holds true for the other classes of games.

Constructivist teachers help students find meaning and relevance to learning, and to specific subject matter content, often through real-life situations and applications, not through decontextualized or contrived learning experiences. For example, a Sport Education season immerses students in the totality of unadulterated sport through the use of roles and responsibilities, team affiliation, competition, and festivity. Outdoor Education moves beyond contrived settings and into real-world application with real-world consequences (orienteering in the wilderness versus on the playground; mountain biking on single track trails instead of sidewalks). Teachers can help students make real-life applications using Fitness Education, including using heart rate monitors and pedometers. In Games for Understanding, tactics and skills are contextualized and embedded in game-like play. Initial game play followed by a series of questions make students aware of tactical problems and help learners connect prior experiences (i.e., initial game play) with new concepts (both tactics and skills) to be practiced.

Additional strategies for teaching constructively include using critical thinking and problem-solving activities. Activities inherent to Adventure Education provide endless possibilities for problem solving and critical thinking, as students create multiple solutions to meet their goal. Having students investigate a real-life and relevant problem or issue situated in their communities or families works to connect students' cultures and biographies with new ideas and concepts. In Fitness Education, for example, investigating the problem of obesity, diabetes, or other cardiovascular-related diseases within one's own culture and community could engage learners on a more critical level (McConnell, Chapter 13). Team members in a Sport Education season could critically explore and report on current and compelling issues in the world of sport and/or physical activity, and the positive and/or negative impact on society. Encouraging students to examine media influence, the lack of accessible and/or safe playgrounds or sidewalks, or time-tracking sedentary activities are just a few other examples.

If learning is constructed by each student, then each student will likely construct different meanings of the same content. If this holds true, then teachers must be very clear about what students understand, as well as what they *do not* understand. Using alternative forms of assessment can inform teachers about what their students know and do not know and, thus, inform the teaching-learning process. Constructivist teachers use various methods of assessment including alternative and authentic, ongoing and continuous, formal and informal. Assessment is for more than sorting students by ability or determining grades (assessment of learning); assessment should help students connect with the content (assessment for learning), and inform the teaching-learning process.

In other words, assessment for learning can be viewed as a mirror, or a tool for reflecting back to students what they have learned. These assessments may or may not be used for grading purposes, but are used to help teachers refine their teaching and extend and refine what it is students practice and learn. A good example of an assessment for learning is provided in Table 5.4. Tracking and self-referencing improvement in healthy behaviors, activity, and/or fitness level, and subsequent reflection on such improvements relative to personal goals could serve as both assessment for and of learning (Fitness Education, Standards 3 and 4). The use of performance assessments (both self and peer) embedded in lessons could connect students with content to be learned, and provide the teacher with real data from which to make adjustments in lessons. Students of various ages and abilities can assess one another on critical elements in a variety of skills, from fly-casting, to use of space and force (Standard 1). Daily self-assessment (rubric and journaling) of personal and social responsibility helps students reflect on their behaviors (assessment for learning), and provide daily point values for the "responsibility" category (assessment of learning) for grading (Standard 5). The Game Performance Assessment Instrument (GPAI; Games for Understanding) captures skillfulness (tactical and skill) in an authentic setting—game play—going beyond shots on goal and assists, to measuring the decisions made by players (i.e., off-the-ball play, appropriate shot selection; Standards 1 and 2).

TABLE 5.4

Culturally Responsive Approach to Assessment *for* Learning

Assessment:
1. Is considered part of effective planning and teaching
2. Is focused on how students learn
3. Considers the many ways students can express what they have learned
4. Is sensitive and constructive due to emotional impact on students
5. Is considerate of learner motivation
6. Is committed to shared learning goals
7. Criteria are clearly defined for learners beforehand
8. Provides constructive guidance for how learners can improve
9. Helps learners take charge of their own learning through self-analysis and reflection
10. Recognizes the need for learners to express the fullest range of their potential achievements

Source: Adapted from Qualifications and Curriculum Authority. (2007). *The 10 principles: Assessment for Learning.* Retrieved May 1, 2009, from http://www.qca.org.uk/qca_433.aspx.

Being sensitive to the public nature of physical education and the resulting effects on performance is critical to providing students a safe place to both learn and demonstrate learning. Some students, in particular some American Indian students, do not fare well in public forums, and may remain silent during teacher-led discussion (Villegas & Lucas, 2002a). Assessing students from other cultures, or those who do not speak English as their primary language, offers particular challenges to teachers. Such challenges may result in teachers mis-interpreting assessment data, and inferring learning deficiencies rather than de-tecting assessment inadequacies. The point here—teachers should recognize the limitations of standardized tests and assessments, and make use of a variety of alternative measures to promote and detect learning. To further amplify this point, to rely on a single assessment (i.e., rules test for any given activity) as demonstration of knowledge and understanding is to disadvantage most, if not all, students.

An Inclusive and Culturally Responsive Teacher Learns About Students and Their Communities

Nieto (2002/2003) worked with a group of public school teachers to explore what kept them in teaching. For these teachers, "teaching [was] first and fore-most about relationships with students . . ." (p. 394). Villegas and Lucas (2002a) remind us of those students who have the most to lose—those most alienated from mainstream practices—and their desperate need for connection with teachers, so much so that such relationships might keep students engaged and in school. Many physical education teachers easily connect with students who are physically skilled and interested in activity; but what about those stu-dents who are less interested, less skilled, physically or intellectually disabled, or overweight or obese? What about limited English proficient or minority stu-dents? Are we connecting with *all* kids, or mostly those just like ourselves?

Requisite to teaching from a constructivist perspective is a depth of under-standing of students' experiences, culture, strengths, and interests, which only comes from getting to know students well. Villegas and Lucas (2002) encour-age teachers to learn about students; students' lives outside of school (family, responsibilities to family financial structure, use of leisure time, language use at home, immigration status); their community life (socioeconomic profile of com-munity, available resources for physical activity, community perceptions of and participation in schools, cultural perceptions of physical activity); students' past experiences with school and in physical education (boring and irrelevant versus meaningful and exciting); and their values and views on specific topics (sport, physical activity, recreation). Making real connections with students themselves, and not working from a set of assumptions that may prove faulty, takes considerable time and effort. Ideally this means going into student homes and meeting with parents or guardians as well as community members, and spending time immersed in a student's culture and community with the intent of increasing one's awareness. A note of caution is appropriate: Proceed respectfully and mindfully, because this is not intended to be a field trip (Kopkowski, 2006). Inviting parents and other community members in as respected partners in education helps foster connections and demonstrates a level of value requisite to trust. Being forever mindful of personal bias toward particular "others," and then deliberately being educated via personal contact, is a logical step toward understanding and developing affirming attitudes for all students.

An Inclusive and Culturally Responsive Teacher Has the Commitment and Skills Necessary to Act as an Agent of Change

Multiple challenges present themselves daily in the work of teaching, and many of those challenges seem oppressive and daunting, so much so that many teachers leave before they barely get started. According to Dickson (2006), about one third of new teachers quit by their third year; one half quit by year five; and one half of teachers in inner city schools quit by year three. Some teachers stay, but consider themselves burned out. But, as John Bennett (2005), past president of AAHPERD (American Alliance for Health, Physical Education, Recreation and Dance) says, the prerequisite to burnout is that you were once on fire to begin with. Agents of change are on fire; they see obstacles as opportunities and have the knowledge and skills to implement change.

A teacher's level of awareness to institutional inequities perpetuated by schools, as well as one's own personal and professional beliefs about schooling and students, is a necessary starting point. An uncritical and unidimensional orientation of "teachers as technicians" is simply not sufficient. The mere fact that teachers are responsible for the growth and development of other human beings implies a moral and ethical obligation, not political neutrality. To remain critically aware and reflective is to clearly envision one's role as teacher and the goals of education, and remain empathetic, hopeful, passionate, and idealistic about education and students. That said, working against a hierarchical and bureaucratic system can be difficult and demoralizing when the ideals of a teacher are challenged daily. For example, the interaction between the No Child Left Behind federal legislation and reduced federal and state funding for education is clearly taking its toll on teachers, students, and schools. That schools have and can continue to be institutions of bias can be disheartening, enough to discourage one from becoming or remaining a teacher, let alone an agent of change. It is also true that schools have, albeit slowly, the ability to change; schools can be the avenue for social justice and change, but only if aspiring and current teachers have an affirming sense of moral purpose surrounding the notion of equitable education. For change to occur, teachers must become involved at all levels—classroom, school, educational system, and community. To truly effect change and feel supported throughout, teachers need to make meaningful connections

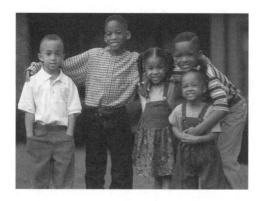

and collaborate with other teachers who are also pursuing social change. As Hargreaves and Fullen (1998; as cited by Villegas & Lucas, 2002a) stated, "hope is the ultimate virtue on which a decent and successful school system depends" (p. 57).

Change in physical education has been difficult historically, as many choose to honor and value tradition more than students. Today, however, with the variety of new and innovative curricular and instructional approaches outlined in this text, physical educators can easily become agents of change. We have a clear opportunity to push past traditional practice, past curricula that serve to disengage and disaffect students. We have before us multiple models that, when implemented with clear and appropriate intent, and coupled with inclusive and culturally responsive teaching practices, can provide both equitable and meaningful physical education experiences for students.

Summary

The intent of this chapter was twofold: 1) to create an awareness and platform for discussion around the notion of inequitable education, and 2) to provide ideas and practical strategies on how to change our practice so *all* students reach their fullest potential. To teach *all kids* is to frame one's thinking and one's teaching in inclusive and culturally responsive praxis. Culturally responsive and inclusive teaching is not a separate instructional method to use sporadically, or only when teaching cooperative activities or a multicultural unit. It is a frame of mind and a commitment to daily teaching practices that cultivates meaningful, affirming, and equitable learning environments, whereby all students are valued members of the educational community. Teaching all kids recognizes that students are the product of their life experiences, including culture, socioeconomic status, race, religion, gender, and sexual orientation. It is our responsibility as teachers to advance teaching practices that INCLUDE all kids (Watson, 2006; see Table 5.5).

TABLE 5.5

INCLUDE All Kids

Intrusive	Send flyers or newletters home with students before parent–teacher conference night as a formal invitation. This is a great way to extend a welcoming hand.
Notable	Take the time to read and learn about different cultures within your school and community.
Curriculum	Rethink how and what you teach. Altering your curriculum and teaching from a different teaching style can benefit all students.
Leaders	Create student leaders or ambassadors to work with new students or English language learners in your classes.
Understand	Just because some kids might look the same and even come from the same country or part of the world, there are regional, religious, and other differences that can be barriers to their participation in your classes.
Display	Display concepts created by students of things they can aspire to while in your class and provide examples (e.g., COOPERATIVE: Helps pick up balls without being asked).
Everyone	Be aware that *you* are facilitating a class climate that will encourage all youth to lead a physically active lifestyle.

Source: Watson, D.L. (2006). Reflections on refugee youth: Potential problems and solutions. *Teaching Elementary Physical Education*, 17, 30–33.

The challenge to care goes beyond lesson planning and content standards, beyond instructional techniques and curricular models. Noddings (1992) calls teachers to consider the inadequacy of traditional curricula and further, calls for a drastic change in vision, in purpose. We must decide what it is that we are actually teaching—what outcomes are imperative for students to become fully contributing members of an equitable, just, and global society. Eisner (2003/ 2004) reminds us of the aim of education—for students to do well outside of school where "the major lessons of schooling manifest themselves" and continues, "we need a radically different conception of what matters in education" (p. 10). A good physical education teacher will be able to implement any number of the curricula presented in this text. However, we argue strongly that little real or substantive improvement will occur in teaching, in student learning, and specifically in the very moral fiber of our lives and the lives of students (and others) without a drastic reconceptualization of our purpose as educators, and specifically as physical educators.

References

Anderson Moore, K., & Redd, Z. (2002 November). Children in poverty: trends, consequences, and policy decisions. *Child Trends Research Brief.* Retrieved January 7, 2004, from http://www.childtrends.org

Bennett, J. (2008, October). *You Can Do It.* Paper presented at AAHPERD Fall Conference, Salem, OR.

Block, M. E., & Conatser, P. (2002). Adapted aquatics and inclusion. *Journal of Physical Education, Recreation, and Dance, 73*(5), 31–34.

Cochran-Smith, M. (2003). Sometimes it's not about the money: teaching and heart. *Journal of Teacher Education, 54*(5), 371–375.

D'Augelli, A. R., & Hershberger, S. L. (1993). Lesbian, gay, and bisexual youth in community settings: personal challenges and mental health problems. *American Journal of Community Psychology, 21,* 421–448.

Dickson, C. B. (2006, May 5). U.S. improving quality of teachers in the classroom. In *Strengthen Teacher Quality*; Department of Education. Retrieved November 3, 2008, from www.ed.gov/admins/tchrqual/learn/nclbsummit/dickson/index.html

Dodds, P. (1983, February). Consciousness Raising Curriculum: A Teacher's Model for Analysis. Paper presented at the Third Physical Education Curriculum Theory Conference, Athens, GA.

Eisner, E. W. (2003/2004). Preparing for today and tomorrow. *Educational Leadership, 61*(4), 6–10.

Evans, J., Davies, B., & Penney, D. (1996). Teachers, teaching and the social construction of gender relations. *Sport, Education & Society, 1*(2), 165–183.

Evans, J., & Penney, D. (2002). Setting the agenda: introduction. In D. Penney (Ed.), *Gender and physical education: contemporary issues and future directions* (pp. 3–12). New York: Routledge.

Fairclough, S., & Stratton, G. (2005). Physical activity levels in middle and high school physical education: a review. *Pediatric Exercise Science, 17,* 217–236.

Fairclough, S., & Stratton, G. (2006). A review of physical activity levels during elementary school physical education. *Pediatric Exercise Science, 25,* 239–257.

Ferguson, R. F. (2003). Teachers' perceptions and expectations and the black-white test score gap. *Urban Education, 38*(4), 460–507.

Futrell, M. H., Gomez, J., & Bedden, D. (2003). Teaching the children of a new America: the challenge of diversity. *Phi Delta Kappan, 85,* 381–385.

Hellison, D. (2003). *Teaching responsibility through physical activity* (2nd ed.). Champaign, IL: Human Kinetics.

Henton, M. (1996). *Adventure in the classroom.* Dubuque, IA: Kendall/Hunt.

Human Rights Watch. (2001). *Hatred in the hallways: violence and discrimination against lesbian, gay, bisexual, and transgender students in U.S. schools.* New York: Human Rights Watch.

Irvine, J. J., & Armento, B. J. (2001). *Culturally responsive teaching: lesson planning for elementary and middle grades.* Boston: McGraw-Hill.

Johnson, L. (2002). "My eyes have been opened"; white teachers and racial awareness. *Journal of Teacher Education, 53*(2), 153–167.

Kailin, J. (2002). *Antiracist education: from theory to practice.* New York: Rowman & Littlefield.

Kasser, S. L., & Lieberman, L. (2003). Maximizing learning opportunities through activity modification. *Teaching Elementary Physical Education, 14*(3), 19–22.

Kopkowski, C. (2006). It's there: talk about it. *NEA Today, 25*(3), 26–31.

Lieberman, L. J., & Houston-Wilson, C. (2002). *Strategies for inclusion: a handbook for physical educators.* Champaign, IL: Human Kinetics.

McCaughtry, N., Bernard, S., Martin, J., Shen, B., & Kulinna, P. (2006). Teachers' perspectives on the challenges of teaching physical education in urban schools: the student emotional filter. *Research Quarterly for Exercise and Sport, 77,* 486–497.

McCaughtry, N., Dillon, S., Jones, E., & Smigell, S. (2005). Sexuality sensitive schooling. *Quest, 57,* 426–443.

McIntosh, P. (1989 July/August). White privilege: unpacking the invisible knapsack. *Peace and Freedom,* 10–12.

Meece, J. L., & Kurtz-Costes, B. (Eds). (2001). Schooling of ethnic minority children and youth [Special Issue]. *Educational Psychologists, 36.*

Nieto, S. (2002/2003). Profoundly multicultural questions. *Educational Leadership, 60*(4), 6–10.

Noddings, N. (1992). *The challenge to care in schools: an alternative approach to education.* New York: Teachers College Press.

Olson, L. (2004 January 8). Enveloping expectations. In Quality counts 2004: count me in: special education in an era of standards. *Education Week on the Web.* Retrieved January 14, 2004, from http://www.edweek.org/sreports/qc04/

Payne, R. K. (1996). *A framework for understanding poverty* (3rd ed.). Highlands, TX: aha! Process.

Redd, S., Brooks, J., & McGarvey, A. M. (2002 August). Educating America's youth: What makes a difference. *Child Trends Research Brief, Child Trends.* Retrieved January 7, 2004, from http://www.childtrends.org

Richards, H. V., Brown, A. F., & Forde, T. B. (2007). Addressing divesity in schools: culturally responsive pedagogy. *Teaching Exceptional Children, 39*(3), 64–68.

Rink, J. E. (2002). *Teaching physical education for learning* (4th ed.). Boston, MA: McGraw-Hill.

Sachs, S. K. (2004). Evaluation of teacher attributes as predictors of success in urban schools. *Journal of Teacher Education, 55,* 177–187.

Siedentop, D. (1994). *Sport education: quality PE through positive sport experiences.* Champaign, IL: Human Kinetics.

Siedentop, D., Hastie, P., & van der Mars, H. (2004). *Complete guide to sport education.* Champaign, IL: Human Kinetics.

Staurowsky, E. J. (1999). American Indian imagery and the miseducation of America. *Quest, 51,* 382–392.

Sykes, H. (2004). Pedagogies of censorship, injury, and masochism: teacher responses to homophobic speech in physical education. *Journal of Curriculum Studies, 36,* 75–99.

Taylor, H. E. (2000). Meeting the needs of lesbian and gay adolescents. *The Clearing House, 73,* 221–224.

Tomlinson, C. A. (2000). Reconcilable differences? Standards-based teaching and differentiation. *Educational Leadership, 58*(1), 6–11.

Tomlinson, C. A. (2003). Deciding to teach them all. *Educational Leadership, 61*(2), 7–11.

U.S. Department of Education, National Center for Education Statistics. (2003). Teacher preparation and professional development. *Digest of Education Statistics, 2002* (NCES 2003–060, Washington, DC), Chapter 2.

U.S. Department of Health & Human Services. (2000). *Healthy people 2010: Understanding and improving health.* Washington, DC: U.S. Government Printing Office.

Villegas, A. M., & Lucas, T. (2002a). *Educating culturally responsive teachers: a coherent approach.* Albany, NY: State University of New York Press.

Villegas, A. M., & Lucas, T. (2002b). Preparing culturally responsive teachers: rethinking the curriculum. *Journal of Teacher Education, 53*(1), 20–32.

Wallhead, T. L., & Ntoumanis, N. (2004). Effects of a sport education intervention on students' motivational responses in physical education. *Journal of Teaching in Physical Education, 23*(1), 4–18.

Watson, D.L. (2006). Reflections on refugee youth: potential problems and solutions. *Teaching Elementary Physical Education, 17,* 30–33.

Weinstein, C., Curran, M., & Tomlinson-Clarke, S. (2003). Culturally responsive classroom management: awareness into action. *Theory into Practice, 42*(4), 269–276.

Weinstein, R. S. (2002). Overcoming inequality in schooling: a call to action for community psychology. *American Journal of Community Psychology, 30*(1), 21–42.

Weiss, M. R., & Chaumeton, N. (1992). Motivational orientations in sport. In T. S. Horn (Ed.), *Advances in sport psychology* (pp. 61–99). Champaign, IL: Human Kinetics.

Additional Resources

Alaska Native Knowledge Network
http://www.ankn.uaf.edu/curriculum/units/index.html

The following leads to a specific 2-week unit on snowshoeing. There is little lesson information for what would be considered physical education content; nonetheless, it is a good place to start when thinking of creating a physical education unit where students learn and engage in snowshoeing, and it honors and respects Native Alaskan culture.

http://www.ankn.uaf.edu/curriculum/units/snowshoe.html

Anti-Defamation League
http://www.adl.org

Center for Multicultural Education
http://education.washington.edu/cme/view.htm

Center for Multilingual, Multicultural Research
http://www.usc.edu/dept/education/CMMR/

Center for Research on Education, Diversity and Excellence
http://crede.berkeley.edu

Crowe, C. (2008). Solving behavior problems together. *Educational Leadership, 66*(3), 44–47.

Electronic Magazine of Multicultural Education
http://www.eastern.edu/publications/emme/themes.html

Fisher, D., & Frey, N. (2008). Releasing responsibility. *Educational Leadership, 66*(3), 32–37.

Gay, Lesbian and Straight Teachers Network
http://www.qrd.org/qrd/www/orgs/glstn/

Learning from a Legacy of Hate
http://www.bsu.edu/learningfromhate/default.htm

Loewen, J. W. (1995). *Lies my teacher told me: everything your American history textbook got wrong.* New York: Simon & Schuster.

Mitra, D. (2008). Amplifying student voice. *Educational Leadership, 66*(3), 20–25.

Moore, A. (2002 November). Children in poverty: new resource with the latest statistics, research and policy options. *Child Trends.* Retrieved January 7, 2004, from http://www.child trends.org

National Association for Multicultural Education
http://www.nameorg.org

National Center for Children in Poverty
http://www.nccp.org

National Education Association
http://www.nea.org/home/MinorityCommunityOutreach.html

New Horizons for Learning
http://www.newhorizons.org/index.html

Poverty and Race Research Action Council
http://www.prrac.org

REACH: Respecting Ethnic and Cultural Heritage
http://www.reachctr.org

Rethinking Schools
http://www.rethinkingschools.org

Teaching Diverse Learners
http://www.alliance.brown.edu/tdl/

Teaching Tolerance
http://www.tolerance.org

Tomlinson, C. (2008). The goals of differentiation. *Educational Leadership, 66*(3), 26–30.

WISE: Working to Improve Schools and Education
http://www.ithaca.edu/wise/index.htm

Yale University Rudd Center for Food Policy and Obesity
http://www.yaleruddcenter.org

Zmuda, A. (2008). Springing into active learning. *Educational Leadership, 66*(3), 38–42.

Main Theme Curriculum Models

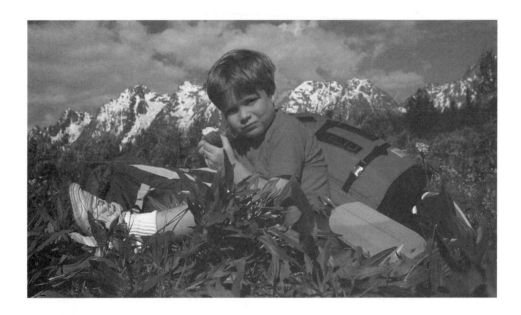

We believe that the main theme curriculum models (Siedentop & Tannehill, 2000; Ennis, 2003), which are the focus of Section II in this book, are the most effective ways to deliver a meaningful and coherent physical education program. Curriculum models are focused, theme-based, and represent a particular philosophy. These models have developed and evolved over time through implementation and revision by teachers and have been adapted to meet the needs of teachers and their learners. The curriculum models focus on specific, relevant, and challenging outcomes that allocate more time for learners to be engaged with learning and that strive toward relevant and challenging outcomes. In some instances the main theme curriculum models are most effectively delivered using a specific instructional strategy and, in fact, might be negatively received or unsuccessful using another. Each model involves the students to varying degrees as active learners, allowing them to be fully involved in their own physical education learning experience.

As noted in Chapter 2, instructional alignment is as important at the curricular level as at the instructional level. When making your curricular decisions, you must ensure that there is alignment between 1) what you believe is of the most value in physical education and 2) the curriculum model you select. If the goal is for students to develop sport skill competence, and working collaboratively in physical activity settings, then Sport Education or Teaching Games for Understanding would be your best choice. For students to gain the ability to cooperate, solve group problems, and strive to work collaboratively as effective team members, you might select Adventure or Personal and Social Responsibility. If your goal is for students to develop the skills and knowledge to develop and maintain an active and healthy lifestyle, then Fitness Education would be a logical choice of models. As you develop your program, it should be recognized that, while each of the main theme curriculum models achieves one or more of the NASPE standards, none of them achieves them all (Siedentop and Tannehill, 2000).

None of the models—alone or within the multimodel curriculum—is intended to be followed like a cookbook. These models, designed to emphasize a clear focus around the content, are developed to meet goals . . . or standards. Teachers must select activities within each model that will allow students to reach learning outcomes as well as to address students' needs and interests and to match resources available to the teacher. As you progress through Section II, you will have the opportunity to learn about the specifics of each curricular model; distinct features and characteristics; the philosophy on which each is built; the standards the models address; the benefits and limitations that impact their use; sample programs, assessments, and instruction ideas; and a discussion of implications for use across K–12. You will begin to recognize that skill themes tend to be used most appropriately with the primary age groups, and fitness is better achieved at the middle and high school levels. Now, this is not always the case and may depend on the focus of your program, the outcomes you choose, and the learning experiences you design. There are examples of each of the models being used effectively and successfully at all levels although admittedly in some cases we see more of some at particular grade levels.

Once you have selected a curriculum model to develop and promote the type of learning you want students to experience, you will determine which instructional model will guide instruction and learning. Metzler (2005) suggests that an instructional model includes a number of strategies, methods, styles, and skills that are used to plan, design, and implement a unit of instruction. As you study the various curriculum models, you will find that in some cases they are most effectively delivered using a particular instructional model.

Multimodel Curriculum

Typically, no one curriculum model will be sufficient for delivering the entire physical education curriculum. Remember, each has a specific focus and theme aligned with what the designer views as most important in physical education. With this in mind, you and your teaching colleagues will need to make difficult decisions about which models will most effectively meet your students' needs and your views on physical education content. Siedentop and Tannehill (2000) introduced the multimodel curriculum (which is not to be confused with the multiactivity curriculum). A multimodel curriculum is made up of a set of well-selected main theme curricula that stand for something important, which focus on students achieving the goals identified as worth their time and energy. It is our belief that if *all* students are to successfully reach *all* the standards of a physically educated person when they exit high school, then a multimodel curriculum would provide the criteria to achieve this goal, doing so in innovative and challenging ways.

A multimodel curriculum supports what Ennis (2003) describes as developing coherent programs based on specific themes. It also is in line with the criteria Beane (1995) proposed for a coherent curriculum: connecting goals and daily learning experiences to develop relevance; designing lessons that clearly connect student learning experiences to facilitate their understanding of how learning accumulates; selecting and designing curricula to reinforce what is meaningful for learners; and providing learners with opportunities to discover how they interpret learning. Yes, it is thinking differently. If we believe in teaching for learning, teaching toward the standards, and teaching in ways that provide coherence and relevance for students, then teaching using main theme curricula is—in our view—the most effective way to design the curriculum. In many cases, it might require teachers to extend their horizons, retool, and step out of their own comfort zones.

As you read about each model you should see your philosophies reflected in different models and come to appreciate what they offer to you as a teacher and to your students as participants. If you recognize that two or more of the models could be used to support the goals and values you have identified as most important in your program, then you will find the multimodel curriculum a useful option for your district curriculum framework. As a collective group of physical educators, use the backward design process previously discussed to determine which models fit and when they should be implemented to achieve what you have identified as most important at each level. When selecting the models, choose those that will allow your students to achieve the standards.

Take a look at how one school district made decisions that resulted in developing a multimodel curriculum across K–12 (Box 1).

You will recall that in the curriculum design process (Chapter 2) we suggested that you determine which of the main theme curriculum models can facilitate student learning and achievement of the standard(s) at each level. Remember, this decision is made only after you, as a collective group of teachers, have come to agreement on shared values, beliefs, and philosophy; after you have unpacked the standards; and after you have identified what should be emphasized at each

---

Box 1

One School District's Effort at Design

As the Vision School District approached the redesign of their physical education curriculum to meet state standards, the district conducted a needs assessment with their students; talked to parents and members of the community; evaluated their current practices; studied what facilities, equipment, and community resources they had access to; attended in-service and summer physical education workshops; and consulted the literature on current practices. They came to terms with the fact that, as a group of educators, they shared some common visions, yet they varied in many aspects of what the program should look like and how all that students should learn. They were, however, able to agree that in order to reach the needs of all students, they must be willing to step outside their own comfort zones for the district's program to be successful.

After discussing their individual beliefs and what they each perceived was critical for students to achieve through the program, they agreed on a program philosophy that left room for their own individual ideas on "how to get there." Students graduating from the district's program will have the skills and knowledge to enjoy physical activity and, as a result of their experiences, will select activity options to pursue. Students will take responsibility for developing and maintaining a physically active lifestyle that is challenging, meaningful, and respects others and the environment.

The educators determined that they can reach these district goals while allowing every student the opportunity to experience physical education through selected curriculum models that they feel capable of delivering (Personal and Social Responsibility, Skill Themes, Sport Education in combination with Teaching Games for Understanding, Fitness for Life, and Outdoor Education in combination with Adventure). Their preliminary work revealed that they can help their students achieve the standards through experiencing the kinds of sports, games, and activities offered within the curriculum models. They also viewed Personal and Social Responsibility as a managerial and instructional strategy that will be a major piece of every program across K–12.

Based on where they believed the standards should be emphasized, the teachers used the backward design process to make curriculum model framework decisions at the district level. They believe that Standard 3: Physical Activity is their major emphasis throughout and is achieved through the other standards.

Continued

Box 1

One School District's Effort at Design—Cont'd

Grade	Standards Emphasis	Curriculum Model(s)
9–12	All standards	Elective program with opportunities for all models
8	Standards 1, 2, 4, & 5	Sport Education (with TGFU) and Fitness for Life
6–7	Standards 1, 2, 5, & 6	Outdoor (with Adventure), Sport Education (with TGFU), and Fitness for Life
3–5	Standards 1, 2, 5, & 6	Skill Themes, Sport Education, and Personal & Social Responsibility
K–2	Standard 1	Skill Themes

Within these curriculum models, teachers made different activity choices based on their own students and facilities. For instance, in Vision SD, they decide that for Sport Education, net games will be introduced in Grades 5 and 8, invasion games in Grades 6 and 8, and target games in Grades 4 and 6. When the focus is on invasion games, teachers may choose between soccer, lacrosse, field hockey, Ultimate, or others; same game–same tactical problems, same off-the-ball movements–different implement, or different on-the-ball skills. Another example can be seen in Outdoor Education, which is offered in Grade 7 and at the high school level as an elective. In Grade 7, teachers may focus more on the adventure aspect of the program, with children learning to work together cooperatively to solve challenge situations and initiatives. They then will move into gaining basic skill in outdoor activities, such as hiking, orienteering, camping, and fishing. As they progress to the high school level, they will have the opportunity to extend their skills and develop other skills through authentic and realistic field trip opportunities. One of the district high schools has access to a swimming pool, so adding kayaking to their program is feasible, especially since the local Y is willing to bring kayaks to the school and assist in teaching. The other high school is adjacent to a huge public park with a nature trail, so they are able to develop the orienteering aspect of the program more thoroughly using a map and compass. The curriculum model framework now allows the teachers within each school to make collective decisions for their own programs that are in line with the district focus.

level. If you do not feel confident implementing one or more of the physical education curriculum models, do not give up—take small steps. Box 2 provides an example of how one school district has chosen to design a multimodel curriculum founded on the principle that a school has the responsibility to educate children and that one of the important goals of education should concern the health and well-being of the child.

Box 3 extends this vision for the middle school level as it highlights the physical education program's responsibility for teaching the skills and knowledge

---

Box 2

A Holistic Curriculum for the Elementary Grades

Elementary School Physical Education: Skill Themes and TGfU

During the early grades (K–2), students will develop basic fundamental motor skills (e.g., locomotor, non-locomotor, manipulative) and basic knowledge to support these skills.

During the intermediate grades (3–5) students will learn several games and activities that allow them to use combinations of fundamental motor skills (e.g., sequence of two or more). Additionally, basic game play strategies will be taught for each of the four categories of games (invasion, net/wall, target, and field) during these small-sided games. Rhythms and gymnastics activities/units will round out the intermediate curriculum.

Health: Health concepts are taught by the school nurse or health education teacher. Children will learn about mental and emotional health, growth and development, relations with others (e.g., friends, family), nutrition, drugs and alcohol, and other related topics. Classroom teachers will reinforce this knowledge with activities that integrate into academic learning.

Fitness: Classroom teachers will be responsible for incorporating activity breaks into their classroom routines (research has shown that children stay more on task with these breaks, thus enhancing learning). Through these activity breaks, teachers will be responsible for delivering the various components of fitness. Teachers will have access to basic equipment to assist with fitness activities (e.g., strength, flexibility, cardiovascular and muscular endurance). Activity breaks can be done in the classroom or outdoors (the school has a rotation schedule so that everyone is not outside simultaneously). One of the fitness components will be the focus of each of the breaks, and every day children will participate in a strength activity, a flexibility activity, a muscular endurance activity, and a cardiovascular activity. Teachers will have a set of activity cards that are developmentally appropriate for these various activities.

Nutrition: The meals offered by the cafeteria are nutritionally balanced. In addition, children are given healthy snacks in the morning and afternoon (e.g., vegetables, fruit, cheese) to keep glucose at a level that will support learning.

Non-school hours: Children will have the opportunity to participate in intramural activities before and/or after school. These activities support the physical education curriculum and involve activities learned in class.

---

that a young person needs to be an active participant in a physically active lifestyle while other areas of the school are responsible for health, nutrition, and fitness. How might a multimodel curriculum be developed at the high school level to address this more holistic focus on wellness and living a healthy lifestyle?

Remember, a curriculum is not stagnant; it is meant to be designed, "lived," evaluated, and revisited. Decisions you make today will not last forever. They

---

Box 3

Middle School Curriculum to Promote Healthy Living

Middle School: Sport Education, Teaching Games for Understanding, Fitness, and Outdoor Education

The focus of middle school physical education is to teach sports and activities that children will be able to do for a lifetime. Activities are sequenced so that they become progressively more difficult at each grade level. For example, for the net/wall games, Grade 6 students will learn pickleball, Grade 7 students will learn badminton, and Grade 8 students will do volleyball. The scope of the activities will include games (e.g., invasion, net/wall, field, target), dance and rhythms, individual activities (e.g., inline skating, tumbling), fitness activities (e.g., yoga, track and field, rope jumping, martial arts, swimming), and outdoor activities (e.g., hiking, camping, orienteering).

Fitness: All students will be assigned to a study hall during the school day. Two days per week, students are required to participate in a fitness workout in the school wellness center. A third day of participation is optional. Students will be tested on fitness at the beginning of the year, two additional times during the year, and at the conclusion of the school year. Those children who are not in the healthy zone will meet with the school nurse and physical education teacher to develop a fitness plan to improve fitness scores.

Health education: Children will enroll in a health class that covers but is not limited to such topics as consumer and community health, sex education, environmental health, and injury prevention and safety (including CPR and basic first aid certification).

Nutrition: The meals offered in the cafeteria are healthy. In addition, all students are required to take a nutrition class in which they learn about eating healthy as well as how to cook.

Non-school hours: Children will participate in at least one intramural sport during the school year. Those students who participate in competitive athletic programs or other types of activity (e.g., dance, gymnastics, swimming) on a regular basis are exempt from this requirement.

---

need to keep pace with what is happening in society while, at the same time, meeting the needs and interests of our youth if we want them to choose to be physically active for a lifetime. Seek supportive resources, access those in the field who can provide you with assistance, locate and attend workshops focused on the model you are seeking to implement, and build slowly—you do not need to conquer the models on the first attempt.

References

Beane, J. A. (1995). Introduction: What is a coherent curriculum? In J. A. Beane (Ed.), *Toward a coherent curriculum* (pp. 1–15). Alexandria, VA: Association for Supervision and Curriculum Development.

Ennis, C. A. (2003). Using curriculum to enhance student learning. In S. J. Silverman & C. A. Ennis (Eds.), *Student learning in physical education: Applying research to enhance instruction* (pp. 109–127). Champaign, IL: Human Kinetics.

Metzler M. W. (2005). *Instructional models for physical education.* Scottsdale, AZ: Holcomb Hathaway Publishers.

Siedentop, D., & Tannehill, D. (2000). *Developing teaching skills in physical education* (4th ed.). Mountain View, CA: Mayfield.

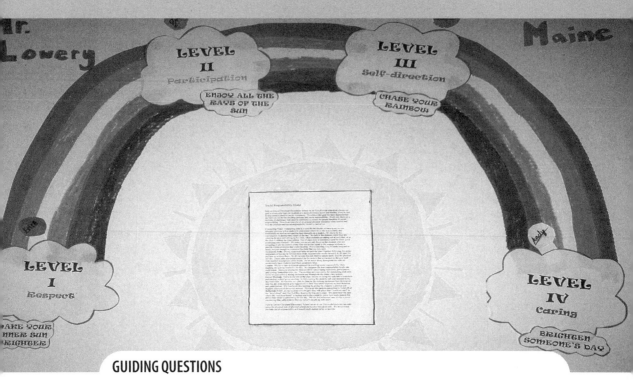

GUIDING QUESTIONS

1 Why teach personal and social responsibility?
2 How is responsibility defined and operationalized?
3 What basic premises underlie teaching personal and social responsibility?
4 Why can personal and social responsibility be considered as both an instructional *and* a curricular approach?
5 What instructional strategies are useful in cultivating and encouraging student attitudes, values, and behaviors that are both personally and socially responsible?
6 Which of the NASPE content standards does the Personal and Social Responsibility curriculum model best support?
7 Why might there be an interest in this curriculum model for contemporary youth?
8 How might this curriculum model be incorporated into the physical education curriculum?
9 How might one assess students while using this curriculum model?

Personal and Social Responsibility

Melissa Parker, University of Northern Colorado
Jim Stiehl, University of Northern Colorado

Envision this: Medium-sized midwestern community. Third period, required physical education class for 9th graders. Fifteen boys and 19 girls; 60% Hispanic and 40% Caucasian. Floor hockey sport education unit. Today the class is being divided into small-sided teams. The first comments are: "I ain't working with no F_____ white girl," followed by "I hate that Mexican."

Why Teach Personal and Social Responsibility?

The above scenario could have occurred three weeks ago at a local high school. We suspect that similar occurrences take place all over the country. Indeed, we are bombarded by the news media with evidence of a multitude of irresponsible behaviors among our youth: violence, vandalism, cheating, delinquency, materialism, peer cruelty and bullying, bigotry, bad language, self-centeredness, and self-injurious behavior such as alcohol abuse, teen pregnancy, drugs, and suicide. When asked, "What place do personal and social responsibility have in physical education?" some would argue that responsibility should be taught at home, not at school. But for a host of reasons, many home and community settings do not prepare students to take more responsibility for their actions and lives. For example, we live in a nation where 9 out of 10 citizens lie regularly (36% intentionally lie to hurt others, and 66% of us believe that there is nothing wrong with telling a lie). In addition, 20% of women are assaulted by their dates, and 83% of us believe that our parents' generation was much more ethical than our own (Patterson & Kim, 1991). These figures suggest circumstances that are less than favorable for young people to develop responsible behaviors and attitudes.

Youth today are exposed on a regular basis to less than empowering messages from a host of sources (news stories, music, television, film, friends, etc.). It is a context that can affect youngsters' lives in ways that are very predictable (e.g., they learn that irresponsibility is acceptable). However, the outcome is not necessarily inevitable. Every teacher has a unique opportunity to create an **educational climate** that causes a shift from what is probable, to what is possible. As teachers we can intentionally invent circumstances that will support children in becoming more concerned about the rights, feelings, and needs of others; where they can become aware of their own behaviors, attitudes, and language; where they can experience making a commitment to themselves and others, live by a set of principles, respect differences, and resolve conflicts peacefully; where they can learn to take better care of themselves, others, and their environment. Physical education teachers *can* make a difference.

Before proceeding, we offer this note of caution. Physical education teachers may not be able to change a child's circumstances, at least not directly. There still may be drugs in the neighborhood, for example, and the temptations to use them may still exist. But, if a child's views of the circumstances and of him- or herself are altered, then that child's resultant actions in those same circumstances might also change. Otherwise, in a world where the future is an extension of the past, the future is quite predictable. Thus, while teachers may not be able to influence what happens in their students' homes and communities, they can influence what happens in their gyms and on their playing fields. This becomes especially important when one considers that some physical educators see more of some children than their parents do—especially during the elementary school years. Although uncertain, it is hoped that the responsible behaviors and attitudes first developed in the physical education class will be used outside the gym, in the home and in community settings. What is certain, however, is that those behaviors and attitudes will not appear if they are not learned in the first place. Stated more strongly, if responsibility doesn't work, then children and adults eventually lose.

Responsibility Defined

The term *responsibility* is as pervasive a word as one can find. In books and magazines, in the newspaper and on television, we hear about fiscal responsibility, legal responsibility, parents' responsibility, full and partial responsibility, shared

educational climate   The emotional ambience or feeling of the gymnasium.

responsibility, and no responsibility. Sometimes responsibility refers to solving problems. Other times, it suggests accepting the consequences of one's choices, acknowledging what one does, or making and keeping agreements. A typical dictionary definition of responsibility involves being called upon to answer for one's acts or decisions, thus putting an emphasis on accountability. This definition aligns with John Hichwa's (1998) notions of obligation and accountability in his book on middle school physical education, *Right Fielders Are People Too*.

In trying to grasp the meaning of what it means to be responsible, while not actually defining responsibility, Don Hellison (2003) asks two very important questions: "What do students need to take responsibility for? And how do they go about taking this responsibility?" (p. 5). Consequently, he decided that students can be responsible for "adopting, modifying, or rejecting" several important values: two related to personal well-being (effort and self-direction) and two related to social well-being (respect for others' rights and feelings, and caring about others). "If I wanted students to remember the values, let alone become involved in trying them out, the values had to be simply stated, concise, and few in number" (p. 6).

For purposes of this chapter, we define responsibility as personal acceptance of being answerable for our conduct concerning others, our surroundings, and ourselves. This includes fulfilling our obligations, keeping our commitments, striving to do and be our personal and moral best, and nurturing and supporting one another. Other qualities can be viewed as specific forms of responsibility (e.g., compassion, cooperation, risk-taking, self-discipline, honesty, and helpfulness, to name a few). The preceding definition is useful because, first of all, it achieves some harmony between principles of self-interest and altruism. It suggests that we can not only explore, develop, and appreciate our own unique potential, but also use our emerging abilities to benefit others and the

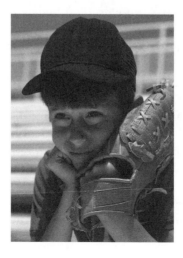

environment in which we all live. Consequently, by becoming responsible, we can reaffirm our own worth, our sense of belonging, and our awareness of place.

This definition also has proven useful because, crucial to developing a program that nurtures responsibility, it incorporates the key notion that responsibility is not imposed from the outside. Rather, it is a voluntary act that involves choice. It is internally motivated, a positive consequence of a positive choice. Taking responsibility means that we acknowledge that we cause our own effects. We are the source of our thoughts, choices, language, and actions. Fundamental to programs that cultivate and encourage responsible attitudes, values, and behaviors is the idea that children are capable, choice-making individuals. We assume that they are capable of understanding their choices, and of accepting the consequences of those choices. In that fashion, children who learn about choices, and how to make appropriate choices, also learn that they can not only cope with future situations, but also often design them.

Premises Underlying Responsibility

The purpose of education in America sometimes feels like a rollercoaster ride. It has peaks and valleys between a place for schooling specific skills, facts, and knowledge, and a venue to develop the whole child. In the 19th century, school was depicted as "professional adherence to narrow scholastic measures of efficiency" (Dewey, 1913, p. vi). Consequently, John Dewey campaigned for "the provision of a school experience wherein the child is whole-heartedly active in acquiring the ideas and skills needed to deal with the problems of 'his' expanding life" (p. vi). Less than a century ago, the Commission on the Reorganization of Secondary Education (Kingsley, 1918) set forth Seven Cardinal Principles of Education. Personal and social responsibility was embedded in three of the principles (worthy home membership, responsible citizenship, and moral and ethical character), and was identified as an active and integral component of education.

Over time, the Seven Cardinal Principles may have been temporarily misplaced. In a parallel fashion, important student needs also might have been temporarily disregarded. In recent years, while some are championing responsibility (e.g., Hellison et al., 2000), and it has appeared cyclically in the educational literature (Haberman, 2000; Sizer, 1992), it has not materialized as an important or deliberate educational undertaking. Included largely as a reaction to societal problems or to classroom management mishaps, responsibility has taken a backseat to teaching basics and to standardized testing. This is unfortunate, because those of us who advocate for a Personal and Social Responsibility model believe that it is fundamental to all that we do. It is an essential component of how we want children to be and to act as a consequence of our education system. Furthermore, because the whole child arrives in our gym, we are obliged (privileged!) to educate the whole child. And by teaching students to assume responsibility for their own behavior and learning, we not only make an important contribution to promoting lifelong involvement in physical activity, but also may be helping to assure the success of our profession.

Greek philosophers identified character as pertaining to thought *and* action—knowing the good, desiring the good, and doing the good (Lickona, 1991). Some would contend that responsibility is a skill that develops naturally, much like walking or running, and doesn't need to be taught. However, Kolberg and Mayer (1972) and Piaget (1962) both postulated that, although individuals progress through stages of moral development and reasoning, not all reach the upper levels. It has been further suggested that young people's problematic behavior is often a sign that they do not know how to act with compassion, empathy, and sensitivity to the needs of others, or in response to conflict (Berman, 1998). Haan, Aerts, and Cooper (1985) contend that although all individuals may in fact *think* in empathetic terms, many still lack skill in *handling* moral conflict. There is strong support for the notion that although responsibility may be an inherent feeling, it is not an inherent behavior. Additionally, the moral development literature is clear on the point that responsibility does not develop naturally, and that it can be taught. When taken together, these contentions illustrate that the most productive educational strategy for developing social responsibility is to teach young people skills in empathy and responsibility (Berman).

The current focus on standards-based education seems to reflect Dewey's previously mentioned concerns about "adherence to narrow scholastic measures of efficiency." Rather than limiting the scope of physical education, current efforts in standards-based school reform provide a manifesto for accomplishing broader educational goals. Considered this way, standards become empowering rather than constricting. For example, National Association for Sport and Physical Education (NASPE) Standard 5, "Exhibits responsible personal and social behavior that respects self and others in physical activity settings" (NASPE, 2004), is not a slogan. This standard gives us the green light to put some teeth into the concept of responsibility. It is our purpose in this chapter to illustrate how these constructs might be both curricular and instructional in nature, and can become an integral part of physical education classes.

Implicit in our definition of personal and social responsibility is that healthy behaviors and successful relationships require each individual to acknowledge and accept certain obligations to others, their surroundings, and themselves. Typical responsibilities in our definition might include keeping agreements, accepting consequences for success or failure, setting realistic goals, finding acceptable solutions to problems, and accepting the fact that we are accountable for our thoughts, choices, language, and actions. Other characterizations of responsibility might include fair play, helping and caring, controlling one's actions, self-direction, empathy, and character development.

Regardless of which specific qualities you choose to identify as "responsibility," these qualities can and should be cultivated in physical education. Although we may not be able to teach responsibility directly, we can adopt deliberate instructional approaches and activities that will foster responsible behavior and attitudes. These approaches and activities must be congruent, an important point to be discussed later in this chapter.

Responsibility is learned and maintained by its consequences. Thus, in order to fully comprehend the meaning of responsibility, children must experience responsible behavior, and must understand and value its product. In other words, children learn responsibility best when they are called upon to be responsible. The gymnasium can be an ideal setting for learning responsibility moving on a continuum from total dependence to independence. Of course, the final test is what youngsters do when they are outside the teacher's influence, not what they do when the teacher is around. Too often, teachers merely become a traffic light for children. In this chapter, we suggest that teachers can provide activities, methods, and encouragement that can empower children to accept responsibility for their actions in the gymnasium and beyond.

In an atmosphere that supports the development of personal and social responsibility, the whole child is greater than the sum of the parts. Such an atmosphere requires the teacher to think and act in ways that promote development of the whole child (i.e., emotional, social, cognitive, and physical aspects). Children are viewed as resources to be developed, not as empty vessels to be filled or problems to be fixed. Accordingly, it is important not only that teachers adopt and apply certain instructional strategies, but also that they embrace "a way of being" (Hellison et al., 2000, p. 45). Inherent in this "way of being" are certain beliefs about children:

- Even with limited experience, children are capable of making appropriate decisions.
- Children and youth have the right to be connected, to be noticed, to have a voice.
- Each child is a unique individual.
- All children have strengths to be nourished.

These beliefs about children are necessary if teachers are to think and act in ways that foster opportunities for personal and social responsibility.

Curriculum and Instruction

Fundamental to including responsibility in physical education is the idea that it is both curricular and instructional in nature. What is taught is inextricably linked to how it is taught. Consider the following in which the anticipated outcome is teamwork; specifically, it is intended that a group of 30 students will be able to work well together. Which of the following strategies (instruction) would promote more responsibility, situation A or situation B? Situation A: teacher assigns each child to one of four similar-size groups. Situation B: students assign themselves to one of the four groups with the following parameters: each group must contain at least two, but no more than four boys; someone wearing the color green must be in each group; at least two members of each group must have the same favorite dessert; and each group must contain at least seven members. Anything that a child should do and can do, but that we do for them, takes away an opportunity to learn responsibility. Furthermore, if students are permitted to make decisions yet, after an unsuccessful attempt, those decision-making "privileges" are withdrawn (a common occurrence when initially trying this approach), a valuable teachable moment may be lost.

For some aspects of physical activity, curriculum and instruction need not be congruent. To illustrate, when teaching a youngster to throw, a variety of instructional formats may be equally appropriate for teaching throwing. Though one approach might be better suited to a particular student, no method would hamper a student's ability to learn. Quite the reverse, when teaching personal and social responsibility, the instructional format can be counterproductive to what is intended to be learned. Hence, the creation of a certain type of atmosphere or climate in physical education is essential.

An atmosphere in which the previously stated beliefs are honored is one where students are empowered to become increasingly self-directed and independent. It is a relational atmosphere where power and control are shared between students and teachers. This means gradually shifting certain decisions from the teacher to the students, and then accepting the students' decisions—being willing to permit students to make and learn from their mistakes. When using this model, teachers introduce it by giving children choices among a few items and then continue to develop these skills by giving children more responsibility and choice during subsequent lessons. This atmosphere is uncommon because many schools are based on a hierarchical system of adult authority, and student submission to that authority. As a result, responsibility is often confused with obedience to adult mandates (e.g., dress this way, do this many push-ups, play a sport for this purpose). The status quo tends to disempower students rather than empower them.

The atmosphere that we are talking about is one that encourages students to be responsible for themselves and others—not for a day or for a unit, but for the entirety of physical education. Just as the successful comedian needs congruence between jokes or material (substance) and style (delivery) and intent (to provoke laughter), so does the teacher who wishes to develop a climate that fosters personal and social responsibility. Admittedly, the lines between curriculum (which we will characterize as substance plus intent) and instruction (delivery) at this point are dotted, not solid; but establishing an atmosphere that accomplishes the goals of teaching personal and social responsibility requires a harmonious blend of curriculum and instruction.

Responsibility as Instruction

Instruction is classically defined as "how" content is delivered to students, so Muska Mosston's spectrum of teaching styles may be instructive here (Mosston & Ashworth, 2002). The "spectrum" is a paradigm of alternative models for teaching and learning. Each of several styles (defined as the decision patterns that take place in a given teaching and learning episode) delineates the specific roles of teacher and student, and each seeks compatibility among the manner of teaching, the desired outcomes, and the subject matter. "Regardless of the preferred activity . . . (i.e., gymnastics, fitness, games, outdoor adventure, aquatics, track and field, dance, leisure, etc.), the selection of styles is determined by what we seek to accomplish in a given episode . . ." (Mosston & Ashworth, 1994, p. viii). Hence the need to align style (instruction) with content and intent (curriculum).

Because the instructional features of a personal and social responsibility model are fundamental to its successful implementation, we present these before curricular considerations. Furthermore, we also highlight some important management aspects of instruction. Comparing personal and social responsibility to baseball (a metaphor borrowed from Judy Rink), managing in ways that permit personal and social responsibility constitutes reaching first base (e.g., choosing a partner). Intentionally emphasizing responsibility by adopting and implementing certain instructional strategies could be considered a double (e.g., providing feedback to a partner). Incorporating some curricular aspects would be a triple; and an interrelated, congruent package of curriculum and instruction is a home run. Figure 6.1 illustrates this concept.

In a climate designed to foster personal and social responsibility, the instructional and managerial approaches are critical. These approaches should empower students by permitting them to take responsibility for their thoughts and actions in incremental steps—starting small and moving toward more complex decisions. The following strategies are largely instructional, yet might be considered to cross the "dotted line" between instruction and curriculum:

- *Including all students.* To practice personal and social responsibility in a meaningful setting, all students must be included. Inclusion means not only that all students have an opportunity to participate, but also that they are engaged at a level appropriate to their interests, skills, and ability. They must be of the opinion that they matter; that their uniqueness is valued. This needs to occur in a climate of safety, acceptance, and where students experience genuine success.

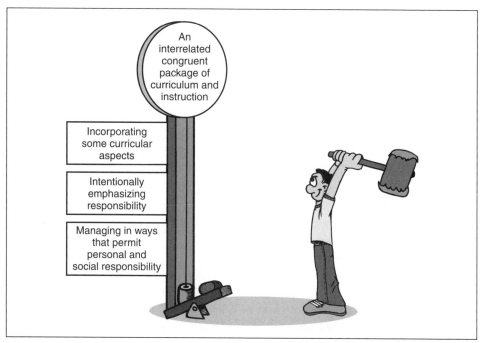

FIGURE 6.1 Ringing the bell when teaching personal and social responsibility.

- *Inviting and making use of student input.* Students have voices that should be heard. They bring to the gymnasium a multitude of experiences—oftentimes different from our own. Their ideas are critical—sometimes more sensible than ours. Moreover, when listened to, students feel a greater sense of ownership in class activities and interactions.
- *Providing choice.* Choice has been said to be the result of mental process preceding action (Lickona, 1991). If that is correct, and if we want students to learn to make appropriate choices, then we must provide adequate opportunities to make choices. We spend too much time telling children to be responsible, and not enough time calling upon them to be responsible. Choices can range from quite simple (e.g., "Can you refrain from name-calling today?"), to more challenging (e.g., "Even though you had a fight with Leo, would you be willing to be his partner this time?").
- *Letting students practice making choices.* Some students are unwilling to make choices. Either they see little need or value, or they perceive themselves incapable or fearful of making appropriate choices. Others simply have limited experience or strategies for making choices. Many are unaware that they already make daily decisions about what to wear, who to spend time with, who to greet and avoid, whether to do homework,

how much (or how little) to smile, and whether to feel sorry for oneself after making a mistake.

Thus, students need to learn about available choices, and then be offered a chance to practice making those choices. For instance, "makes me" language is irresponsible ("The teacher makes me so angry"; "She made me do it"; "It wasn't my fault"); it says that you are not responsible. As a matter of fact, it tells you that someone or something else is in control. Some youngsters need to practice alternative ways of speaking, such as "I'm choosing to be angry," or "I let myself be angered by her." Although it may be easier to place responsibility for their feelings or reactions onto someone else (i.e., they can blame others), they may lose in the long run because they will convince themselves that they are not in control. In addition to practicing new ways of speaking, they may also practice ways of acting (for example, by setting personal goals and then proceeding to achieve those goals).

- *Allowing for reflection about the choices made.* For students to learn about decision making, they must make decisions and reflect on the consequences of those decisions, both positive and negative. By encouraging children to examine the payoffs and benefits for making responsible choices, responsible children emerge. At first, choices may be minor, accompanied by relatively unimportant consequences. But as choices become more challenging, and the consequences less trivial, consideration of the outcomes will enhance a child's preparedness to make important choices later.
- *Being student centered.* All youth need to know that there is a caring adult in their lives who will not desert them, who values them, and who considers them worthwhile. All children want to be loved and cared for—some more than others. If they are being asked to practice personal and social responsibility, children need to know that their attempts will occur in a climate where there is a supportive adult who is genuinely concerned about their best interests, and who preserves their dignity and worth.

There are many strategies for promoting personal and social responsibility. A few are presented here, and each relates to conceptions about "how a class should operate." For example, although all students have a need to belong, many do not feel *included* or connected to others in their physical education class. And yet, in order to promote responsibility, students must value and accept one another. Ways to accomplish this are not difficult. First, do away with traditional elimination games. Nothing does more to reinforce a student's perceptions of inadequacy than being eliminated from a game. Second, design activities in ways that ensure that all students will play an integral part—by forming small-sided teams, or by modifying rules such as all students get a chance to touch the ball before anyone takes a shot. The power of strategies such as these cannot be underestimated; no student will learn responsibility when alienated from the class.

On a managerial level, students can provide *input* on everything from class rules and consequences, to what to do with equipment when the teacher is talking. Students can play a part in structuring their practice time and in selecting the content they want to learn. To accomplish this, teachers might ask students about their preferred warm-up activities, and then integrate those with teacher-designed ones. On outdoor trips students might be encouraged to decide what time they want their day to begin. And at the beginning of a marking period, students may propose what they want to learn, and the two suggestions most favored by the group are then included with the teacher-designed content for that time period.

Besides inclusion and input, the importance of *choice* cannot be overstated. Choice is fundamental to creating a climate that will foster personal and social responsibility. By providing choices to students, teachers gradually shift power and control from themselves to those students. Initial choices should be well within the capacity of the students. Typically, this involves simple choices followed by a slow progression to more complex choices. Simple choices can be initiated through organizational and managerial aspects of class—choosing partners or groups, which piece of equipment to use, or when to get a drink of water or use the restroom. "Teaching by invitation" (Graham, Holt/Hale, & Parker, 2010) allows for simple choices of content. When teaching by invitation, students are able to individually adjust the parameters of a task by deciding how they want to participate. An example would be, "You may want to continue dribbling in self-space, or you may want to begin dribbing and walking in general space."

More empowering (and complex) choices tend to shift from instructional to curricular in nature, and might include options regarding what kind of warm-up to do, which type of game to play, or what content will be learned. Some teachers may have difficulty with the notion of children making decisions about what they will do in class. Likewise, many children may have little experience in making decisions, and thus may need guidance and *practice* in that area. Independent decision making is critical to the development of the whole child, and is certainly vital to developing personal and social responsibility. Another technique for enhancing students' independent decision-making abilities is by asking them to establish personal goals, and to try to achieve those goals. Children are very accustomed to having adults make decisions for them—thus, either disempowering or enabling those students. However, most students can establish goals about a variety of curricular options in physical education. On the simplest level they can decide, for instance, how many push-ups or crunches are necessary for them to achieve a health-enhancing fitness level, and how many they need (or want) to do on any given day. Students can set goals regarding their own fitness, or how high they want to climb on a climbing wall.

So that students are able to assess the results of their decisions, *reflection* is critical to acquiring personal and social responsibility skills. Reflection can occur, for example, by means of a simple "thumbs up" or "thumbs down" to questions at the end of class, or by exit slips that allow for written reflections about specific goals for the day. Some teachers always write back to children in their reflections, and others simply talk to them. Whatever method is chosen, students need feedback about the choices and decisions they made.

Student-centeredness means that, first and foremost, each child's welfare should be the primary concern in any physical education setting. It means that students are more important than the content. It means knowing the students in your classes. The idea of getting to know one's students seems simple; yet, in reality it often does not occur. On the simplest level, know and use students' names. Some teachers play with students prior to the beginning of class (be careful about during class, because it takes away from some of your ability to teach). Find out something about them—what they like, what they don't like, what scares them, what makes them laugh. Be available to them—many students simply want someone who will listen to them. Open doors are always inviting.

Thus, major elements that empower children to develop responsible attitudes and behavior are a sense of being valued, having a voice, receiving choices accompanied by opportunities for practice and reflection, getting frequent and specific feedback, and knowing that a caring adult will provide ongoing support. Conversely, adult behaviors that reinforce irresponsibility include vagueness in identifying what responsibility means, enabling or rescuing children by making excuses for them, not encouraging them to make decisions or to become more autonomous, and simply telling them to be more responsible.

Responsibility as Curriculum

Responsibility as curriculum is complex. Returning to the metaphor of a comedian, curriculum includes both material and jokes—the content, the subject matter, the "what"—and the purpose or intent (to provoke laughter). Frequently, curriculum is simplistically defined as subject matter irrespective of intent. However, although subject matter (e.g., basketball) can be separated from intent (e.g., tactics, fitness, character development), it seems to make more sense to combine these when discussing curriculum.

The most widely known framework for teaching personal and social responsibility in physical education is the work of Don Hellison (2003). Using his approach as an example of instruction and curriculum, Hellison provides field-tested strategies (instruction) for fostering responsibility through physical activity (curriculum). In terms of instruction, he offers students guidelines for their behavior, outlines expectations, and invites greater participation in learning. Regarding curriculum, Hellison identifies personal and social responsibility in terms of principles or goals: respecting the rights and feelings of others, participation and effort, self-direction, and helping others and leadership. Respect and helping others are social responsibilities, while effort and self-direction are personal responsibilities. Representing a "hierarchy of values" (Hellison et al., 2000, p. 40), these goals are arranged in an informal progression of levels. Two goals, respect (level 1) and effort (level 2) are necessary for establishing the type of positive learning climate that will support working independently (level 3) and contributing to the well-being of others (level 4). An important fifth level, "outside the gym," involves transferring the other four levels to school, home, and neighborhood.

Hellison's levels of responsibility or goals can be used to plan, to teach, and to evaluate student learning. However, success in achieving those goals will depend not only on instructional strategies, but also on the careful integration of responsibility and physical activity content. In other words, he uses a specific lesson format and certain strategies to present his curriculum, which can be considered a thoughtful blend of activities and goals.

Our depiction of instruction as strategy, and of curriculum as content and intent, deserves brief expansion. John Goodlad suggests that it may be impossible to distinguish the method from the message (Hellison, 2003, p. 55). Similarly, it may be difficult to distinguish goals from activities, because the latter must at least complement, if not enhance, the former. For example, a certain style of teaching might be useful in promoting fitness through aerobic dance and swimming. The style of teaching cannot easily be separated from the intent (fitness); nor can we readily disengage the activity (dance or swimming) from that intent. No matter how first-rate one's teaching strategies are, the desire to promote fitness is unlikely to occur through chess. Similarly, despite excellent instruction, the most ambitious attempts to cultivate responsibility may be undercut by inappropriate activities. Thus, although we argue for a deliberate combination of instruction, content, and goals, for purposes of discussion we have distinguished instruction from curriculum, and have characterized the latter as intent (goals) and content (physical activity).

Hellison's instructional method includes a specific lesson format (e.g., counseling time, an awareness talk, the physical activity lesson, a brief group meeting, reflection time) and precise strategies (e.g., modified tasks, self-paced challenges, goal setting, self-grading, student coaches and other leadership roles). His curriculum includes explicit goals (levels of responsibility) coupled with specific content (physical activity). In our opinion, if teachers want to promote responsibility through physical activity, they must attend to both goals and content.

Finally, from an instructional and curricular perspective, it may be helpful to discuss priorities. If responsibility is viewed predominantly from an instructional perspective, then teaching physical activity (content) is at least as important as promoting responsibility (e.g., giving students a voice, shifting decisions from teacher to student). However, if responsibility is viewed from a curricular perspective (i.e., constitutes the primary "what" to be learned), then other aspects of physical activity (e.g., skill acquisition, fitness, regular participation in physical activity, self-expression, and enjoyment) become secondary to responsibility. Although the lines between instruction and curriculum are imprecise, the point is that goals, substance, and delivery are important considerations, and their harmony may be more important for this model than with other instructional and curricular models.

The Standards and Personal and Social Responsibility

Standard 5 ("Exhibits responsible personal and social behavior that respects self and others in physical activity settings") is the obvious standard related to this model. However, the National Content Standards are not designed to be detached from one another. Perhaps more than anything, responsibility is not a stand-alone concept. It is our belief that the strength of the standards is their integration and interconnectedness. Just as a child is multidimensional, so are the standards. If we focus on one or two standards to the exclusion of others, we have done a huge disservice to the potential of physical education, and have denied exciting possibilities. In teaching personal and social responsibility, we have the opportunity and obligation (the responsibility!) to enhance all other standards.

Standard 1 ("Demonstrates competency in motor skills and movement patterns needed to perform a variety of physical activities") also connects directly to the concept of responsibility. Physical activity is our prime medium

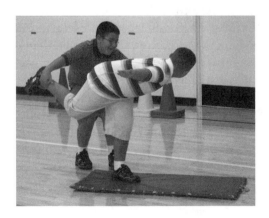

through which to teach responsibility. Because of its dynamic interactive nature, physical activity is replete with opportunities for students to practice and learn responsibility. Of course, if responsibility is to make sense or be credible to children, then the medium (physical activity) must be taught well. If motor skills, games, dance, outdoor pursuits, or gymnastics activities are used to teach responsibility, then those activities must be presented in ways that allow students to become more proficient in those activities.

Standard 2 ("Demonstrates understanding of movement concepts, principles, strategies, and tactics as they apply to the learning and performance of physical activities") is a by-product of assuming more responsibility for one's own actions. As students become more involved and responsible for their own learning, they learn more. For example, if in an effort to teach cooperation and helping, a teacher designs peer teaching activities that require students to provide feedback to one another, they not only learn to provide feedback, but also learn the critical cues of the skills being practiced. Additionally, as students start to learn more in class, they may seek to learn outside of class.

Standard 3 ("Participates regularly in physical activity") and Standard 4 ("Achieves and maintains a health-enhancing level of fitness") are similar to Standard 1. They, too, can become the medium through which responsibility is learned, and they also must be taught well.

Standard 6 ("Values physical activity for health, enjoyment, challenge, self-expression, and/or social interaction") becomes a logical by-product when teaching personal and social responsibility. If students learn to take responsibility for their actions in a physical activity setting, they also may learn to value the various benefits of engaging in regular physical activity.

Benefits, Compromises, and Limitations

Benefits

In our estimation, the benefits of teaching personal and social responsibility outweigh any considerations. Promoting a child's sense of responsibility will be vital to his or her success and fulfillment, and the betterment of society. Urgent societal problems, serious conditions in schools, and an ominous future all call for programs that support children in adjusting to the larger cultural and societal context. Physical education teachers have an exciting opportunity to engage students in positive, goal-directed activities that can enhance their skills and lessen the likelihood of engaging in risky behaviors.

No child arrives in physical education class with singular needs, and their needs certainly are not relegated to motor skills and fitness. Many carry with them the baggage of previous experiences in physical activity—both positive and negative. Some bring questions about their own competence. Still others turn up with few basic social skills, and devoid of strategies for dealing with conflict and caring. By cultivating and nourishing responsibility, we can begin to address these and other significant issues. We can provide a safe atmosphere where children can make decisions without the fear of making mistakes. We can create opportunities for belonging and connectedness. We can reduce class management issues while also allowing students to grow in ways not often seen in school. We can ensure a climate where every child can be healthy, creative, self-disciplined, curious, caring of others, able to work with others, concerned about the community and environment, and possess a playful spirit. Is this type of setting desirable? Most would say, "Yes." Without our intervention, is it probable? In all likelihood, no. Is it possible? Absolutely, yes!

Compromises

Teaching for personal and social responsibility takes time. For those who measure "time-on-task" as the time associated with learning motor skills, the time devoted to teaching responsibility may compete with the time assigned to teaching physical skills—at least initially. However, as youngsters assume more responsibility for their own learning, traditional "time-on-task" may become more efficient and effective; that is, the more students can take responsibility for their own behavior, the less they need to be prompted or reminded by the teacher to use their time effectively.

Limitations

The only bona fide limitation to this model is the teacher. There is no "quick fix," and teaching personal and social responsibility can be very demanding. We must be willing to try new possibilities, to devote time to activities that promote responsibility, to commit to persevering over an extended time period, and to attempt language that supports shifts in student attitudes and behaviors. Of major importance is the teacher's belief that teaching responsibility is important and worth doing.

The value of teaching responsibility lies in answering this question: "What is possible for my students, and what is my responsibility in creating opportunities for that to occur?" Nurturing personal and social responsibility may require observing and trying to understand children from a different perspective. It requires transferring some control to students. For most of us this differs from how we were taught, or were taught to teach. For example, when learning discipline or management techniques, we are encouraged to develop an authority relationship with students. Although seemingly efficient at first glance, this relationship may encourage obedience rather than responsibility. This, in turn, may reinforce victim behavior, powerlessness, and rebelliousness. As stated earlier, obedience can be a deterrent to responsibility and independence.

Finally, teaching responsibility requires personalizing and operationalizing responsibility for ourselves and our students, and teaching in a manner that deliberately promotes responsibility. In other words, successfully promoting responsibility sometimes requires new, and often different, ways of thinking and acting. It may not be comfortable, and it may not be easy; in fact, it can be tricky and taxing.

Implementing a Responsibility Approach

In-School Responsibility-Based Program

Many programs employ, to varying degrees, aspects of the personal and social responsibility model. Although there are recent efforts to incorporate Hellison's Personal and Social Responsibility model into school physical education as the primary focus of the physical education program (Wright & Burton, 2008), in most school physical education programs, responsibility is rarely presented as a solitary model. More than likely it is combined with other models in this book (e.g., developmental elementary physical education, sport education, and outdoor education). What is likely to be found in school physical education are instructional approaches that support the development of personal and social responsibility, combined with some curricular aspects. The emphasis in these classes is the process or method used. Although extended day programs do exist (e.g., Hansen & Parker, 2009; Hellison, 2003; Martinek, McLaughlin, & Schilling, 2004; Stiehl & Galvan, 2005) that adhere more clearly to the curricular model, what is presented here are in-school examples. Unlike in other chapters, you will not find a complete sample lesson plan, but instead a series of activities that you will be able to incorporate into existing or other lessons.

Class Setting

In an elementary physical education class that is using a developmental skill theme approach, partners are practicing overarm throwing and catching. The teacher is focusing on two responsibility constructs simultaneously: 1) helping others, and 2) self-direction and respectful behavior to others. Because the class practices as partners, the next task is to combine with another pair (of the students' choice—with whom they can work productively). Each pair receives two coaching cue cards (see Figure 6.2). The task is for one pair to observe the other, and to indicate on the cue card whether the throwers have demonstrated the cues. The pairs then switch roles. After both pairs have observed each other, they provide feedback to one another, and design practice tasks that will allow each of them to improve.

At the end of the class, the teacher distributes exit slips (Graham, Holt/Hale, & Parker, 2010), and each child responds to the questions that probe responsible actions, such as: "What did you do to help someone else today? Were you on task by listening when others were talking? What goal did you set for yourself?" The roles assigned to each student allowed them to practice

<table>
<tr><td colspan="4">Coach's checklist</td></tr>
</table>

Coach: _____	Player: _____		
Steps forward on opposite foot	Yes	No	Sometimes
Faces target	Yes	No	Sometimes
Arm way back	Yes	No	Sometimes
Eyes on target	Yes	No	Sometimes
Follows through	Yes	No	Sometimes

FIGURE 6.2 Cue card.

responsibility, first by providing feedback to another pair, then by designing tasks that will allow them to practice the requisite skills, and finally by reflecting on what they actually did. Additionally, these same roles can be used as formative assessment tasks.

As an additional opportunity for promoting responsibility, children in the same class are allowed to get a drink of water and go to the restroom without asking the teacher. The guidelines are: no one else at the water fountain, and the "key" to the restroom is on the wall (similar to a service station). If guidelines are not followed, instead of immediately removing the option, either a class discussion is held to remedy the situation or a private discussion occurs with those who are not working productively. For more examples of ways to incorporate responsibility constructs into the gymnasium, see Hellison (2003), and Parker, Kallusky, and Hellison (1998).

At the secondary level, warm-up/fitness activities are one venue that provide prime opportunities to allow students to practice responsibility constructs. In a middle school class, students are initially taught about the constructs of fitness, specifically cardiovascular warm-ups, stretching, and abdominal and upper body strength. During the first week of class, the teacher leads the class through a multitude of different fitness activities that would be appropriate for the identified constructs. After that, a reminder about the areas of fitness that need to be addressed are posted (e.g., aerobic, stretching, and abdominal strength). When the students arrive in the gym, they have 15 minutes to complete their warm-up. They may choose any appropriate activity, and carry out the activity with a partner/group of their choice. The teacher can attend to the details of the beginning of class, and interact with students as they are accomplishing their warm-up. At the end of class, the students complete an exit slip that asks what activities they did to accomplish each aspect of the warm-up. Additionally, they are asked to set goals for themselves with respect to abdominal and upper body strength.

On a larger scale, the entire Sport Education Model (see Chapter 11) provides multiple and varied opportunities for students to be engaged with learning responsibility. In the model, students are first and foremost responsible to their team. Thus, they must be in class and be ready to play. If a player is absent for a critical game, the entire team suffers. (And, in our experience, the other players are quick to let the missing player know they have let the others down.) Second, within a team specific duties are assigned (e.g., equipment manager, statistician, and trainer). These tasks allow students to practice individual responsibilities that allow the entire team to function smoothly. Each person contributes a piece. Finally, the "duty" team has a chance to practice responsibility as they officiate and make decisions that affect others. If these responsibility items are also included on the score sheet in the team folder, it provides a chance for reflection on what is working well for a team, and what needs attention.

Assessment

The goal of standards-based curriculum is student learning. In the case of personal and social responsibility, it is the learning of affective skills—which are notoriously difficult to measure. However, if we are true to the underlying principle of authentic assessment, and the primary client of assessment is the student, and the primary purpose of assessment is feedback to the student, it might not be as difficult as originally perceived.

Assessment of personal and social responsibility is most appropriately formative in nature. As previously stated (Parker & Hellison, 2001), to grade on a construct such as responsibility defeats the purpose of teaching it. But, if one subscribes to the tenet that the purpose of formative assessment is to provide feedback to the student, then multiple types of assessment are possible within the model. Assessment items would be developed to provide feedback to the student about how he or she was progressing within the constructs being taught. The following should serve as examples. The first example (Figure 6.3) is a checklist that asks students to reflect on their actions during any given lesson. The checklist presented here has its basis in Hellison's (2003) framework, but has been adapted for an elementary class that was having problems paying attention and working independently. Figure 6.4 shows two exit slips, one 4th and one 6th/7th grade, that again ask students to reflect upon their day in physical education. However, this time they are asked to identify what they did, and the focus is shifting to helping and caring, not just paying attention. The key to both of these assessments is that the teacher must provide written or verbal responses to students (versus collecting information and giving no reply). That way the relational nature of personal and social responsibility is developed.

My self-control

_____ I did no name-calling   _____ I listened to the teacher

_____ I didn't trip people   _____ I stopped when the teacher said stop

_____ I didn't push   _____ I held equipment still

Other things I did:

_____

My effort and participation

_____ I worked the whole time   _____ I tried new things

_____ I stayed on task   _____ I tried things that were hard

Other things I did:

_____

My self-direction

_____ I worked even when the teacher wasn't looking

_____ I followed directions   _____ I practiced on my own

Other things I did:

_____

My caring and helping

_____ I helped someone who didn't understand

_____ I told someone they did something right

_____ I helped teach someone something

Other things I did:

_____

FIGURE 6.3 Personal checklist.
Source: Adapted from Hellison, D. (2003). _Teaching personal and social responsibility through physical activity._ Champaign, IL: Human Kinetics.

At the unit level, teachers might wish to actually observe the development of personal and social responsibility. The observation of personal and social responsibility should reflect the definitions of responsibility that were provided to the students and that they were able to practice. Figure 6.5 is an example of a teacher observation of personal and social responsibility as conceptualized for an indoor vertical wall middle school climbing unit.

4th grade

What is one way that someone showed respect to you during your lesson?

What is one way that you showed someone respect during the lesson?

What is one way you helped someone today?

Adelante journal (6th/7th)

What is one thing you practiced today to make you a better climber?

What is one thing you did to help someone else?

FIGURE 6.4 Exit slips.

Summative assessment of personal and social responsibility can occur at the end of a course from information collected over time. Figure 6.6 represents several categories of responsibility for the extended canoe trip portion of an outdoor education class. In this evaluation, information is collected over a 2-week period and reported on a rubric-like form. Once again, it is important to note that responsibility has been specifically defined for this course and is woven throughout every course component.

Student Name	Respects Self	Respects Others	Respects Equipment	Communicates Well	Works Cooperatively	Comments

Respects self

!   Remains positive; participates and works to best ability

+   Sometimes down; occasionally not working at full potential or participating with effort (student is simply going through the motions of the activity)

−   Acts in a less than serious manner by not working to best ability or participating with effort

Respects others

!   Helps others when in need; open to others' ideas; listens

+   Sometimes helps other; sometimes open to others' ideas; occasionally listens

−   Lets others struggle; not open to others' ideas; interrupts others when they are speaking

Respects equipment

!   Appropriate use of equipment; returns equipment to its proper place when done

+   Sometimes uses equipment appropriately; sometimes returns equipment to its proper place

−   Total disregard for equipment (throws equipment on the ground, does not return it to its proper place)

Communicates well

!   Learned correct commands and used them appropriately; continued communication with partner throughout climb

+   Sometimes used incorrect commands; sometimes did not communicate with partner during climb

−   Never used correct commands; never communicated with partner during climb

Works cooperatively

!   Takes turns with partner; worked with partner to create a successful climb

+   Mostly took turns with partner; did not always work with partner to create a successful climb

−   Never took turns with partner; never worked with partner to create a successful climb

FIGURE 6.5 Teacher observation rubric for personal and social responsibility.

Outdoor Education—Canoeing
Trip Evaluation

Student _____   **Teacher** _____

Directions: Rate student on each of the six criteria below. Use a five-point rating scale. The five descriptors under each of the six criteria (Accomplishing Tasks, Human Relations, etc.) depict what a 5, a 4, a 3, a 2, and a 1 rating would likely be for each criterion.

A. Accomplishing Tasks

5. You show responsibility by following through on all tasks, coming prepared with gear, having necessary gear and equipment readily available (e.g., map, compass, and raingear), seeking extra responsibility, following the safety policy, and volunteering to do work that needs to be done.

4. You show responsibility by doing all tasks when asked, having necessary gear and equipment available (e.g., map, compass, and raingear) but you aren't quite sure about where it is, following the safety policy, and volunteering occasionally.

3. You follow the safety policy. You do tasks, but only when asked. You tend to not have necessary gear and equipment readily available (e.g., map, compass, and raingear). You rarely volunteer and/or frequently need to be reminded of responsibilities.

2. You quit on tasks requiring perseverance, only doing what is asked. You do follow the safety policy. You do not have necessary gear and equipment available (e.g., map, compass, and raingear). You do not volunteer and/or you fail to meet obligations.

1. You fail to follow the safety policy.

Comments:_____
_____
_____

B. Human Relations

5. You demonstrate positive human relationships through being cooperative, contributing positively to the group, and being open to suggestions.

4. You demonstrate an awareness of positive human relationships through being cooperative.

3. Human relations are characterized by the downside. The trip seems like a burden to you, and there is recurrent, though sometimes subtle, complaining. Your attitude has the potential to pull the group down.

2. You often grumble over decisions of others, do not accept criticism, become a burden to the group, and do not cooperate with leaders.

1. You are a burden to the group by doing very little work and letting others complete most of the tasks.

Comments:_____
_____
_____

FIGURE 6.6 Summative assessment of personal and social responsibility in an outdoor class.

Continued

C. Leadership

5. You demonstrate leadership through showing initiative and responsibility in unfamiliar situations and encourage leadership in others.

4. You take leadership when asked.

3. Little or no leadership is taken.

2. You often do not complete assigned tasks.

1. You make work for others to do.

Comments:_____

_____

_____

D. Skill Development

5. You try to improve skills by asking for help and attempting all skills.

4. Skill development is shown through attempting all skills.

3. Skills are worked on only when the leader is watching or you are constantly reminded.

2. Little is done to improve skills, and the same errors are repeated over and over.

1. You do not work on skill development and are satisfied to get through the trip.

Comments:_____

_____

_____

E. Environmental Awareness

5. You demonstrate an awareness of the factors affecting the ecology of the area by showing an appreciation of the outdoors, using the environment carefully and being willing to inconvenience yourself for the environment.

4. You demonstrate knowledge of the factors affecting the ecology of the area, and are willing to inconvenience yourself somewhat for the environment.

3. Your environmental awareness and actions are permeated with carelessness and lack of concern.

2. You resent inconveniences and merely comply with the ethic.

1. You are unwilling to be inconvenienced or comply with practices recommended by the minimal impact/environmental ethic.

Comments:_____

_____

_____

Figure 6.6—Cont'd   *Continued*

Source: Developed by and adapted from: Parker, M., Young, A., & Ramsey, T. (2001). For the Department of Recreation and Leisure Studies. Cortland, NY: State University of New York Cortland.

F. Overall Contribution

5. Overall, you are instrumental in making the trip a success by being cheerful and pleasant whenever things may be hard or uncomfortable, being alert and attentive to the needs of others, respecting the rights and feelings of others, and helping others without being asked. You really seem to enjoy being on the trip rather than just being part of a class that you have to complete.

4. You are instrumental in making the trip a success through a positive attitude, being alert and attentive to the needs of others, and respecting the rights and feelings of others. Overall, you are an engaged follower. You help others and seem to enjoy being on the trip even if it is not your first priority.

3. Overall, you do not respect the rights and feelings of others and help others only when asked. It seems as if "the glass is half empty," and you are just getting through the trip.

2. Overall, you complain a lot, have few positive comments, and have a low morale. You do not help others and are on the trip only because you have to be.

1. Overall, you clearly do not want to be on the trip and let everybody know it.

Comments:_____

_____

_____

FIGURE 6.6—CONT'D

Summary

If, after reading this, you choose to include personal and social responsibility in your physical education program, the following core principles of the responsibility model may guide your work.

- *Relational.* The teacher–student relationship is perhaps the most important factor in implementing this model. Curriculum guides loom overwhelmingly and, with all the concentration on content, it is easy to become consumed with something other than our primary focus—the student. Yet, "without a certain kind of relationship, nothing else . . . will work very well" (Hellison, 2003, p. 97). In order to implement the responsibility model successfully, students must be viewed and treated in certain ways: as resources to be nourished, not problems to be fixed; as having a voice that must be heard; as having ideas, needs, interests, and concerns to which we must pay attention. Students themselves should receive top priority, not the curriculum (kids are sacred, activities are not). The nature and quality of the relationship we establish with our students is paramount to the success of any model, but especially this one. As a colleague once said, "Kids won't care how much you know, until they know how much you care."

- *Congruency.* Instruction must match curriculum (intent and content). How we teach cannot undercut what we teach, or why. For purposes of discussion, we have portrayed curriculum as including both the aims (intent) and substance (content) of our programs. What's more, we have made a distinction between curriculum and instruction; yet, we readily admit that the lines between these various aspects of teaching are more dotted than solid. If the objective is to cultivate responsible attitudes and behaviors, then we ought to assure consistency between well-intentioned goals and our ability to carry them out. Stated differently, we can ill afford to employ instructional strategies or to introduce content and activities that contradict the very skills and attitudes we are trying to inspire.

- *Choice.* The practice of offering choices to our students serves several purposes: decision-making capabilities and confidence are reinforced; students' needs for input and control in their lives are addressed; potentially disruptive behaviors are frequently prevented; and the magnitude of students' sense of ownership in the program and their commitment to themselves and one another are strengthened. In addition, students become *empowered* to meet their own needs, without hurting, disturbing, or depriving anyone else. They also learn to act in their own best interests when an adult is not around to tell them what to do.

  Finally, offering choices in no way undermines an authority relationship. The teacher still decides what is and is not negotiable, and offering choices does not necessarily imply putting students in charge. For example, students may not be given a choice about whether to participate in an activity or not; but they may be provided opportunities to choose the way in which they might participate on any given day. Karl Rohnke suggests "Always offer choices. A coerced player is no longer a player" (Rohnke & Grout, 1998, p. 15). Only in a win-lose gymnasium does empowering students mean disempowering teachers.

- *Climate.* The success of our instructional interactions with our students depends, to a large degree, on the climate we develop. Working toward a positive climate—even if temporarily at the expense of the content—can help keep us from being sabotaged by negative attitudes, weak learning behaviors, unrealistic self-expectations, and less than desirable student interactions. If we are to foster a climate that encourages risk-taking, initiative, and personal commitment to learning and to others, then we must assure that students feel physically and emotionally *safe*, that they have a sense of *belonging*, and that they experience genuine *success*.

- *Relinquishing control.* The undercurrent from many schools warns that control is the goal. However, if responsibility is misperceived as one more discipline or behavior management technique, then the likelihood of generating responsible, caring attitudes and behaviors is next to nil. Control brings about obedience, which is often a deterrent to responsibility and independence. For some, surrendering some control may be difficult. This is especially true for those of us who believe that control is effective (even if only temporarily), or who have modeled our teaching behavior after our role models (perhaps leaving us short on options), or were advised not to "smile before Christmas"—advice that, when heeded, sometimes leaves little room to enjoy being a teacher. Yet, if we are to promote responsible attitudes and behaviors in our students, we may need to let go of some familiar attitudes and needs, develop new techniques, and learn new behaviors ourselves.

No one said teaching personal and social responsibility is easy—in fact it can be downright difficult. Yet, the power of teaching personal and social responsibility cannot be underestimated. Children are capable of accepting responsibility for their own actions, and for the consequences of their own behavior. They can learn to take better care of others, their surroundings, and themselves. When we create a climate that supports the development of responsible attitudes and behavior, we can produce unprecedented results.

References

Berman, S. H. (1998). The bridge of civility: empathy, ethics, and service. *School Administrator, 55*(5):27–32.

Dewey, J. (1913). *Interest and effort in education.* Boston: Houghton Mifflin.

Graham, G., Holt/Hale, S., & Parker, M. (2010). *Children moving* (8th ed.). New York: McGraw-Hill.

Haan, N., Aerts, E., & Cooper, B. (1985). *On moral grounds: the search for practical morality.* New York: New York University Press.

Haberman, M. (2000). Urban schools: day camps or custodial centers. *Phi Delta Kappan, 82,* 203–208.

Hansen, K., & Parker, M. (2009). Rock climbing: a lesson in responsibility. *Journal of Physical Education, Recreation and Dance, 80*(2), 17–23, 55.

Hellison, D. (2003). *Teaching personal and social responsibility through physical activity.* Champaign, IL: Human Kinetics.

Hellison, D., Cutforth, N., Kallusky, J., Martinek, T., Parker, M., & Stiehl, J. (2000). *Youth development and physical activity: linking universities and communities.* Champaign, IL: Human Kinetics.

Hichwa, J. (1998). *Right fielders are people too.* Champaign, IL: Human Kinetics.

Kingsley, C. (1918). *Cardinal principles of secondary education.* Washington, DC: Department of the Interior, Bureau of Education, Bulletin No. 35.

Kolberg, L., & Mayer, R. (1972). Development as the aim of education. *Harvard Educational Review, 42*(4), 449–496.

Lickona, T. (1991). *Educating for character.* New York: Bantam Books.

Martinek, T., McLaughlin, D., & Schilling, T. (2004). Project effort: teaching responsibility beyond the gym. *Journal of Physical Education, Recreation and Dance, 74,* 33–39.

Mosston, M., & Ashworth, S. (2002). *Teaching physical education* (5th ed.). San Francisco: Benjamin Cummings.

National Association for Sport and Physical Education. (2004). *Moving into the future: national content standards in physical education.* St. Louis, MO: Mosby.

Parker, M., Kallusky, J., & Hellison, D. (1998). High impact, low risk: ten strategies to teach responsibility in physical education. *Journal of Physical Education, Recreation and Dance, 70*(2), 26–28.

Parker, M., Young, A., & Ramsey, T. (2001). For the Department of Recreation and Leisure Studies. Cortland, NY: State University of New York Cortland.

Patterson, J., & Kim, P. (1991). *The day America told the truth.* Englewood, Cliffs, NJ: Prentice Hall.

Piaget, J. (1962). *Play, dreams, and imitation in childhood.* New York: Norton.

Piaget, J., & Inhelder, B. (1969). *The psychology of the child.* New York: Basic Books.

Rohnke, K., & Grout. J. (1998). *Back pocket adventure.* Needham Heights, MA: Simon and Schuster.

Sizer, T. R. (1992). *Horace's school: redesigning the American high school.* Boston, MA: Houghton Mifflin.

Stiehl, J., & Galvan, C. (2005). School-based physical activity programs. *Journal of Physical Education, Recreation, and Dance, 76*(9), 25–31.

Wright, P., & Burton, S. (2008). Implementation and outcomes of a responsibility-based physical activity program integrated into an intact high school physical education class. *Journal of Teaching in Physical Education, 27,* 138–154.

Additional Resources

Coles, R. (1993). *The call to service.* Boston: Houghton Mifflin.

Debusk, M., & Hellison, D. (1989). Implementing a physical education self responsibility model for delinquency prone youth. *Journal of Teaching in Physical Education, 8,* 104–112.

Hastie, P. A., & Buchanan, A. M. (2000). Teaching responsibility through sport education: prospects of a coalition. *Research Quarterly for Exercise and Sport, 71,* 25–35.

Hellison, D., & Martinek, T. (2006). Social and personal responsibility programs. In D. Kirk, D. MacDonald, & M. O'Sullivan (Eds.), *The handbook of physical education* (pp. 61–62). Thousand Oaks, CA: Sage.

Laker, A. (2000). *Beyond the boundaries of physical education: educating young people for citizenship and social responsibility.* New York: Routledge Falmer.

Li, W., Wright, P., Rukavina, P., & Pickering, M. (2008). Measuring students' perceptions of personal and social responsibility and the relationship to intrinsic motivation urban physical education. *Journal of Teaching in Physical Education, 27,* 167–178.

Martinek, T., Shilling, T., & Johnson, D. (2001). Transferring personal and social responsibility of underserved youth to the classroom. *Urban Review, 23*(1), 29–45.

Mosston, M., & Ashworth, S. (1994). *Teaching physical education* (4th ed.). New York: Macmillan.

Parker, M., & Hellison, D. (2001). Teaching responsibility in physical education: standards, outcomes and beyond. *Journal of Physical Education, Recreation and Dance, 72*(9), 25–27.

Parker, M., Stiehl, J., & Hansen, K. (2000). *Climbing club.* Paper presented at Central District Association for Health, Physical Education, Recreation and Dance, Des Moines, IA.

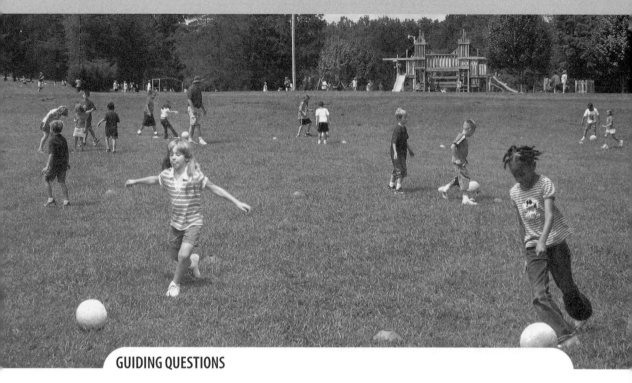

GUIDING QUESTIONS

1 What is a skill theme approach to physical education?
2 Why is the skill theme approach described as developmental physical education?
3 Describe the four phases of skill theme curriculum development.
4 What is the goal of content selection in physical education? How is that goal determined?
5 Why is the skill theme approach considered a standards-based curriculum?
6 How are the standards both by-products and products of a skill theme curriculum?
7 Outline the three steps in planning a skill theme.
8 Describe assessment within a skill theme curriculum.

The Skill Theme Approach to Physical Education

Shirley Holt/Hale, Linden Elementary School, Oak Ridge, Tennessee

Developmental Physical Education

The skill theme approach to physical education is often referred to as a "developmental model" for curriculum development. Several factors during the timespan between the 1960s and 1980s contributed to this developmental approach to elementary physical education. Prior to this time, elementary physical education in the United States, if it existed as a separate discipline, was a curriculum of games of low organization and/or a somewhat simplified version of secondary sports. However, physical education in England was viewed as separate from recess with a curriculum of movement experiences that were appropriate for young children. During the 1970s many physical educators in the United States, including this author, traveled to England to observe and teach in this program.

About this same time, physical education professionals in the United States were beginning to discuss appropriate activities for children. Research in motor development was focused on developmental stages of skills (e.g., throwing, jumping, kicking). Hoffman, Young, and Klesius (1981) authored a text entitled, *Meaningful Movement for Children: A Developmental Theme Approach to Physical Education*, describing developmental physical education as:

- Physical education with a focus on the whole child
- Physical education experiences related to developmental tasks and stages
- Activities chosen to facilitate a theme, not just for development of the activity

David Gallahue (1987) authored the first of his elementary texts entitled *Developmental Physical Education for Today's Elementary School*

Children, defining developmental physical education as content chosen to match children's stages of motor development and motor learning rather than chronological age or grade level.

Levels of motor skill proficiency provided the basis for the design of appropriate physical education experiences for children of different skill abilities in *Children Moving* (Graham, Holt/Hale, McEwen, & Parker, 1980). The design of curriculum that is developmentally and instructionally appropriate for children, reflecting the needs and interests of children, is "developmental physical education."

Rudolf Laban and the Movement Analysis Framework

A child-centered skill theme approach to elementary physical education has its curricular foundation in the work of Rudolf Laban. Born in Hungary in 1879, Rudolf Laban was fascinated by what he called "the rhythm of movement." Laban's study of human movement led him from the Berlin State Opera in the mid-1920s as choreographer of ballet, to the study of the efficiency of movement and human capacity in industry in Britain. In the 1940s, he returned to the study of movement and dance with the establishment of the Laban Art of Movement Guild in England. From Rudolf Laban's work, we have the **movement analysis framework** (Table 7.1).

With Laban's theories of movement and the principles governing control of human movement as the construct base, physical education for children in England began to focus on the acquisition of skill and the principles that affected movement control, with strong emphasis on the **movement concepts** that affect actions and skills. Movement education/physical education derived its content from the four major components: body awareness, space awareness, effort, and relationships.

The Skill Theme Approach

With the movement analysis framework as the core from which all curriculum would be drawn, the British model faced several barriers in the United States. Although dance for children seemed to be universal, and gymnastics became educational gymnastics, the focus on the games skills of English children was not as applicable for children in the United States. Creative dance faced its own challenges as teachers attempted to "dab, flick, and flutter," as described in the British texts. The framework itself was confusing, with very little direction about

> **movement analysis framework** A framework developed by Rudolph Laban for the classification of the components of movement (i.e., skills and concepts) and divided into four categories: body awareness, space awareness, effort, and relationships.

TABLE 7.1

The Movement Analysis Framework

MAJOR CATEGORIES OF MOVEMENT AND THEIR IMPORTANT SUB-DIVISIONS
USED FOR DESCRIPTION AND CONTENT SELECTION

BODY AWARENESS	SPACE AWARENESS	EFFORT	RELATIONSHIP
1. Whole body: stretch curl, twist	1. General space	1. Time: sudden/ sustained	1. With objects: manipulative, non-manipulative
2. Parts of the body: alone, in combination, initiating/following, stretch/curl/twist, meeting/parting	2. Personal space	2. Weight: heavy/ light	2. With people
3. Weight bearing: support, transference of weight, balance	3. Direction in space	3. Space: direct/ flexible	
4. Actions: locomotion, elevation, turns	4. Levels in space	4. Flow: bound/ free	
5. Body shapes: round, narrow, wide, twisted	5. Pathways in space: floor/air		
6. Symmetrical/ asymmetrical use of the body	6. Extensions in space: far, near, large, small		

Source: Adapted from Stanley, S. (1969). *Physical education: a movement orientation* (pp. 36–75). Toronto: McGraw-Hill of Canada Limited.

where to begin the selection of content, what scope and sequence was best to follow, and what was developmentally appropriate for children of varying skills and experiences. In the mid 1970s, the concept of "teaching by skill themes" was first conceptualized, resulting in the publication of a text entitled, *Children Moving: A Reflective Approach to Teaching Physical Education* (Graham, Holt/Hale, McEwen, & Parker, 1980). Inspired by the work of Sheila Stanley, the authors believed that movement education provided a curricular and instructional format that could be effective for all children, with the modifications that would Americanize the best that movement education had to offer. The curriculum would be rich in movement experiences for children in the early environments of physical education; multiple experiences would be provided for each task. Basic skills and concepts would be studied in many **contexts**, with

contexts   Experiencing the skill in a variety of environments and situations, rather than experiencing the skill in only one setting (e.g., jumping and landing in its many forms), and in different settings, rather than in the singular, narrow setting of a particular sport.

diversity in approaches to solving movement challenges. This richness and versatility would continue into the application of skills in games/sports, educational gymnastics, and dance.

Definition and Characteristics

Teaching by themes establishes the focus of physical education on the acquisition of specific skills and the use of those skills in a variety of contexts (Graham, Holt/Hale, & Parker, 2010). The skill theme approach is characterized by curriculum design that promotes competence in a variety of locomotor, nonlocomotor, and manipulative skills, and provides **developmentally appropriate experiences** and **instructionally appropriate experiences** reflecting the needs and interests of students over the span of the elementary school years.

Teaching by skill themes is not:

- Selection of a sport and teaching the skills of the sport followed by playing *the* game
- Selection of an activity for the day
- Physical education as a feeder program for middle school physical education and sports
- A "busy, happy, good" curriculum (Placek, 1983), with success measured by no injuries and no student sent to the principal's office

Teaching by skill themes is:

- Teaching skills and concepts for understanding, mastery, and application
- Selection of content appropriate for children at their developmental levels, recognizing a variety of developmental levels within a single class
- Selection of skills that leads to physically active lifestyles, the development of competency in those skills, and confidence in self
- Combining skills and **movement concepts**, building bridges between skill acquisition and application

developmentally appropriate experiences Matching the curricular experiences to the developmental level of the child (cognitive, social, physical, and emotional).

instructionally appropriate experiences Matching instruction to the developmental levels of the children being taught in physical education.

movement concepts Concepts that are the enhancers and the enrichers of the skill; they tell us how, where, and in what relationships the movement is going to take place.

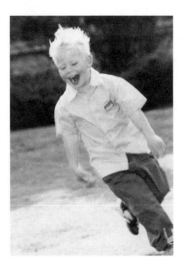

Curriculum Content

The basic skills of elementary physical education include traveling, jumping and landing, balancing, transferring weight, dribbling, catching, throwing, kicking, volleying, and striking. Skills are the action verbs of physical education, the movements to be performed. The students will kick, catch, balance, transfer weight. Concepts are the components of the physical education framework that indicate where the action takes place, how the body moves, and if the action takes place alone or with others, with or without equipment. Movement concepts are often categorized as body awareness, space awareness, effort, and relationships. Concepts are the modifiers of the action verbs—the adverbs; they describe how the skill is to be performed. They expand the skill beyond its simplest form and provide richness to the movement. Movement concepts include directions, levels, partner relationships, body shapes, force, and speed, to name only a few. A listing of the basic skills and movement concepts can be found in Table 7.2.

When first introduced to children, movement concepts and skills are taught as single lessons. When skills are first taught, they are introduced and practiced in isolation (i.e., the focus is on a single variable). For example, dribbling is first taught as dribbling in self-space without the addition of traveling, moving in relation to others, or a game situation. As students demonstrate mastery of the basic skill appropriate for their developmental levels, concepts are added to provide variety and breadth to the skill. When concepts are first taught, the movement concept is the focus for that lesson; all tasks center around students understanding that single concept. Adverbs modify verbs only after they have been studied in isolation. For example, the concept of pathways is taught for

TABLE 7.2	
Movement Skills and Concepts	
Skills	**Concepts**
Traveling, chasing, fleeing, dodging	Self and general space
Jumping and landing	Directions: forward, backward, right, left, up, down, clockwise, counterclockwise
Transferring weight, rolling	
	Levels: high, medium, low
Balancing	
	Pathways: straight, curved, zigzag
Kicking and punting	
	Extensions: near, far, large, small
Throwing and catching	
	Time: fast, slow, sudden, sustained
Volleying and dribbling	
	Force: heavy, light
Striking with rackets and paddles	
	Flow: bound, free
Striking with long implements	
	Actions: stretching, curling, twisting, turning
	Body shapes: round, narrow, wide, twisted
	Relationships: objects, people

Source: Graham, G., Holt/Hale, S. A., & Parker, M. (2010). *Children moving: a reflective approach to teaching physical education.* (8th ed.). New York: McGraw-Hill. Reprinted with permission.

understanding before students are asked to dribble and travel in different pathways.

Movement concepts can modify any number of skills. For example, children can balance at low, medium, and high levels; they can throw and catch at high, medium, and low levels. They can travel at different levels. Children can dribble forward, backward, to the right, and to the left. They can travel in different directions. A gymnast, a dancer, and a basketball player all travel in different pathways. The movement analysis framework, depicted as "The Wheel" (Graham, Holt/Hale, & Parker, 2010), clarifies the concept of movement concepts as adverbs modifying different skills as verbs. A visual spinning of the outer circle moves the concepts in place to enhance and expand the contexts in which the skill will be studied (Figure 7.1).

Curriculum Development

Teaching by skill themes is the teaching of skills, the combining of skills and concepts, to achieve the selected purpose or outcome.

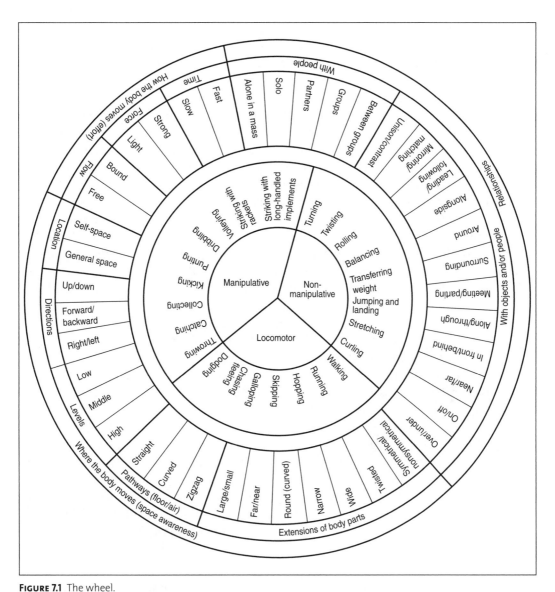

FIGURE 7.1 The wheel.

Source: Graham, G., Holt/Hale, S. A., & Parker, M. (2010). *Children moving: a reflective approach to teaching physical education.* (8th ed.). New York: McGraw-Hill. Reprinted with permission.

Phase One: The **skill theme** begins with the study of the basic skill—**cognitive and performance understanding** of the concept, mastery of the skill at the level appropriate for this age, for these children. Elementary age children are not expected to demonstrate mastery of throwing and catching equal to the throwing and catching of middle and secondary school students. Kindergarten children are not expected to dribble—hand, foot, or implement—with the same degree of skill as 4th graders. Mastery is measured by the achievement of the critical elements of the skill, in a progression leading to a mature pattern. Dribbling is in self-space with a pushing action, and proper forward/backward stance. Jumping and landing is a performance of proper take-off and landing—jumping for height and distance.

Phase Two: Following the introduction of the basic skill and mastery of the **critical elements**, movement concepts and/or other skills are added. Dribbling is combined with directions, pathways, traveling, and body positions. Jumping and landing is combined with turns, shapes in the air, and one- or two-foot take-offs. The wheel now becomes multidimensional as skills are combined and a number of concepts are added to a single skill (e.g., travel and dribble while changing directions, pathways, and speed).

Phase Three: Skills, and their combinations, are practiced in a variety of contexts to expand the possibilities for **application** of the skill. Dribbling is performed with music for a rhythmic beat, against a defense, and in sequences of combination skills and concepts. Jumping and landing is performed as an expressive gesture, and to convey feelings/actions, combined with transferring weight and balance for explosive sequences, and practiced in the specific skills of lead-ups to spikes in volleyball, jump stops in basketball, and split-steps in tennis. Experiencing the skill in a variety of contexts and in combinations leads to the selection of the particular content area for application of the skill.

Phase Four: Following mastery of the basic skill, the combination of the skill with movement concepts, the combination of the skill with other skills, and the experiencing of the skills in different contexts, the application of the

---

skill theme   The selection of a skill and all of the variables that accompany that skill for a study; the variables that accompany the skill (e.g., concepts, contexts, combinations) provide enrichment, breadth, and depth.

cognitive and performance understanding   The combination of 1) the ability to demonstrate mental understanding for recall and verbalization and 2) the ability to translate cognitive understanding into performance/movement.

critical elements   The components determined to be the most critical pieces for attainment of the performance outcomes and mastery of the skill.

application   Using a skill in a new or more complex environment or using a skill in a dynamic (rather than a practice) and controlled situation.

skill/the culmination of the theme is in the chosen area: gymnastics, dance, games/sports. Figure 7.2 illustrates the development of a theme for the skill of dribbling. Figure 7.3 provides the template for the development of the theme of jumping and landing.

It is this combination of skills and movement concepts, with experiences in a variety of movement contexts, that makes this a skill theme approach to

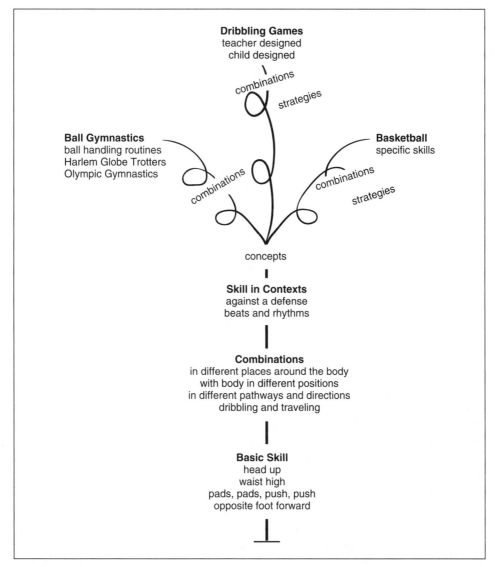

FIGURE 7.2 A sample skill theme.

Source: Graham, G., Holt/Hale, S. A. & Parker, M. (2010). *Children moving: a reflective approach to teaching physical education.* (8th ed.). New York: McGraw-Hill. Reprinted with permission.

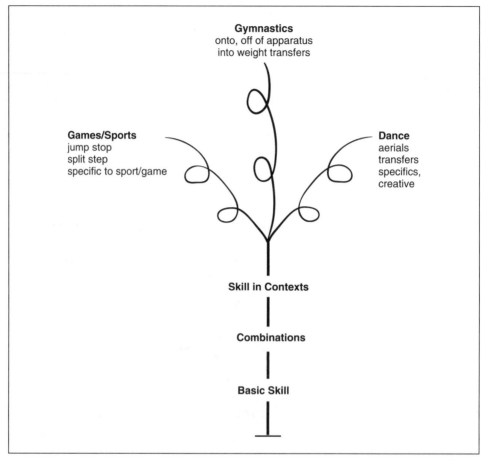

FIGURE 7.3 A template for skill theme development.

curriculum for physical education. This development of curriculum can perhaps best be illustrated by Figure 7.4, first presented by Kate Barrett, University of North Carolina at Greensboro, a pioneer in the development of movement-based physical education in the United States. The movement skills and concepts from the movement analysis framework are the core for curriculum development in elementary physical education. Following the teaching of the basic skills and concepts, and the achievement of student learning, the teacher may choose the application of the learning in games/sports, educational gymnastics, or dance. Some skills may be applied in either content area, with the culmination of the skill theme being games, gymnastics, or dance. Other skills are specific to one or two content areas only. For example, jumping and landing as a skill theme is applicable to games/sports, gymnastics, and dance. Throwing and catching as a skill theme is applicable to the games/sports area only.

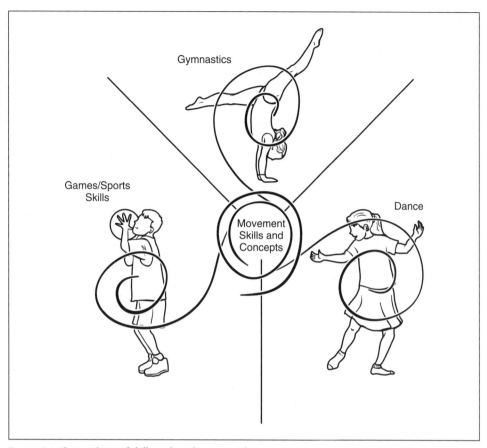

FIGURE 7.4 The teaching of skills and application in the content areas.

The concept area for application of the skill, following the study of the skill in a variety of contexts, will guide the selection of additional concepts, skills, combinations, and strategies needed for successful application of the skill in the **culminating activity**.*

> **culminating activity**   The ending activity for the lesson, the series of lessons, or the study of the theme; the activity that brings together the skill components and concepts that were the focus of the lesson or theme.

---

*The skill theme of dribbling will be used throughout this chapter for purposes of illustration.

Contributions to Student Learning

Content selection in physical education is based on the following beliefs:

- Student learning is the goal of physical education.
- Student learning is definable and is measurable.
- Student learning is defined by the **national content standards** (National Association for Sport and Physical Education [NASPE], 2004).
- Student learning and experiences in physical education do impact continued participation in physical activity and the adoption of an active lifestyle.

A skill theme approach to physical education shares those beliefs. Student learning is *the* key component of physical education. Student learning in physical education is defined by the skills and knowledge one must have to successfully participate in selected physical activity. Successful participation comes from the development of skills necessary for that participation. Student learning in physical education is definable and measurable. Student learning is not synonymous with student activity; what the students did in physical education today is not necessarily the same as what the students learned in physical education today. All content selection and all teaching of physical education must be done with student learning as the measurable outcome. Student learning in physical education is defined by the national content standards. Those standards lead to a physically educated individual—one who has the skills, knowledge, and dispositions necessary for successful participation in physical activity.

Each skill theme developed, and each lesson taught, is designed with student learning as its goal. Students will dribble, kick, catch. Students will demonstrate cognitive and performance understanding of directions, levels, pathways. Having fun is a by-product of well-designed lessons; enjoyment in physical activity is a by-product of skill competency and confidence in self as a result of that competency.

The skill theme approach provides students with competency in the basic skills of physical education, and a working knowledge of movement concepts. The skill theme curriculum progresses from mastery of basic skills and **fundamental movement patterns** to combinations of skills and concepts in a

national content standards   The standards developed by NASPE (2004) to specify the curricular content for physical education—what students should know and be able to do in physical education.

fundamental movement patterns   Two or more basic and fundamental skills combined for a movement pattern with a progression from basic motor skills to fundamental skills to movement patterns.

variety of contexts (elementary). Patterns and combinations lead to **specialized skills,** more complex *skills* (upper elementary and middle school), which lead to the application of those skills in the authentic settings of games/sports, gymnastics, and dance (secondary school physical education). Although **game-like experiences** are included throughout the theme development (e.g., teacher-designed, child-designed games; one-on-one, two-on-two challenges), they are designed with a developmental and instructional match, reserving *the* game/sport beyond the years of elementary physical education due to the group/peer dynamics, rules, and scoring of the sport/game, and the complexity of play.

Skill Themes and the National Standards

A standards-based curriculum, as outlined in Chapter 1, begins by identifying the skills, knowledge, and dispositions that students should demonstrate to meet the standards. The standards are statements of "what students should know and be able to do." For physical education, those standards are the national content standards developed by NASPE (2004), the standards that define a physically educated person.

A skill theme approach to physical education contributes significantly to all six of the national standards (NASPE, 2004), as illustrated in the Curriculum Model table developed by Tannehill and Lund (see this book's Introduction).

Standard 1: Demonstrates competency in motor skills and movement patterns needed to perform a variety of physical activities.

Physical education with a skill theme approach links directly to Standard 1 through the development of mature patterns/competency in the skills of physical education (Figure 7.2). A skill theme curriculum is designed to develop competency—not introduction—to the skill. Competency is developed through the mastery of skills in their static form, followed by performance of skills in dynamic situations, and finally application of skills in unpredictable, everchanging environments (i.e., competency). For example, the skill of dribbling is initially performed in self-space, with demonstration of the critical elements of a mature pattern. Dribbling is then combined with traveling and studied in a variety of contexts. Finally, the skill of dribbling is performed in

---

specialized skills   The skills of a particular sport or activity (e.g., dig or bump in volleyball).

game-like experiences   Experiences designed by the teacher to move students beyond the practice-in-isolation to dynamic, unpredictable situations; designed by the teacher to control the number of variables and the complexity of the movement experience.

dynamic game-like situations, leading to application in games/sports that utilize the skill. Mastery at each level leads to competency in the performance of the skill.

Standard 2: Demonstrates understanding of movement concepts, principles, strategies, and tactics as they apply to the learning and performance of physical activities.

A skill theme curriculum contributes to Standard 2 as children develop a functional understanding of movement concepts (Figure 7.2). After children attain a "working" knowledge of the concepts, the concepts are combined with skills to provide a breadth of understanding and experience with the skill. For example, after children explore and demonstrate an understanding of pathways, directions, time, and space, they are presented experiences combining dribbling and traveling with changes in directions, pathways, locations in space, and speed of movement. At a more advanced level of skill performance and understanding, children are introduced to the strategies and tactics of dribbling against opponents, in dynamic situations, and in game-like environments.

Standard 3: Participates regularly in physical activity.

*Standard 4: Achieves and maintains a **health-enhancing level of physical fitness.***

A health-enhancing level of physical fitness is attained through a quality program of physical education. In a skill theme physical education program, children do not do formal exercises or run laps for endurance. Time is not set aside for fitness. Muscular strength, flexibility, and cardiovascular endurance are achieved through lessons that maximize participation, time on task, and individual challenges while developing skill. Enjoyment and challenge come as children experience tasks and activities appropriate for their developmental skill levels. Because tasks are developmentally appropriate, children experience success in activity, leading to increased enjoyment and a desire to participate in further physical activity. Equipped with the skills for participation in physical activity, and the success that comes from developmentally appropriate physical education experiences, children become eager participants in physical activity, well on their way to becoming lifelong movers.

Standard 5: Exhibits responsible personal and social behavior that respects self and others in physical activity settings.

health-enhancing level of physical fitness   The fitness and level of fitness needed to be "healthy" in each of the categories considered critical for good health: muscular strength and endurance, flexibility, cardiovascular efficiency, and body composition; criteria is referenced as compared to norm-referenced physical fitness.

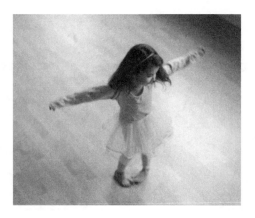

A skill theme "classroom" is rich in opportunities for the development of personal and social responsibility. Responsibility and respect for self and others are critical components of the skill theme approach. With children functioning at different skill levels, the gymnasium is often viewed as "organized chaos." The teacher is a facilitator of learning, moving throughout the activity with **cues** and feedback—to refine, to reteach, to challenge the student to a higher level of performance—always to maximize student learning. Students teach, assess, and assist other students in an environment where responsible personal and social behavior is expected. Is responsible behavior an automatic product of a skill theme physical education program? No, it is a standard that is taught through specifically planned activities, a standard that is promoted by a positive, emotionally safe learning environment for all children. Responsible personal and social behavior is critical for student learning in the independent, multi-level environment of a skill theme approach to physical education.

Standard 6: Values physical acitvity for health, enjoyment, challenge, self-expression, and/or social interaction.

Although Standards 3–6 are by-products of a skill theme approach to physical education, they are also outcomes of the program (Figure 7.5). The goal of a skill theme physical education program is physically educated individuals. Those individuals, when they leave the elementary school program, have a broad base of skills, with accompanying movement concepts and principles, from which they may select activities for specialization. They possess a health-enhancing level of fitness, and have a foundation for responsible personal and

cues   The simple phrases—the 2 to 3 words—that give children the cognitive reminder of what is needed to perform the skill correctly (e.g., pads, pads, push, push—push, don't slap the ball).

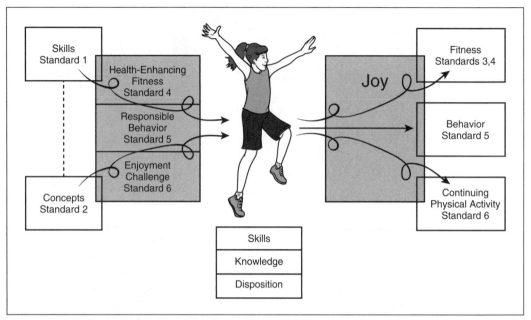

FIGURE 7.5 The skill theme approach and the national standards.

social behavior in physical activity. With a solid skills base, developmentally appropriate challenges, and positive interactions with others in physical activity, they know the joy of participation in activity. The product of developmental physical education with a skill theme approach is students with competence, confidence, and a love of movement, eager to participate in further physical activity.

Implementation of the Skill Theme Approach: A Sample Theme

A skill theme curriculum is a developmental curriculum, with the focus on providing developmentally appropriate physical education for children. With that philosophical base, there is no pre-set curriculum per grade level. A skill theme is a progression from simple to increasingly complex skills without established grade-level exit objectives, as compared to classroom content areas where each grade level has established student expectations and exit objectives in preparation for the next grade. Table 7.3 illustrates a skill theme progression. The national standards themselves are based on this philosophical base, and are therefore void of grade-level benchmarks. The national content standards provide sample

TABLE 7.3

A Skill Theme Progression

Proficiency Level
Small-group basketball
Dribble/Pass Keep-Away
Dribbling and throwing at a target
Making up fancy dribbling/passing routines
Dribbling and passing in game situations
Dribbling while dodging
Dribble Tag
Now You've Got It, Now You Don't
Dribbling against opponents group situations

Utilization Level
Dribbling against an opponent: one on one
Dribbling and passing with a partner
Mirroring and matching while dribbling
Dribbling around stationary obstacles
Dribbling in different pathways
Starting and stopping while changing directions
Dribbling while changing directions
Dribbling and changing speed of travel

Control Level
Moving switches
Dribbling and traveling
Dribbling in different places around the body while stationary
Dribbling with the body in different positions
Switches
Dribbling and looking
Dribbling at different heights
Dribbling like a basketball player
All the time dribble

Precontrol Level
Dribbling and walking
Bouncing a ball down (dribbling) continuously
Bouncing a ball down and catching it

Source: Graham, G., Holt/Hale, S. A. & Parker, M. (2010). *Children moving: a reflective approach to teaching physical education* (8th ed.). New York: McGraw-Hill. Reprinted with permission.

performance outcomes as indicators across a three-year grade range, and **exit ex-pectations** at the end of each three-year period. While this permits the teacher to truly present a developmentally appropriate curriculum for the class and individuals within each class, it requires pre-planning, reflection, and on-going planning for the teacher.

An activities-based curriculum requires the teacher to choose an activity for the day—a game, equipment, or activity that will be the focus of the lesson, with class time devoted to the activity itself. The emphasis is on the activity and children's enjoyment of the activity. A unit approach to curriculum requires the teacher to choose the unit to be presented—sport, gymnastics, dance—and outline the skills to be taught to the class during the unit. Emphasis is on the sport, the dance, or the gymnastics skills, and class participation in *the* game.

A skill theme approach requires the teacher to select the skill for the theme, and plan a series of tasks that he or she thinks are developmentally appropriate based on age and past experiences of the children. After each class is taught, the teacher must then reflect on the match between his or her selected tasks, and the children's abilities. Only then can planning for the next lesson take place. The emphasis is on these children, this class, this child. This time spent in planning and reflection results in the development of skill and enjoyment of physical activity for all children, not just the highly skilled.

Planning the Theme

Each theme begins with the selection of the skill to be taught. Once a skill theme has been selected, a task analysis must be done to identify all the components of the skill to be taught in the theme. This process begins with a brainstorming of ideas, everything students should "know and be able to do." A skill theme progression represents the full spectrum of a skill, from simple to complex, often with application in more than one content area. The full progression is not intended to be taught as a single unit or at a single grade level. The teacher must now make decisions regarding the depth and the breadth of the theme to be presented. Decisions must be made regarding what students should know and be able to do in relation to the skill in order to reach performance and cognitive competency.

---

performance outcomes   Student behaviors that demonstrate progress toward achieving the standards.

exit expectations   What learners are expected to know and be able to do when they exit a series of lessons, or, in the case of the national standards, when they exit a particular grade range.

The second step of planning for teaching a theme involves placing the ideas in a progression from simple to complex. Each item that is necessary for mastery of the skill, and progression toward application of the skill, is coded as essential (E) (e.g., dribbling with the critical elements of pushing, not slapping the ball; proper stance; heads up when traveling; dribbling and traveling while others are traveling). Many of the ideas on the listing would be fun for the children and would add variety to the theme, but they are not absolutely essential to the development of the skill. The skill level of the students, their past experiences with the skill, and the number of days per week they have physical education will greatly impact what is coded as essential for the theme. Those items coded as essential become the focus of individual lessons.

The third step of planning for teaching the theme, and probably the most difficult in the beginning, is the assignment of the "essentials" to grade levels. This process begins with the establishment of the exit goal (i.e., what students should know and be able to do when they complete their last study of the theme in elementary physical education). Once the exit goal has been established, student performance outcomes are developed for each descending grade level in the process of backward design, as discussed in Chapter 2. Using the content standards' student expectations as guidelines (K–2, 3–5, 6–8), performance outcomes can be established for each grade level. Grade-level outcomes are not absolutes. They are targets for students to attain in their progress toward the established standards. The assignment of grade-level performance outcomes appears at first glance to be in contradiction to the developmental, skill theme approach to learning in physical education. Although *the skill theme curriculum is not grade-level specific*, it is important to have performance outcomes for each grade level in order to assure progress toward the exit expectations at the end of each 3-year interval (i.e., Grades 2, 5, 8) and toward the exit goal (i.e., a mature pattern of skill execution in both planned and unplanned situations). Table 7.4 illustrates grade-level performance outcomes.

Given the performance outcomes for each grade level, the teacher still must determine the skills, concepts, and combinations needed to achieve those outcomes, and more importantly, the range from entry to exit for each grade level. It is important to remember that, whatever range is established for a given grade level, a number of children will be functioning above and below the range, thus the concept of developmental physical education—matching the curriculum to the child.

Assessment in the Skill Theme Process

The goal of physical education is student learning. That learning is definable and measurable. Student learning cannot be assumed; it must be measured. A skill theme approach to curriculum assessment centers on the student's progress in

TABLE 7.4

Grade-Level Performance Outcomes

Kindergarten
Dribble a ball (multiple contacts) in self-space

Grade 1
Dribble with one hand in self-space for a designated number of times

Grade 2
Dribble in self-space with control of the ball
Dribble in self-space with feet in forward/backward stance
Dribble and travel in general space by walking with control of the ball
Recognize the correct stance for dribbling

Grade 3
Dribble in self-space with preferred hand demonstrating mature pattern (finger pads/push, opposite foot forward, waist high)
Dribble and travel in general space at slow to moderate speed without losing the ball or bumping others
Evaluate selected critical elements of self-dribbling—stationary and traveling
Identify the critical elements of a mature dribble
Dribble in time with a 4/4 rhythm and with other students in a teacher-designed group routine

Grade 4
Dribble in self-space with both preferred and non-preferred hand demonstrating a mature pattern (finger pads/push, opposite foot forward, head up, waist high)
Dribble and travel with control of body and ball
Combine dribbling with traveling and shooting baskets
Combine dribbling and passing to a partner while traveling
Analyze dynamic games situations and apply concepts of open space, speed, and directions while dribbling
Evaluate dribbling skill of partner to determine performance of components of mature pattern
Create a ball gymnastics routine combining dribbling and ball handling skills

Grade 5
Dribble in dynamic situations, demonstrating a mature pattern with the preferred hand
Demonstrate offensive and defensive strategies in a game-like situation

Grade 6
Create a small group game combining dribbling, throwing and catching, and moving toward a target
Dribble in a one-on-one keep-away game involving shooting or moving toward a goal
Combine dribbling, throwing and catching, and shooting baskets or throwing at a goal in a two-on-two game-like situation.

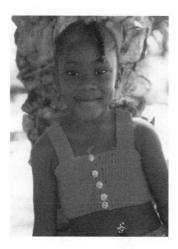

skill development, and the student's cognitive and performance understanding of the skill, movement concepts, combinations, and applications. For too many years assessment in elementary physical education was nonexistent. Grades were placed on report cards by classroom teachers, provided as a "blanket satisfactory" for every student, or given based on participation and/or behavior. As was true for curriculum content with no student learning for too many years, the days of no assessment are in the past. Student learning is the goal of physical education; assessment is the measure of that learning.

A skill theme approach to physical education is a rich environment for authentic performance-based assessments. (See Chapter 6 for a discussion of authentic, alternative, and performance-based assessments.) Skill theme assessments include teacher and peer observations, student projects, journal entries, exit slips, portfolios, and cognitive tests for knowledge and analysis. Student learning in each theme studied includes at least three assessments: teacher observation of critical elements; a cognitive assessment; and an event task, student project, and/or assessment of critical elements in a game-like performance.

- Student learning in a skill theme curriculum is assessed by teacher observation of the critical elements being developed within the theme. This observation is easily completed during task-related "instant activity." Observations are completed each day of the theme, thus providing multiple entries for each student on each critical element.
- Event tasks and exit slips provide formative assessments, as measures of student and class learning throughout the theme. Exit slips can focus on the psychomotor or the affective domain (Figure 7.6).
- A student project (individual, partner, group) provides the summative assessment for the theme of study; when complete these projects (digital recordings, routines, sequences, and dances) are placed in the student's

portfolio. *PE Metrics* (NASPE, 2008) and *Creating Rubrics for Physical Education* (Lund, 1999) are excellent resources for the design of rubrics and evaluation of student projects.

- Cognitive understanding and/or analysis of the skill is attained through brief written responses—sometimes individual, sometimes with a partner. (Children love this opportunity to "take a test together.")

(A)

What was your favorite practice task today?
What skill do you hope to improve?

(B)

Did you encourage or help someone today? How did you encourage or help?
Did someone encourage or help you today? How did they encourage or help you?

FIGURE 7.6 Sample exit slips for physical education.

Assessment within skill themes is perceived by the students as a natural part of the teaching/learning process. Pre-tests, post-tests, and lengthy written tests are not part of assessment in a skill theme curriculum. Assessments take only a small portion of class time and are often combinations of focus areas. Figure 7.7 is an example of a combination assessment—cognitive, affective, and performance. Student learning is ongoing; assessment should be ongoing and should complement learning. The national standards are the touchstone for both.

Dribbling Skills Test

Name: Homeroom:

                                         Date:

Test for Understanding

1. The critical cue for dribbling is: _____ , _____ , _____ , _____ .

2. The critical cue for dribbling and traveling is: _____ _____ .

Self-Evaluation of Dribbling Skill

	I still need to practice at this skill	I'm pretty good at this skill	I'm very good at this skill
1. Dribbling in self-space with preferred hand			
2. Dribbling in self-space with other hand			
3. Switches of hands and feet			
4. Dribbling and traveling			

My favorite station for dribbling was:

I liked this station best because:

FIGURE 7.7 Self-assessment for dribbling.
Source: Adapted from Holt/Hale, S. A. (2004). *On the move: lesson plans to accompany children moving.* New York: McGraw-Hill. Reprinted with permission.

Summary

Teaching by skill themes establishes the focus on the acquisition of specific skills, and the use of those skills in a variety of contexts (Graham, Holt/Hale, & Parker, 2010). Teaching by skill themes is the teaching of skills, the combining of skills and movement concepts to achieve the selected purpose or outcome. That outcome is established by the national standards for physical education (NASPE, 2004). The skill theme curriculum progresses from mastery of basic skills and movement patterns, to combinations and use of skills in a variety of contexts. From combinations and contexts, the skill theme progresses to the specialized skills of games/sports, gymnastics, and dance, and to application in real-world settings.

The skill theme approach to physical education derives its curriculum from the movement framework, composed of skills and movement concepts. At the elementary level, the curriculum progresses from basic skills to combinations, to skills in a variety of contexts to attain mastery and versatility in the use of the skill. Basic skills and concepts are studied in many contexts, with diversity in approaches to solving movement challenges. This broad base provides students with options for application of the skill. Students gain competency in the skill and the breadth of the skill through the richness and versatility of movement experiences. They are then able to 1) apply the skill in games/sports, gymnastics, and dance and 2) perform the skill in predictable and unpredictable situations. This breadth, coupled with the depth of skill, or the mastery, broadens the options for students as they pursue physically active lifestyles.

Within a skill theme approach, the progression of skill development is not in a lock-step manner, but rather in the development of performance outcomes leading to the goal for each grade level, and the exit goal for the school's physical education program. Once that exit goal has been determined, backward design provides the grade-level performance indicators to attain the goal.

Planning is a critical part of a skill theme approach to physical education. There are no card files, no activity notebooks to provide the curriculum, no texts to provide grade-level expectations. Themes of study are chosen based on student needs and interests. The length and breadth of the theme will be impacted by the skill level of the students, their past experiences with the skill, and the number of days per week they have physical education. Student learning is the goal of physical education and the goal of the skill theme approach to physical education. That student learning is defined by the national standards. Student learning in physical education consists of the skills, knowledge, and dispositions for a physically active, healthy lifestyle. That learning is measurable and must be assessed.

The skill theme curriculum, while content by definition, greatly impacts the teaching of physical education. As a developmental approach to physical education, the teacher of skill themes must focus on children—what is appropriate for this class, for this child. This focus on developmentally and instructionally appropriate experiences for children eliminates a prescribed curriculum; daily lessons must be based on previous learning. Teaching must meet the needs and developmental levels of the students being taught.

The skill theme approach to physical education requires a focus on children and the teaching that leads them to the acquisition of skills, knowledge, and dispositions. It is that focus on children and their learning, with appropriately designed lessons, that provides the competence and confidence that leads to a joy of movement and the pursuit of physical activity outside the physical education classroom and continuation beyond the formal school years.

References

Gallahue, D. (1987). *Developmental physical education for today's elementary school children.* New York: MacMillan.

Graham, G., Holt/Hale, S. A., McEwen, T., & Parker, M. (1980). *Children moving: a reflective approach to teaching physical education.* Mountain View, CA: Mayfield.

Graham, G., Holt/Hale, S. A., & Parker, M. (2010). *Children moving: a reflective approach to teaching physical education* (8th ed.). New York: McGraw-Hill.

Hoffman, H. A., Young, J., & Klesius, S. E. (1981). *Meaningful movement for children: a developmental theme approach to physical education.* Boston: Allyn and Bacon.

Holt/Hale, S. A. (2004). *On the move: lesson plans to accompany children moving.* New York: McGraw-Hill.

Lund, J. L. (1999). *Creating rubrics for physical education.* Reston, VA: NASPE.

National Association for Sport and Physical Education. (2004). *Moving into the future: national standards for physical education* (2nd ed.). Reston, VA: NASPE.

National Association for Sport and Physical Education. (2008). *PE metrics: assessing the national standards.* Reston, VA: NASPE.

Placek, J. (1983). Concepts of success in teaching: busy, happy and good? In T. Templin & J. Olson (Eds.), *Teaching in physical education* (pp. 46–56). Champaign, IL: Human Kinetics.

Stanley, S. (1969). *Physical education: a movement orientation.* New York: McGraw-Hill.

Additional Resources

Holt/Hale, S. A. (1999). *Assessing motor skills in elementary physical education.* Reston, VA: NASPE.

Lambert, L. (1999). *Standards-based assessment of student learning.* Reston, VA: NASPE.

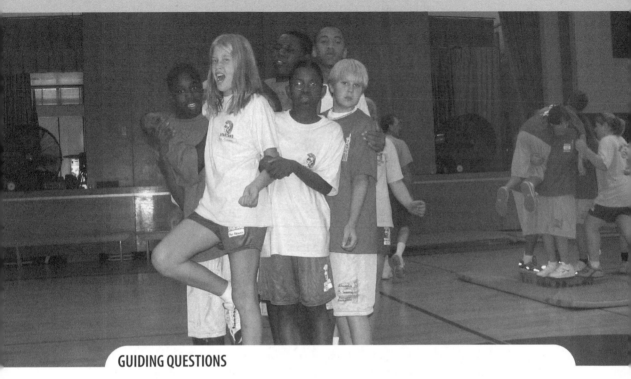

GUIDING QUESTIONS

1 How can Adventure Education be incorporated into a physical education program?
2 Can I teach Adventure Education in my regularly scheduled classes?
3 How does Adventure Education incorporate the national standards?
4 How can I assess Adventure Education activities?
5 How can I convince fellow teachers or school administration to support the implementation of Adventure Education in my physical education program?
6 How do I design a sequence of tasks that are safe, purposeful, and motivating for students?
7 What might interest young people about the Adventure Education curriculum model?

Adventure Education in Your Physical Education Program

Ben Dyson, The University of Memphis
Mike Brown, The University of Waikato

Imagine the scene: One group of students is scaling a climbing wall, another group is involved in a trust fall from a height of 5 feet, a group of eight students in a circle has eight balls in the air simultaneously, and another group of students is building a human pyramid. The instructor is at the trust fall, but scans the room frequently. There is a great deal of calling and shouts of encouragement coming from the students, and all students seem to be involved in some form of activity. Students are challenging themselves, solving problems in a variety of activities, taking risks while receiving support from peers, and developing trust as they strive toward a group goal. The teacher's objectives for this lesson are for students to: challenge themselves by trying new things (by extending themselves, physically, mentally, or emotionally), provide positive feedback to each group member, and work as a team so that all teammates contribute to the task. Is this an Outward-Bound program in Colorado? No, this is a middle school physical education class in Memphis, Tennessee. Eighty percent of the students are African American, 15% are Hispanic, and 5% are Caucasian; 90% of the students are on free or reduced-priced lunches. And, it's working. Adventure Education has these students engaged in learning about themselves and their peers, striving to accomplish group tasks, and challenging themselves in physical activity experiences that are not often seen in your traditional physical education lessons. If it works here, maybe it could work in your gymnasium! What is **Adventure Education**? By the end

> **Adventure Education**   Involves activities that encourage holistic student involvement (physical, cognitive, social, and emotional) in a task that involves challenges and an uncertainty of the final outcome. Activities are carefully sequenced to ensure student safety while allowing them to take ownership of their learning.

of this chapter, you will have a good understanding of this curricular approach, be able to describe features and characteristics of Adventure Education, and understand its possible contributions to enhance learning in physical education. You will be able to explain the philosophy and instructional goals of Adventure Education. In addition, resources for teaching will be provided. First, we will briefly define Adventure Education, and then discuss more thoroughly the role of experience and reflection in this curriculum model prior to looking in more detail at the components of an adventure program.

Adventure Education

Adventure education is primarily concerned with the development of interpersonal and intrapersonal relationships through the use of holistic learning experiences (Priest, 1999). A more formal definition has been provided by Bailey (1999):

> *Adventure education . . . uses kinesthetic learning through physical experience. It involves structured learning experiences that create the opportunity for increased human performance and capacity. There is conscious reflection on the experience and application that carries it beyond the present moment. (p. 39)*

When the authors of this chapter think of experiences in Adventure Education, several words come to mind. The activity may be uncertain, mysterious, explorative, inquisitive, interesting, curious, analytical, surprising, quizzical, or motivating for students. The teacher, as facilitator, is trying to create a situation where the challenge is at the students' level, and the physical activity is combined with appropriate opportunities for reflection under thoughtful supervision. Adventure Education emphasizes the value of the "process" of students participating in a physical activity, such as a cooperative activity, an initiative problem, or a challenge task, and de-emphasizes the outcome of the activity. Through an atmosphere of cooperation, challenge, trust, self-expression, and problem solving, students are encouraged to think independently while working with others. The experiences are designed to be holistic, and provide opportunities for creative reflection and the future application of learning with questions such as, *What happened in the lesson? Why was this important?* In this student-centered approach, the teacher tries to develop student interdependence through collaborative tasks and personal goal setting. The broader goals are to encourage students to become reflective learners and become active members of the school and local community. Central to an understanding of Adventure Education is the importance of conscious reflection on experience in the learning process. Adventure Education has its roots in the experiential education movement.

Experiential Education

The founder of **experiential education**, John Dewey, was interested in making it possible for students to connect abstract notions to concrete life experiences. Dewey (1938) was concerned that the quality of the experience be planned and structured in a way that encouraged students to reflect on and learn through their engagement in activity. Central to the experiential approach is the belief that learning will happen more effectively if the student is as involved as possible in the activity. This student participation could include involvement in the planning, performing, reflecting on, and assessment of the experience. Involvement is maximized if students are required to commit themselves to the activity mentally, emotionally, and physically. Essential to the experiential process is the opportunity for reflection and "meaning-making" that connects the experience(s) to the students' world. Thus an activity moves from being an isolated endeavor and is consciously integrated into the lives of the individuals and the group.

Adventure Education in Physical Education

The principles of Adventure Education are often referred to as **Adventure-Based Learning**. Adventure-Based Learning is the purposeful use of sequenced adventure activities such as games, trust activities, and problem-solving initiatives for the physical and social development of students (Cosgriff, 2000). Perhaps the most widely known program for integrating adventure into the physical education curriculum is **Project Adventure**. As a student-centered curriculum, Project Adventure (PA) is physically exciting with a philosophical orientation toward the education of the total person. Karl Rohnke (1986) suggested that PA learning goals promote a holistic educative process. The intent of PA is to increase the student's sense of personal confidence, increase mutual support within the group, develop an increased level of agility and physical coordination, and develop an increased appreciation in one's physical self while interacting with others (Rohnke, 1986). Project Adventure utilizes challenging or novel activities to promote learning by developing each student's cognitive, physical, emotional, and social capabilities to assist in the development of "rounded" citizens who can participate as effective members of society (Project Adventure, 1991).

experiential education   Involves the purposeful planning and implementation of direct experiences coupled with the facilitation of reflection and responsibility.

Adventure-Based Learning   An alternate term to describe Adventure Education in the physical education curriculum.

Project Adventure (PA)   A student-centered curriculum that integrates adventure in physical education.

Figure 8.1 presents the five philosophical concepts on which Project Adventure is based: challenge, cooperation, risk, trust, and problem solving. The Adventure Education philosophy uses physical activity as the medium through which students learn how to challenge themselves, cooperate on tasks, take real or perceived physical or emotional risks (making a mistake with the support of others), trust in oneself and others, and solve problems with others' help and guidance. The learning "process" of the physical experience is at the center of Adventure Education. The specific wording of these definitions comes from Devonshire and Cedarwood Elementary Schools in Ohio, two schools that have infused PA as a curriculum focus throughout their school programs (Dyson, 1994, 1995; Dyson & O'Sullivan, 1998).

Students can set personal goals for challenge, cooperation, trust, risk, and problem solving in different content areas. In physical education, this could mean challenging oneself to climb to the top of a climbing wall, or walk a mile every second day; in language arts, it could be taking a risk such as standing up in front of the class with a personal journal, trusting the group not to ridicule you; and in math, this could mean problem solving, or cooperating when working in a group. Students can be encouraged to self-assess their experiences, such as those found based on the PA concepts. Students can be asked to respond to the questions in Figure 8.2 in their adventure journal.

Adventure-Based Learning can be exciting; it can engage and it can challenge. It has the ability to be a student-centered approach to learning in physical education where students can negotiate tasks and, with guided reflection, derive meaning from their own experiences rather than have meaning imposed by others in positions of authority.

---

1. *Challenge:* The students will view physical and mental challenges as an adventure to be attempted and experienced.

2. *Cooperation:* Through group work and a supportive group atmosphere, the students will learn to work together cooperatively. Students will communicate thoughts, feelings, and behaviors effectively.

3. *Risk:* Students will make a commitment to take a risk, display their talents and limitations, and realize that they will be accepted in a positive, safe environment.

4. *Trust:* Through attempting activities that involve some physical or emotional risks, students will trust their physical or emotional safety to others.

5. *Problem Solving:* Group members will effectively communicate, cooperate, and compromise with each other through trial-and-error participation in a graduated series of problem-solving activities.

FIGURE 8.1 Project Adventure philosophical concepts.
Source: Dyson, B. P. (1994). *A case study of two alternative elementary physical education programs.* Unpublished doctoral dissertation, Ohio State University.

How did you solve problems today?

_____

How did you take risks today?

_____

How did you cooperate with each other today?

_____

How did you challenge each other today?

_____

How did you trust each other today?

FIGURE 8.2 Student reflection prompts on Project Adventure concepts.

Essential Practices of Adventure Education

We present three essential practices that distinguish Adventure Education from other physical education instructional models: the experiential learning cycle, the full value contract, and challenge by choice.

We want to emphasize that Adventure Education should be thought of as a process, and not an outcome-based curriculum model. As Dewey (1938) contended, experience is learning—learning occurs through, and in, experience. The experience or set of activities that the students participate in is the medium through which students learn to cooperate, problem solve, risk, trust, and challenge themselves. Thus teachers' planning of experiences should focus more on how the particular activities enable participation and appropriate student decision making, and provide meaningful feedback through direct (and manageable) consequences rather than on the "novelty" or "thrill" value of the activity. As McKenzie (2000) has reported, it is the qualities of the activities (challenging and engaging) that are responsible for the success of Adventure Education programs rather than the activities themselves. Thus, there is no "magic" activity—rather the process and the relationships (student–student and student–teacher) contribute to program effectiveness.

Experiential Learning Cycle

Several experiential learning cycles have been popularized in the literature; however, Kolb's (1984) four-stage model of the experiential learning cycle is perhaps the most widely used in Adventure Education.

The four stages are:

- The experience
- Observations and reflections
- Abstract concepts and generalizations
- Applying or transferring

THE EXPERIENCE. Once the learning objectives have been identified (for example, solving a problem, challenging oneself, taking a physical or emotional risk, team-building, or cooperation), many types of activities can be selected. For example, as stated in our adventure scenario at the beginning of the chapter, students could be scaling a climbing wall, involved in a trust fall from a height of 5 feet (Table 8.1 and Table 8.3), in a circle playing Pattern Ball (Table 8.2), or building a human pyramid.

OBSERVATIONS AND REFLECTIONS. "What happened?" Reflection provides an opportunity to integrate the new experience with past experiences. In the reflection stage, the intention is that the student will reflect back on and examine what occurred during the experience. This group discussion might give rise to differing student interpretations and descriptions of events. For example, students would be encouraged to describe their experiences of climbing the gymnasium wall. The teacher might ask probing questions like: Did you find this activity challenging? Why was this so? Did you take a physical or emotional risk? Why was this risky? Who took responsibility for which jobs? Did you feel safe? What made you feel safe? An alternative approach might encourage the students to express their thinking through art, movement/drama, or a short musical piece utilizing a contemporary genre. The teacher should be careful to avoid the trap of asking predictable questions, which are met with an equally predictable response (e.g., "What did you learn?" "Trust").

ABSTRACT CONCEPTS AND GENERALIZATIONS. "So what?" "What does this mean for me and for the group?" At the third stage, students share what they felt, observed, and thought during the experience, and make connections between ideas and experience. The intention at this point is to assist students to take abstract concepts related to what happened at different stages during the activity, and form some generalized statements about what made the activity successful, or less than successful. For example, students are asked to reflect on what climbing the gymnasium wall meant to them. The teacher might ask probing questions like: So, how were you feeling about the level of risk in the group? What did you learn about trusting others in this experience? Does the experience here apply to other situations in your life? Do you think your group was sharing responsibility for everyone's safety? Again care needs to be taken to avoid formulaic question–answer responses.

APPLYING OR TRANSFERRING. "Now what?" "How can I apply what I have learned?" For the experience to be considered worthwhile, students should be given opportunities to apply what they have learned in one situation to other

---

TABLE 8.1

Adventure Education Block Plan

Learning activity 1: Ice-breaker or acquaintance activities Task 1: Introduction Task 2: Daily journal guidelines Task 3: Ice-breakers 1) Meet and greet, 2) Human treasure hunt, 3)Pattern ball Task 4: Group processing Assessment: Pattern ball rubric and daily journal after class Standards: 1, 2, 5, & 6	Learning activity 5: Decision making/problem solving Task 1: Traffic jam Task 2: Group processing Assessment: Daily journal after class Standards: 5 & 6
Learning activity 2: De-inhibitizers activities Task 1: Speed ball Task 2: Group processing Assessment: Adventure log and daily journal after class Standards: 1, 3, 5, & 6	Learning activity 6: Responsibility (individual and social) Task 1: Spider's web Task 2: Group processing Assessment: PSRM assessment and daily journal after class Standards: 1, 2, 5, & 6
Learning activity 3: Communication activities Task 1: Swamp crossing Task 2: Group processing Assessment: Daily journal after class Standards: 1, 2, 5, & 6	Learning activity 7: Trust/empathy activities Task 1: Set personal goals; choose groups Task 2: Trust lean Task 3: Three-person pendulum Task 4: Quick group processing Task 5: Trust fall Task 6: Debrief/group processing Assessment: Three-person pendulum checklist Standards: 1, 2, 5, & 6
Learning activity 4: Decision making/problem solving Task 1: Tarp flip Task 2: Group processing Assessment: Daily journal after class Standards: 5 & 6	Learning activity 8: Application activities Task 1: Create your own initiative Task 2: Take time to write in your daily journal Assessment: Group processing and share journal Standards: 1, 2, 5, & 6

Note: Planning and flexibility are in constant tension in Adventure Education; you need to provide sufficient structure to ensure a supportive learning environment, but you also need to be able to "think on your feet" as the students make their own choices and discoveries.

---

settings. During this phase, students think of ways to put into practice the general principles that they identified in the previous stage, that is, to transfer experiences to other real-life settings. The application of what has been learned feeds back into the next experience, to continue the cycle of learning. For example, students are now encouraged to think of the messages and lessons from an activity like scaling a climbing wall that might be useful at home. The

TABLE 8.2

Ice-Breaker Activities for Adventure Education

These three activities are in the block plan in Table 8.1 Learning activity 1: Icebreaker or acquaintance activities. These activities can be used at all school levels and are examples of activities that could start your Adventure-Based Learning. The activities focus on emotional and social skills development.

Standards that should be met by students: 5 & 6.

Instructional goals:

1. Students get to know each other's names.
2. Students will express themselves in an appropriate manner.
3. Students will talk to each other.
4. Students will demonstrate positive interdependence—rely on each other to catch the ball.
5. Students will learn to be considerate of others when throwing a ball/object to them.

Task 1: Meet and Greet
Many students do not know each other's names. This task has a dual purpose for all participants to use each other's names and for the teacher to use students' names. So the first task is to meet and greet as many participants as possible in 2 minutes. Students walk around saying, "Hi I'm Sam" and shake hands. A modification could be for each student to find a novel way to greet another (e.g., create a special handshake or method of greeting someone).

Task 2: Human Treasure Hunt
This is an icebreaker activity that asks students to find someone for each of the facts the teacher has typed on a sheet of paper. For example, find someone who: can swim a mile, wears glasses, can play a musical instrument, walks to school, was born in another country, etc. Participants write down the name of a student next to each fact.

Task 3: Pattern Ball
Arrange six to eight students in a circle and tell them the purpose of the activity is to create a pattern while throwing balls or objects in the air to other teammates. Students start with one hand in the air and drop their hand when they have thrown the ball. This ensures that students know who has received a ball or object from another student. The instruction is to create a pattern by repeatedly throwing a ball to the same member of the group and catching a ball from another member. (A simplified example would be Sam throws to Juan, Juan throws to Lily, Lily throws to Marquis, and Marquis throws to Sam.) Specific suggestions to improve success:

- Ask the students to throw crisscross so that you are not throwing to someone beside you.
- The ball or object is always thrown in the same pattern.
- The intent is to start with one ball or one object, then add more.
- Have students use other students' names before throwing.

Objective: Develop a throwing pattern and get as many balls/objects in the air simultaneously as there are people in the group (for example, eight people throw eight balls).

Continued

TABLE 8.2

Ice-Breaker Activities for Adventure Education—Cont'd

Equipment: A variety of balls and objects.

Group Processing: Once the activity has been attempted, the teacher can ask questions to help facilitate the experience for students: What do you need to do to be successful? What does the thrower need to do? What does the catcher need to do? Then the students can try pattern ball again. We have used pattern ball in a variety of groups: 1) with 90 middle school students in one gymnasium in groups of six to eight students; 2) with fourth grade students as a warm-up in their classroom for the school day, with instructions such as "throw the bean bag and ask a multiplication question"; 3) in a high school rugby practice starting with one ball and adding as many as the group can handle.

Task 4: Turning over a New Leaf

Have 8–12 students stand on a tarp ("leaf") stretched out on the ground. Each student should write down a potential problem they could have participating in an adventure activity (e.g., poor listening skills) on a piece of masking tape and place this on the leaf. The task is to turn the tarp over while all students have two feet on the tarp. Students need to avoid touching the toxic ground (poison peanut butter) around them. This task is difficult and requires that students design a creative solution, so it could take them an hour to complete. The intent is that the group will turn over the leaf and in the process metaphorically "turn over a new leaf." Once the leaf is turned over the students are to create a solution to their problem and write it on another piece of masking tape and place that on the turned-over leaf. A solution to poor listening skills could be to always look at the person you are talking to. The intent would be for the students to openly reflect after the experience using the experiential learning cycle: What happened? So what? Now what? A positive outcome for the students would be to transfer this experience and practice good listening skills in other situations.

---

teacher might ask probing questions like: How does climbing the wall relate to your life at home or on the playground? Now that we know that we need to encourage each other to be successful, what are we going to do about it? What new personal goals can you set for yourself? Are you able to challenge yourself to take more risks after this experience? What kinds of risks are you going to take now? The four stages of the experiential learning cycle are interrelated and there should be interaction among them (Luckner & Nadler, 1997).

These four stages are the basis for the Adventure Education practice of **group processing (debriefing)** of learning activities. Group processing of an experience is considered desirable within the experiential framework because it

group processing (debriefing)   The practice of encouraging students to reflect on and communicate with other group members about their feelings, observations, and experiences during an activity.

TABLE 8.3

Lesson Plan for Learning Activity Four: Progressive Trust Activities

Here is a practical example that has been taught at the middle school level (Standards that will be met by students are 1, 2, 5, and 6). The activities are designed to enhance students' psychomotor, cognitive, and affective capabilities by using adventure activities. The intent of this lesson is to provide you with an example and framework for using adventure activities in your physical education program. The three-person pendulum checklist (Figure 8.5) can also be used as a form of peer assessment. Adapt this to suit your context, your instructional goals, and your students' needs.

Instructional goals:

- Students will trust others when falling from a height in a state of physical and emotional anxiety.
- Students will understand mechanical principles that relate to the trust fall: mechanical principles of balance, force absorption, and Newton's first law (a body will maintain a state of rest or constant velocity unless acted on by an external force that changes the state).
- Students will demonstrate spotting and falling techniques and cues.
- Students will demonstrate positive interdependence to enable themselves and other students to fall and catch with appropriate technique and safety.

Trust Fall Spotter Learning Cues
1. Ready (alert) position
2. One foot in front of the other (wide base of support)
3. Knees bent
4. Arms and hands slightly bent ready to catch

Faller Learning Cues
1. Arms crossed across the chest
2. Feet planted solidly on ground or platform
3. Body stiff as a board

Commands for Trust Fall
1. "Ready position"
2. "Ready to catch"
3. "Ready"
4. "Falling"
5. "Fall on"

Task 1: Cognitive and Affective Task
Students decide on pair groupings. Students set one physical and one social/emotional goal for the lesson. (For example, students will work together to achieve the task.)

Task 2: Initial Task—Trust Lean
Task: In groups of two, students lean/fall to a partner who catches them. Students should have three to five attempts at each position, and then rotate. *The teacher should demonstrate with students before they practice spotting and falling.*

Continued

TABLE 8.3

Lesson Plan for Learning Activity Four: Progressive Trust Activities—Cont'd

Goals:

- For students to freely lean or fall to a spotter.
- Gain confidence in leaning/falling in a small controlled manner.
- All students must lean/fall, and all must practice the cues for spotting and leaning/falling.
- Lean/fall spotter will use the cues listed above for the leaner. Faller or leaner will use the cues listed above for the faller.

Commands: The faller should use 1) "ready to catch" and 2) "falling/leaning." The spotter should use 1) "ready" and 2) "fall/lean on."

Task 3: Three-Person Pendulum

Task: In groups of three, all students choose new groups. This fall involves two spotters so that the faller can fall backwards or forward. The teacher should demonstrate again with two spotters and a faller. There should be three to five attempts at each position and then the students should rotate.

Goals:

- Students need to use all of the learning cues for both the faller and the spotter as well as the commands.
- Three-person pendulum spotter will use the same cues listed above for the trust fall spotter. Faller or leaner will use the same cues listed above for the faller or leaner.

Commands: The commands are the same as those listed above as the commands for the trust fall.

Task 4: Quick Group Processing

The teacher poses questions and leads students in a discussion.

- Q: What do you need to do when spotting?
- Q: What do you need to do when falling?
- Q: Did you trust your spotter? Why? Why not?
- Q: Do you feel physically and emotionally safe? Why? Why not?

Note: Students and teachers should use a specific assessment of the students' ability to spot and fall before they move onto the trust fall from a height of 4 or 5 feet (outlined in Standard 1).

Task 5: Trust Fall

Task: To fall from a height of 4 or 5 feet into the arms of catchers. In student groups of nine with a minimum of eight catchers and one faller. This is a challenge by choice activity. There may be students who choose not to fall—they should be encouraged to fall, but not made to feel that they have to fall. This fall involves eight spotters so the faller can feel safe. The teacher should demonstrate with a student who has a "good stiff body" when falling.

Briefing: Teachers should tell students that this trust fall puts into practice many of the skills learned with the trust leaning/falling activities. It is very important that everyone follows directions and pays attention throughout the activity.

Continued

TABLE 8.3

Lesson Plan for Learning Activity Four: Progressive Trust Activities—Cont'd

Caveat: A teacher must be able to trust students, and, therefore, it is highly recommended that several adventure activities have occurred before the fall is attempted. Safety is a primary concern. All students should feel physically and emotionally safe. One attempt, with a stiff body, is success.

Directions: Practice securing your arms across your chest. Climb carefully up to the platform. Stand in a steady position and keep your body in a rigid position throughout the fall. Sitting is not an option, and is unsafe.

Faller or leaner cues are the same as those used before for the faller or leaner. The teacher prompt should be "remember to be stiff and rigid."

After catchers are ready, the faller's heels can move to the edge of the platform. Practice the commands before falling.

Commands: The faller should use 1) "are you ready to catch?" and 2) "falling." The spotter should use 1) "ready to catch" and 2) "fall on."

Directions for spotters/catchers: Stand shoulder-to-shoulder with the person next to you. Arms are outreached and palms are up and at a 90-degree angle; your fingertips should meet the elbows of the person across from you. Remove all jewelry. Create a zipper with your arms—each person should have one arm of another person between their two arms. Do not clasp hands or elbows with anyone. Stand with one foot in front of the other (wide base of support), and knees bent. Tip your head back slightly—feet can fly. Watch the faller at all times. Follow the command initiated by the faller. Be ready to respond: "ready" and "fall on." If you are not ready say, "not ready." When the faller falls, do not reach for him/her, but allow him/her to land in your arms. Once you have caught the faller, gently lower him or her to the ground feet first. Rotate positions so that you are not always standing in the middle where the largest impact occurs.

Spotter cues are the same for the trust fall listed above with the addition of the following: a zipper formation.

Variation: If there is a large class and only one teacher, you can have the entire class form the catching line, and after the faller lands, have the faller passed to the end of the line. This can be a fun levitation exercise for the faller, and it keeps everyone involved. Ideally, two platforms should be set up with alternate falling from different platforms. Or a teacher's assistant/parent can supervise the other falling station.

Task 6: Cognitive and Affective Task

Group processing (this is a debrief of the activities):

• What were your physical and social/emotional goals today—how did they go?
• What are most important mechanical principles for falling and catching?
• How can these principles apply to other sports?
• What were the physical and emotional risks of the activity?
• What are some of the risks that you take in life?

Assessment: Answer the above questions in your adventure journal.

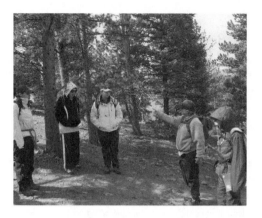

helps the student to sort and order information in a meaningful way, and therefore aids in learning that is lasting and transferable. The goal of processing the activities is for students to focus on relevant issues arising from the experience, increase self-change, verbally reflect and analyze the experience, and promote the integration of what is learned in students' lives in other situations (Gass, 1993). Care should be taken to avoid overprocessing activities. Teachers need to be careful to give students opportunities to move beyond the simple question–answer format so students can do more than merely respond to teacher-directed questioning (Brown, 2004). There is an obvious tension in physical education related to time allocation of activity time versus reflective time. We suggest that you start with short, 5-minute briefings/debriefings at the beginning and end of your lessons, using several key points. For example, before a lesson ask: "What actions might you take today to make the lesson a success?" "What's one positive thing you will do for a classmate today?" After a lesson, ask the previous questions: "What happened? So what? Now what?" For the purist adventure educator, this is too "quick and dirty," so you must be careful not to diminish the value of the open dialogue or reflection with students (Sugarman, Doherty, Garvey, & Gass, 2000). To be successful, students must consider and share ideas, accept each other, communicate in positive ways, and value social interaction and self-expression. The role of reflection and analysis following an activity, or as more recently recommended, preceding an activity through **frontloading,** is a central feature of the experiential learning process in Adventure Education (Dyson & Pine, 1996; Sugarman et al., 2000). Frontloading emphasizes key learning points prior to the activity, rather than reviewing learning after the activity has been completed (Priest & Gass, 1997).

frontloading   Emphasizes the key learning points of an activity before beginning, rather than simply reviewing after the activity is completed.

Full Value Contract

Another essential practice in Adventure Education is the **full value contract** (**FVC**). FVC is the social contract that members of a group agree to adhere to with regard to personal behavior and their interactions with other group members. This contract can be made in writing or simply stated verbally. Ideally, groups will be able to spend time to develop a contract of behavior that supports their goals (both individual and collective). However, in short-duration programs or with groups who lack the maturity to articulate their goals clearly, some assistance may be required from the teacher. The FVC provides a framework for students to refer to in their dealings with others. It also encourages students to set and work toward individual and group goals, to agree to follow certain safety guidelines, to agree to give and receive feedback (both positive and constructive), and to agree to work toward changing behavior when it is appropriate (Schoel, Prouty, & Radcliffe, 1988). An example for a class contract can be as simple as: "I agree to follow the safety rules agreed to by the class, and I will set one personal goal for myself before each activity." The key part of any social contract is the need for students to feel a sense of ownership. So, it is important that the FVC is seen as a "living" and meaningful expression of the group's desires. Students can reword the contract to suit their specific physical or emotional goals for the lesson. By using an FVC, student behavior or actions (individual or collective) that become either emotionally or physically risky can be stopped and questioned with reference to the guidelines established. So, it is not up to the facilitator to "discipline" students; rather the facilitator uses the contract that has been collectively created to draw attention to behavior that is not appropriate. Students, as group members, take ownership to ensure that they act appropriately. An example of an FVC used at a nonprofit organization Bridges Inc. in Memphis, Tennessee, appears in Figure 8.3.

Challenge by Choice

The third essential practice for achieving an Adventure Education learning environment is the concept of **challenge by choice**. This teaching practice can be

full value contract (FVC)   A social contract that members of a group adhere to in regards to their behavior/actions both as individuals and in their interactions with others. The essence of FVC is built on three commitments: 1) to work together as a group toward individual and group goals; 2) to adhere to safety and behavior guidelines; and 3) to give and receive feedback to help change behavior (Schoel, Prouty, and Radcliffe, 1988).

challenge by choice   Students have options to choose from, depending upon their comfort levels related to physical and emotional safety, and students are unable to opt out of participation before beginning the activities.

This FVC was created and agreed upon by seventh grade students:

Play Hard
Play Fair
Be Safe
Have Fun

Each of these phrases has a physical sign that goes along with it:
Play hard: Hands up showing your strong muscles.
Play fair: Bow at waist with palms pressed together, like a Japanese greeting.
Be safe: Use the baseball umpire's "safe" signal.
Have fun: Hands raised like a winner and give a shout.

You can use this FVC in your gymnasium or classroom.

FIGURE 8.3 An example of the full value contract from BRIDGES, Inc., Memphis, Tennessee.
Source: Dyson, B., Seed, A., Pickering, M., Stover, B., Snowden, H., & Willis, L. (2007). *BRIDGES to quality: report on 1st year implementation of 7th grade immersion and leadership development.* Memphis, TN: Center for Research and Educational Policy.

interpreted as a challenge with choices, that is, students can choose from an array of different activities with different levels of physical and emotional challenge and associated risk. The teacher develops a unit or sequence of activities that allows students to make different choices of levels of participation in different lessons. Challenge by choice does not offer the student an avenue to automatically opt out of participation before the activity begins; it is an invitation to participate in an appropriate challenge of the student's choice. The intent is to offer students the opportunity to try a potentially difficult challenge in a caring and supportive environment; the opportunity to "back off" if anxiety or self-doubt becomes too great, knowing that an opportunity for a future attempt will be available; an opportunity to attempt a challenge, recognizing that the attempt/process is more important than the outcome; and the opportunity to respect other individuals' ideas and choices. For example, a student might attempt a trust lean or three-person pendulum fall, described in lesson one (Table 8.3), but may decide not to complete a trust fall from a height of 5 feet. However, the student would be expected to be a spotter for other students in the trust fall, and otherwise participate fully in the activity. It is important that students understand they will not be forced into situations that are dangerous or humiliating. At the same time, students must recognize that if they are not confronted with a challenge, then they may not experience the thrill of achieving the seemingly impossible task, and the associated joy of stretching their potential.

Because Adventure Education is frequently thought of and referred to as a philosophy rather than merely a set of activities, the experienced Adventure Education teacher can teach any content using an adventure approach. With sport, dance, or aerobic activities, the teacher can focus on cooperation, trust, risk, problem solving, and challenge. The teacher can use these principles as instructional objectives for the class. The experiential cycle can be used as the framework for the lesson, using the pattern of activity followed by in-depth group processing. The students and teachers can develop a full value contract that would say, for example, "We will abide by the rules, and we will set a physical and/or emotional goal for the lesson." In addition, challenge by choice or invitation can be built into the cooperative (not competitive) game. The potential of many adventure activities is limited only by one's own creativity and imagination.

How Adventure Education Can Address the National Standards

How does your program meet the required national standards for physical education? By aligning the adventure program with the national standards, we can provide written documentation regarding the goals of the program, and identify how the program aligns with the total education of the student. (Refer to the Standards Table in the Introduction.) The standards that your students achieve will depend on the specific emphasis in your program and the instructional goals in your lessons and unit plans. Standards 5 and 6 are the major foci of Adventure Education because of the emphasis on personal and social behavior, respect, challenge, self-expression, and social interaction. That is why many physical educators use Adventure Education activities to build students' emotional and social skills.

Standard 5: Exhibits responsible personal and social behavior that respects self and others in physical activity settings.

The intent of Standard 5 is for students to develop self-initiated behaviors to promote personal and group success. "Key to this standard is developing re-

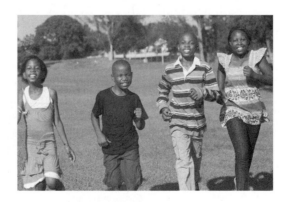

spect for individual similarities and differences through interaction among students in physical activity" (National Association for Sport and Physical Education [NASPE], 2004, p. 14). Adventure Education, by its very nature, is based on the tenets of cooperation, risk, trust, problem solving, and challenge. The icebreaker activities in Learning Activity 1 (Table 8.1) start the students off by working on cooperation and problem-solving activities and provide challenges for students.

An example of a necessary personal and social behavior is trust. However, before students can be expected to trust each other they must participate in a number of activities. The block plan (Table 8.1) shows a sequence of activities that leads to Learning Activity 7, a sequence of trust activities. In addition, progressive activities that facilitate students' building trust are outlined in the lesson plan (Table 8.3). First, trust is briefed as the focus for the tasks for the day. It is connected to Standard 5 with a discussion referring to the need for trust in relationships, and how trust can foster respect for self and others. The trust lean is the first physical task. Students are in groups of two. Students practice falling to a partner who catches them. Correct spotting technique is demonstrated and practiced with students. The next progression is a three-person pendulum, with two students spotting one student leaning or falling. Again, correct spotting technique is practiced and emphasized with students. This is followed by a short debrief or group processing session where students are encouraged to talk about their feelings concerning their physical and emotional safety (which is another aspect of Standard 5) related to trust falls. Issues relating to what it means to trust another person can be explored in detail. Alternatively, where difficulties are observed by the facilitator, questions can be posed in a non-threatening manner to guide appropriate behavior. Before the trust fall is attempted, students should be assessed on their spotting and falling skills (Figure 8.4). The final physical task is the trust fall. Students fall from a height of 4 or 5 feet into the arms of student catchers. Correct spotting technique is demonstrated and practiced with students so that students trust each other. In the final task, the students and the teacher/facilitator discuss the physical, emotional, and social challenges of the trust activities, and determine the level of trust developed by the group. To be successful in any Adventure Education activity, students must interact positively with each other, which is the intent of Standard 5.

T-charts (Figure 8.5) can be used to enhance social skills when using adventures in the classroom or gymnasium (Henton, 1996). **T-charts**, originally

T-charts   Help students visualize appropriate behavior by asking students to write down what a certain behavior "sounds like" and what a certain behavior "looks like."

Name: _____

Name of Peer Assessor: _____

Competent: Good technique, safe
Needs Work: Poor technique, unsafe

	Competent	Needs Work
Spotting cues		
Ready (alert) position		
One foot in front		
Knees bent		
Hands ready to catch		
Falling cues		
Arms crossed across the chest		
Feet planted solidly on ground		
Body stiff as a board		

Group processing

1) What happened?

2) So what?

3) Now what?

FIGURE 8.4 Three-person pendulum checklist.

Looks like	Sounds like
a thumbs up	"good job"
a high five	"nice pass"
a pat on the shoulder	"big extension"

FIGURE 8.5 T-chart for encouraging positive reinforcement.

developed in cooperative learning by Johnson and Johnson (1998), ask students to write down what a certain behavior "sounds like," and what a certain behavior "looks like." For example, to encourage students to provide positive comments and reinforcement to others, students might write: It sounds like "good job," "nice pass," and "big extension," and it might look like a thumbs up, a high five, or a pat on the shoulder. The T-chart can be included on the student task sheet, or used as a starting point for group processing of a problem or issue. The content of the T-chart in Figure 8.5 comes from a fourth grade class at Madbury Elementary in New Hampshire (Dyson & Rubin, 2003).

Standard 6: Values physical activity for health, enjoyment, challenge, self-expression, and/or social interaction.

Standard 6 is achieved when students develop an awareness of the intrinsic and extrinsic values and benefits of participating in adventure activities. The adventure activities should, and often do, provide students with enjoyment, challenge, self-expression, and social interaction, and in so doing, directly pertain to Standard 6. "These benefits develop self-confidence and promote a positive self-image, thereby enticing people to continue participation in activity throughout the life span" (NASPE, 2004, p. 14). Learning activities from the Adventure Education block plan (Table 8.1) present a number of tasks that when taught effectively can be used to meet the requirements for Standard 6. Examples would include the human treasure hunt, pattern ball, and the trust fall.

Two possible ways to assess Standard 6 are the use of group processing and an assignment asking students to create their own initiative or event task (NASPE, 1995). Group processing involves using debriefing as a means of informal assessment (What happened? So what? Now what?). A journal entry of the debriefing could provide a more formal assessment (Figure 8.6). To create their own activity or task, students can work in cooperative groups to develop their own initiative, and then teach their initiative to other classmates. This challenge allows students to be self-expressive and take ownership for their own creation. In a group, students would identify the skills and tactics that they need to accomplish their initiative. In addition, students would make a list of necessary equipment. The skills and tactics need to be chosen carefully to ensure that all students in the group are able to perform parts of the initiative. The culminating event and potentially motivating project should be completed in a 40- to 50-minute period. "When students take ownership for their learning, they tend to become more engaged and interested" (Lund & Kirk, 2002, p. 209).

Standard 2: Demonstrates understanding of movement concepts, principles, strategies, and tactics as they apply to the learning and performance of physical activities.

Front-loading questions before the experience:

1. What is your physical goal for this experience?

2. What is your social goal for this experience?

Reflective questions after the experience:

1. What was your physical goal for this experience? Did you reach your goal? Why or why not?

2. What was your social goal for this experience? Did you reach your goal? Why or why not?

FIGURE 8.6 Prompts to enhance group processing.

Although Standards 5 and 6 are fore-grounded in Adventure Education, Standard 2 can also be achieved in an adventure curriculum. The national standards were developed as a guide for teachers, and we believe that Standard 2 should be connected to each of the other standards and become an integrated part of every physical education lesson.

Adventure Education provides a wide variety of activities to achieve the cognitive focus in Standard 2, such as mechanical principles of balance, force absorption, and Newton's first law (a body will maintain a state of rest or constant velocity unless acted on by an external force that changes the state). These principles can be the focus of a trust fall progression (Table 8.3), when a teacher's instructional goals require an understanding of absorption of force and stability. During Adventure Education activities, an emphasis can be placed on "applying and generalizing these concepts to real-life physical activity situations" (NASPE, 2004, p. 12). Since adventure activities require cognitive understanding of mechanical principles, with challenging and problem-solving tasks, these activities can help students achieve Standard 2. Developing an understanding of physical education skills and tactics is a minor focus for Adventure Education. Nonetheless, in an integrated middle school physical education and science unit, integrating and applying principles of force and recognizing the need for a solid base of support for spotting could provide a cognitive focus for the trust fall experience. The activities listed in the block plan (Table 8.1) provide examples of tasks that require students to understand the activity and the movement patterns involved in order to be successful at completing the tasks in addition to decision making and problem solving, which require higher order thinking (e.g., Table 8.2, Turning over a new leaf). Students can demonstrate knowledge related to Standard 2 through the use of an adventure journal, in which students are encouraged to write about their Adventure Education experience.

To be able to write an adventure journal or role-play a scenario, students must first have an understanding of the purpose of the adventure activity. Although the focus of the journal is typically related to students' feelings and social interactions (Standard 5), it can also have a technical focus on climbing skills and tactics, or falling and catching techniques related to mechanics (e.g., trust fall). In the adventure journal, students will write about their Adventure Education experience. Guiding questions to enhance the journal could be: What are some of the skills and tactics for climbing or belaying? In the trust fall, why does the catcher have a low center of gravity and a wide base of support? How do the mechanical principles we have learned apply to other sports? When possible and appropriate, to showcase a student's journal, it should be published in the school newspaper, or used as an artifact in a student's portfolio.

There are several other ways that students could demonstrate knowledge related to Standard 2. A role-play could follow an initiative task where students have completed the challenge to "climb the wall" as a cooperative group. Two students could assume the roles of Edmund Hillary and Tenzing Norgay as they approached the summit of Mount Everest in 1953. Students could describe how they felt as the summit grew closer, and explain the technical skills used to reach the summit. A student reporter could interview classmates about the event. Students could write a technical climbing report for the class and the school newspaper, and/or a local newspaper (adapted from NASPE, 1995,

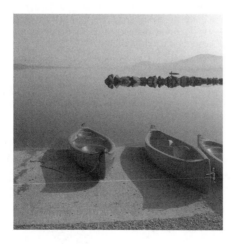

p. 120). These examples relate to Standard 2 when the teacher discusses the skills and strategies of climbing, stability, center of gravity, and how muscles fatigue under stress.

Assessment

Adventure education provides a unique set of challenges for assessment. If, as stated earlier, we perceive adventure activities as the medium through which we learn the affective values and ideas of physical education, then Standard 5 and Standard 6 (NASPE, 2004) should be apparent in our teaching. Our intent, then, is focused on the students and how we can help them gain an understanding of the Adventure Based Learning process and gain a better understanding of themselves. Assessment then becomes part of the teacher's instructional strategy and the teacher uses it to provide feedback to their students and themselves about their students. Any assessment can be a labor-intensive endeavor for the physical education teacher who is teaching 500 or more students per week. To be realistic, you can start small with group processing self-reflection (Figure 8.6) and build from that point. Students talk about their experience in a reflective discussion and then write down their responses in their journals.

Earlier in the chapter we presented two assessments: PA concepts reflection (Figure 8.2) and the three-person pendulum checklist (Figure 8.4). Figure 8.7

Level 4
Calls other group members' names when throwing and catching. Reaches for the ball or object when catching. Consistently performs a leading pass; movement is smooth, and ball or object is easy to catch. Gives accurate and positive feedback to other students. Accepts corrective feedback from others, and attempts to make improvement in throwing and/or catching skill.

Level 3
Often calls other group member's names when throwing and catching. Generally reaches for the ball or object when catching. Frequently performs a leading pass; movement is smooth, and ball or object is generally easy to catch. Gives positive feedback to other students. Accepts corrective feedback from others.

Level 2
Sometimes calls other group members' names when throwing and catching. Infrequently reaches for the ball or object when catching. Infrequently performs a leading pass; movement is rushed, and ball or object is difficult to catch. Does not provide positive feedback to other students. Ignores corrective feedback.

Level 1
Does not call other group members' names when throwing or catching. Does not reach for the ball or object when catching. Does not perform a leading pass; movement is jerky and rushed. Frequently makes negative comments to other students. Is upset when corrected by other group members.

FIGURE 8.7 Pattern ball rubric.

shows the rubric for the pattern ball. An example of another reflection/assessment is used again at The University of Memphis with Physical Education Teacher Education (PETE) majors after a 2-day adventure experience. This student reflection after the Adventure Based Learning involves an integration of Kolb's (1984) experiential learning cycle and Tsangaridou and O'Sullivan's (1994) levels of critical reflection (Figure 8.8). The students are asked to reflect at three levels—description, justification, and critique—and then set appropriate goals. These levels of reflection are matched to Kolb's cycle. We find that this process encourages students to critically reflect on their experience. The instructor carefully reads the student's reflection and provides feedback to each student. This reflection becomes part of the instructional strategy and informs future instruction; that is, it becomes a planning tool to create appropriate goals and to create future activities or tasks, and therefore the reflection or formative assessment becomes an integrated part of the instructional program. The intent is to create a planning, teaching, and reflective cycle (Figure 8.9).

Another excellent way of achieving authentic assessment is by using a portfolio. With Adventure Education units, we recommend a group portfolio so that the work is manageable for students (Melogano, 2000). Portfolios can document students' progress, improvement, and individual performance; help students take responsibility for their own learning; encourage students' self-evaluation and reflection; and motivate both students and teachers. The teacher needs to specify the explicit goals to be met in the portfolio.

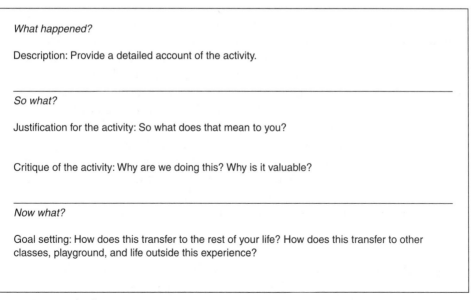

FIGURE 8.8 Crtical reflection in experience.

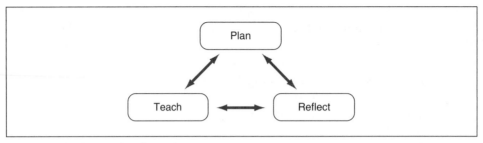

FIGURE 8.9 The plan, teach, reflect cycle.

Examples of entries for a portfolio could be: write a daily log of activities, write specific physical and social/emotional goals, evaluate your effort and experience, or explain how this experience relates to the rest of your life. Students could select artifacts from those described in the previous standards section of this chapter: adventure journal, rubrics, T-charts, and adventure log. In Adventure Based Learning, students can keep track of their physical activities using an adventure log. The idea of a logbook is not exclusive to Adventure Education (it is often used in fitness programs), but it can be used to demonstrate to teachers and parents that students are indeed being physically active. An adventure log requires students to keep a basic record of their perceived effort and ability in Adventure Education. Students are encouraged to develop personal physical activity goals and determine whether their goals are met. This log is submitted to the teacher each week, who should provide specific feedback to students frequently.

If you use the group portfolio, students can become **positively interdependent** on each other to provide their "best work." Students need to carefully select appropriate items for their portfolio based on a sound rationale, that is, a judgment of the quality of their work. Through careful selection, students critique their own and other group members' work, and make decisions about the best way to show how it meets the goals and standards of the unit. The portfolio is an assessment that can represent several of the national standards listed above, because the portfolio consists of the different assessments and assignments carried out in the unit. The portfolio has the potential to demonstrate how much students "know and are able to do," relative to the goals, tasks, and assessments from the unit at hand. The portfolio can be assessed on a three-level rubric of awesome, developing, or needs improvement. The teacher

positively interdependent   Group members depend on each other, as each individual's part is essential to the entire group completing its task.

should identify required entries for students to put in their portfolio and offer the choice for students to add at least one new entry that they believe is valuable.

Why Is Adventure Education Appealing to Youth?

Adventure Education is made up of novel tasks that may be unlike anything students have done in the past. Many activities are designed to be fun. It requires a different set of physical and social skills than a regular physical education class would require. This may allow a student who is not skilled at, for example, basketball to excel or show leadership during a problem-solving initiative. The instruction is not just "drill and kill" like many sport and physical education practices, but rather unpredictable and challenging. Participants feel a sense of accomplishment after completing a task that appeared to be impossible. Students get excited during Adventure Based Learning and encourage each other more vocally than they normally would. The activities promote face-to-face interaction (working in close proximity to each other) rather than individual practice. The tasks are designed to promote positive interdependence, with students relying on each other to complete the task. In addition, the activities should be user-friendly, that is, students can take them out of the class and play them with on their own. Adventure Based Learning promotes character development, personal growth, cooperation, and leadership skills.

Summary

The use of adventure activities or Adventure Based Learning in physical education offers physical educators the opportunity to experiment with an innovative curricular strategy. The use of a holistic student-centered approach that embraces the learner physically, cognitively, emotionally, and socially can help teachers meet national standards (NASPE, 2004). Research suggests that both teachers and students report favorably on the use of Adventure Education (Brown, 2006; Dyson, 1995; Prouty, Panicucci, & Collinson, 2007). Adventure Education experiences provide students with challenges, support, and the oppoturnity to build trust, solve problems, and cooperate. Student-centered pedagogy, which is integral to the Adventure Education approach, enables constructive changes in student relationships, and by focusing on the process of learning, can help improve student enjoyment and help develop a positive learnng environment in physical education. It also enables the teacher to assume a different role from that traditionally occupied by educators; the teacher has the ability to facilitate peer learning situations and cooperative activities rather than being the "expert" who supplies answers.

We would encourage physical education teachers who are interested in developing a program that includes adventure activities to begin slowly, and progressively expand their repertoire of activities as they become more familiar with "letting go," and allowing students to take control of their learning. Often the reluctance to "let go" is a result of a concern that chaos will reign; however, our research suggests that by carefully structuring activities and inducting the students into the process through briefing and debriefing sessions, a smoother transition from teacher-directed to student-directed learning will occur (Dyson, 1994, 1995; Dyson & O'Sullivan, 1998).

This transition will require time and effort with reflection from both students and their teacher. We strongly recommend that you consult with colleagues and your professional association to build a network of like-minded professionals who are seeking to revitalize physical education. The suggestions in this chapter may not transfer immediately to your context—"your world in your gymnasium"—without modification and adaptation, and trial and error. You will need to seek out training, on-going professional development, and local expertise, and you will need to convince other physical educators and administrators that this is a worthwhile curriculum. The outcomes have the potential to achieve the national standards, improve your physical education program, and most importantly, improve the experiences for K–12 students. It is our hope that your students will experience the joy of physical activity, and the value of teamwork and cooperation in a non-competitive environment that will enhance not only their physical development, but also their social relationships with their peers and you, their teacher.

References

Bailey, J. (1999). A world of adventure education. In J. Miles & S. Priest (Eds.), *Adventure programming* (pp. 39–42). State College, PA: Venture.

Brown, M. (2004). "Let's go round the circle." How verbal facilitation can function as a means of direct instruction. *Journal of Experiential Education, 27*(2), 161–175.

Brown, M. (2006). Adventure education in physical education. In D. Kirk, D. MacDonald, & M. Sullivan (Eds.), *Handbook of physical education* (pp. 685–702). London: Sage.

Cosgriff, M. (2000). Walking our talk: adventure based learning and physical education. *Journal of Physical Education New Zealand, 33*(2), 89–98.

Dewey, J. (1938). *Experience and education.* New York: Collier.

Dyson, B., Seed, A., Pickering, M., Stover, B., Snowden, H., & Willis, L. (2007). *BRIDGES to quality: report on 1st year implementation of 7th grade immersion and leadership development.* Memphis, TN: Center for Research and Educational Policy.

Dyson, B., & O'Sullivan, M. (1998). Innovation in two alternative elementary school programs: why it works. *Research Quarterly for Exercise and Sport Science, 69,* 242–253.

Dyson, B., & Pine, S. (1996). Start and end class right. *Strategies, 9,* 5–9.

Dyson, B., & Rubin, A. (2003). How to implement cooperative learning in your elementary physical education program. *Journal of Physical Education, Recreation, and Dance, 74,* 48–55.

Dyson, B. P. (1994). *A case study of two alternative elementary physical education programs.* Unpublished doctoral dissertation, Ohio State University.

Dyson, B. P. (1995). Student voices in an alternative physical education program. *Journal of Teaching in Physical Education, 14,* 394–407.

Gass, M. A. (1993). *Adventure therapy: therapeutic applications of adventure programming in mental health settings.* Boulder, CO: Association for Experiential Education.

Henton, M. (1996). *Adventure in the classroom.* Dubuque, IA: Kendall Hunt.

Johnson, D. W., & Johnson, R. T. (1989). *Cooperation and competition theory and research.* Edina, MN: Interaction Book.

Kolb, D. (1984). *Experiential learning.* Englewood Cliffs, NJ: Prentice-Hall.

Luckner, J. L., & Nadler, R. S. (1997). *Processing the experience: strategies to enhance and generalize learning* (2nd ed.). Dubuque, IA: Kendall Hunt.

Lund, J. L., & Kirk, M. F. (2002). *Performance-based assessment for middle school and high school physical education.* Champaign, IL: Human Kinetics.

McKenzie, M. (2000). How are adventure education program outcomes achieved? A review of the literature. *Australian Journal of Outdoor Education, 5*(1), 19–27.

Melogano, V. J. (2000). *Portfolio assessment for K–12 physical education.* Reston, VA: National Association for Sport and Physical Education.

National Association for Sport and Physical Education. (1995). *Moving into the future: national standards for physical education: a guide to content and assessment.* St. Louis, MO: Mosby.

National Association for Sport and Physical Education. (2004). *Moving into the future: national standards for physical education* (2nd ed.). Reston, VA: National Association of Sport and Physical Education.

Priest, S. (1999). The semantics of adventure programming. In J. Miles & S. Priest (Eds.), *Adventure programming* (pp. 111–114). State College, PA: Venture.

Priest, S., & Gass, M. A. (1997). *Effective leadership in adventure programming.* Champaign, IL: Human Kinetics.

Project Adventure. (1991). *Adventure programming workshop manual.* Dubuque, IA: Kendall Hunt.

Prouty, D., Panicucci, J., & Collinson, R. (Eds.), (2007). *Adventure education: theory and applications.* Champaign, IL: Human Kinetics.

Rohnke, K. (1986). Project Adventure: a widely used generic product. *Journal of Physical Education Recreation and Dance, 57*(6), 68–70.

Schoel, J., Prouty, D., & Radcliffe, P. (1988). *Islands of healing: a guide to adventure based counseling.* Hamilton, MA: Project Adventure.

Sugarman, D., Doherty, K., Garvey, D., & Gass, M. (2000). *Reflective learning: theory and practice.* Dubuque, IA: Kendall Hunt.

Tsangaridou, N., & O'Sullivan, M. (1994). Using pedagogical reflective strategies to enhance reflection among pre-service physical education teachers. *Journal of Teaching in Physical Education, 14,* 13–33.

Additional Resource

Parker, M., & Hellison, D. (2001). Teaching responsibility in physical education: standards, outcomes, and beyond. *Journal of Physical Education Recreation and Dance, 72*(9), 25–27.

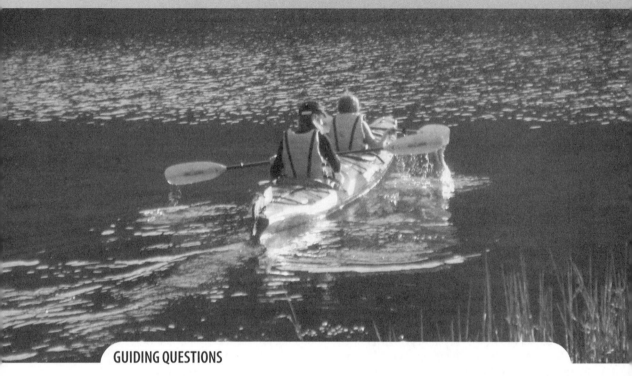

GUIDING QUESTIONS

1 Why the increased interest in outdoor activities?
2 How are "outdoor" activities conceptualized?
3 What activities might an outdoor education curriculum utilze?
4 Are there unique or important instructional considerations that must be taken into account when implementing an outdoor curriculum?
5 How can participation in outdoor activities contribute to student learning?
6 What are some examples of successful outdoor programs?
7 What might a typical outdoor lesson look like?
8 How do instructors select activities for an outdoor curriculum?
9 Which of the NASPE standards does an outdoor curriculum best support?
10 Why might there be an interest in outdoor education for contemporary youth?
11 How might an outdoor education curriculum be incorporated into the physical education curriculum?
12 Describe assessments that are used in an outdoor education curriculum.

Outdoor Education

Jim Stiehl , University of Northern Colorado
Melissa Parker, University of Northern Colorado

Although not as prominent as the more traditional lifetime or "carry-over" activities (e.g., golf, tennis, bowling, and badminton), outdoor activities are increasingly appearing in public school physical education programs. Although the major purpose of this chapter is to discuss outdoor curriculum, before proceeding, it is important to note our conviction that curriculum (what a student experiences) and instruction (how the experiences are presented) are inextricably woven together. Although curriculum is often discussed as detached and distinct from instruction, the reason for doing so is more often one of practicality than reality. Good content that is poorly delivered, and good intentions with weak or inappropriate content, will produce similar unfavorable results. This is especially true in the outdoor realm. Associated with the natural environment are a considerable number of safety issues (Dougherty, 1998) that, in turn, demand unique qualifications and experience on the part of the teacher. Thus, although our emphasis will be on curriculum, we cannot ignore instructional considerations, and will occasionally include them throughout this chapter.

The Appeal of Outdoor Activities

Activities that provide excitement, challenge, and sometimes a degree of risk appeal to many youngsters. Children also favor activities where winning or losing holds little importance compared to cooperating and facing the challenges of a natural environment. Outdoor activities that incorporate these elements include backpacking, rock climbing, orienteering, cross-country skiing and snowshoeing, winter camping, white-water paddling, and mountain biking, among others—all of which may involve making choices with sometimes weighty consequences.

   As illustrated throughout this chapter, it is easy to imagine how outdoor activities can address each of the physical activity content standards as a basis for curriculum development. For example, the vigorous nature of many outdoor activities requires a health-enhancing level of physical fitness. Outdoor activities also call for acquiring and applying new and enjoyable skills, often leading to increased participation in physical activity. Furthermore, successfully navigating and enjoying the outdoors demands a responsible and tolerant attitude. That is, individuals must be concerned about their own welfare as well as the welfare of others and their surroundings, and also must become tolerant of the adverse and uncertain conditions that sometimes accompany forays into the outdoors. Finally, outdoor activities afford opportunities for successfully including a wide range of abilities in a supportive, inclusive environment. Coupled with occasions to practice leadership, to respect and nurture human differences and commonalities, and to make important choices, outdoor activities lend themselves readily to the broad outcomes expected in a quality physical education program. Most physical activity educators (Ziegler, 2003), including us, do not consider outdoor activities as a replacement for more traditional physical education activities. Rather, we view outdoor activities as a means of curriculum extension and enrichment.

Conceptualizing Outdoor Activities

For the purposes of this book, outdoor activities are set apart from adventure activities, yet elements from one may appear in the other. As noted in Chapter 8, adventure programs typically emphasize communication, cooperation, trust, and group problem solving, most often in a developed setting (e.g., gymnasium, playground, challenge ropes course, nearby athletic field). This occurs by means of structured experiences, often simulating obstacles and situations that occur in everyday life. These structured experiences are presented in ways that allow students to deal with them in a manner that is enjoyable, creative, and productive. In an effort to gain new insights that can be applied to future problems and situations, students reflect upon and interpret these structured experiences. The responsibility of the teacher is to facilitate individual and group achievements, and to ensure that the entire process occurs in a physically and emotionally safe environment.

A similarity between adventure and outdoor activities is their focus on personal and group development. Indeed, concepts that are promoted in adventure activities (e.g., teamwork, trust) often precede students' visits to the outdoors. One important difference, however, is that outdoor activities occur in natural settings, with little to no control imposed on the environment, and where hazards may sometimes be beyond the participants' control. Though discussed in more detail later in this chapter, such hazards might include adverse weather (e.g., lightning), wildlife, insect bites, contaminated drinking water, and uneven or wet terrain. Therefore, teachers and students must understand possible hazards in the natural environment, and they must exercise appropriate judgment in attempting to minimize such hazards.

Also, taking students into an outdoor setting affords plentiful opportunities to inspire students to alter their outlook on the environment. For example, students in outdoor activities must be especially mindful of minimizing their impact on fragile habitats. How often when walking on a trail have we seen undesirable evidence of human behavior (e.g., litter, trail erosion, soap scum in water)? These and other patterns of behavior that ignore our impact on the environment may result in rapid deterioration of the "natural" character of an area, the quality of its natural resources, and its capacity to support recreational use. Teachers can help students acquire an appreciation of and concern for the natural environment, while also heightening their sensitivity to the impact of their actions on others.

Several other features of outdoor education distinguish it from other curricula. For example, in contrast to adventure education, outdoor education places greater emphasis on skill development. Whereas adventure education emphasizes symbolic activities such as challenge ropes courses and new games, outdoor education focuses more on explicit knowledge and skills that are pertinent to a specific outdoor activity (e.g., hiking, caving, canoeing, or snowboarding). Another feature of outdoor education, which differentiates it from most other curricula in physical education, is its instructional approach. Based on the century-old belief of John Dewey, that all genuine education comes through experience, much of the learning that occurs in an outdoor setting is experiential, with activity (the "do" aspect of learning) supporting more formal instruction. Yet another distinctive feature of outdoor education is its affective component.

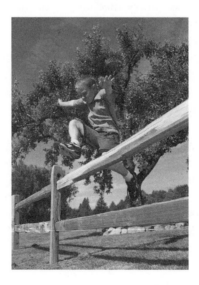

Natural settings often provide a valuable backdrop for identifying and resolving real-life problems (e.g., talking behind someone's back, failing to respect classmates, avoiding work, having an excuse for everything, and blaming others), and for acquiring knowledge and skills with which to enjoy a lifetime of creative, physically active living, through wholesome outdoor pursuits.

Instructional Considerations

Some outdoor activities can be physically and mentally challenging, occurring in an environment where weather, terrain, and group makeup can demand careful planning, communication, and teamwork. Teachers and students alike must be safe, competent, and responsible participants in the outdoor setting. Flawed judgment, poor planning, inadequate technical and medical skills, or misuse of equipment can quickly and easily jeopardize a venture into the outdoors. For teachers who regard outdoor activities as a possibility for their curriculum, several considerations may be worth contemplating. Depending on the extent and setting of an outdoor experience, additional training and expertise beyond that normally expected of physical activity educators may be necessary. At one end of the continuum, for example, urban orienteering (conducted in areas near a school) may involve acquiring some new knowledge and a few new skills (e.g., map reading, compass use, selecting proper clothing). Challenges and risks afforded by the natural environment and the use of outdoor skills are relatively unimportant for this activity. At the other end of the continuum, however, extended trips into remote wilderness areas offer an environment with a high degree of challenge and risk. This setting will demand more self-reliance and may call for a basic knowledge of backcountry medicine, land navigation, weather, hazard evaluation, trip planning, and other skills and experiences essential to creating safe and enjoyable learning opportunities for students. As one progresses along the continuum from an urban to a wilderness experience and setting, a teacher's need for technical skills, knowledge, and judgment increases. In an outdoor setting, the environment becomes more variable and less structured, programmatic time frames become more extensive (moving from hourly classes to days, perhaps weeks of continuous impact). The demands for general and specific instructional supervision become greater in an outdoor classroom, because students are less likely to possess skills and knowledge necessary for effective coping.

An outdoor curriculum can demand "extensive training and experience beyond that expected of" most physical activity educators (Stiehl, 2000, p. 68), and we would be remiss not to mention them here. Although few colleges and universities prepare students with all of the skills essential for developing an outdoor curriculum component, the following skills and competencies should be taken into account to assure an appropriate consistency between instructor qualifications and program goals:

1. *Technical* (e.g., orienteering; paddling; knot tying; rope handling and **belaying**; edging with skis and snowshoes; crossing swift water, snow, and rockfall)
2. *Outdoor living* (e.g., packing a pack, selecting a campsite, operating and caring for a stove, cooking and baking, finding routes, sanitation)
3. *Safety* (e.g., inspecting and repairing equipment, water treatment, weather interpretation, wilderness first aid, risk management and emergency procedures, animal habitat precautions)
4. *Environmental* (e.g., minimum-impact travel, trail etiquette, **leave-no-trace** camping)
5. *Organizational* (e.g., planning expeditions and routes, securing permits, arranging transportation and equipment, planning rations and nutrition)
6. *Instructional* (e.g., developing teaching progressions; analyzing tasks, matching teaching strategies to learner characteristics; selecting instructional sites and methods, such as demonstrations, lectures, discussions, skits, visual aids, journals; recognizing and effectively using opportunities for "teachable moments")
7. *Facilitation* (e.g., fostering productive group dynamics, resolving conflicts, cultivating personal trust and group cooperation, providing opportunities for individual and group decision making, conducting effective briefing and debriefing sessions)
8. *Leadership* (e.g., sharing decisions; establishing a clear decision-making process; employing a democratic, delegating, or autocratic style as appropriate to a situation or to the developmental phase of the group; providing opportunities for using good judgment)
9. *Environmental ethics* (e.g., developing and applying appropriate standards of outdoor ethics, to include a vision for a clean, sustainable environment, as well as extending the notion of community to include the land and other life forms; relying less on our ability to spend and consume than on our ability to do and save)

In addition to these competencies, a teacher's knowledge of the following can greatly enhance students' outdoor experiences: ecology and habitats, individual species, mammal tracking, constellations and useful astronomy, meteorology, and geology. Thus, if our job is to enthuse our students about the many ways they can move and be healthy, then appropriate outdoor experiences coupled with sufficient teacher expertise can assist in achieving that aim.

belaying   Using the system for—or the act of—managing the ropes to protect the climber.

leave-no-trace   A widely accepted code of outdoor ethics and minimum-impact principles designed to shape a sustainable future for wildlands.

Two additional considerations for some outdoor activities are cost and student–teacher ratio. Orienteering, for example, is a relatively inexpensive activity that can be supervised by a single teacher. Kayaking, on the other hand, can entail considerable cost, as well as the need for a much smaller student–teacher ratio in order to conform to principles of safety.

Contributions to Student Learning

As mentioned earlier, a wide spectrum of ages and abilities can be served through outdoor activities. These activities range from less to more challenging (orienteering versus white-water paddling), involve negligible to substantial risk (hiking versus rock climbing), and require nominal to extensive teacher knowledge and expertise. Bearing in mind this range of options, outdoor activities lend themselves to addressing all of the standards in a standards-based curriculum. Of course, not unlike more traditional activities and models, certain standards may be more primary in some outdoor activities than in others. For instance, acquiring competency in movement skills and patterns (Standard 1) may be better addressed through paddling than through hiking. However, hiking may emphasize responsible personal and social behavior (Standard 5) more than paddling does. Both paddling and hiking, however, give emphasis to participating regularly in physical activity (Standard 3), respecting self and others, and recognizing the joy and challenge of healthy movement experiences, especially with others (Standard 6). Hence, the selection of activities in an outdoor education curriculum has a direct impact on the degree to which the content standards are met.

Thus, for some outdoor activities, some standards may play a major role, whereas for other outdoor activities, those same standards may play a minor role. Regardless, the primary or secondary role of each standard is intentional; that is, skill acquisition is a deliberate intention in paddling or rock climbing. However, some standards may relate to an activity, yet are not deliberate. Rather, they might better be regarded as a by-product of participation. For instance, in both paddling and rock climbing, achieving a health-enhancing level of fitness (Standard 4) might not be intentional, yet frequently occurs as a consequence of taking part in those activities.

The benefits of including outdoor activities in a standards-based curriculum are presented in the following table, according to the six content standards for physical education. At the outset, however, we must express three of our opinions about standards. First, standards will not soon vanish, nor should they. When used properly, standards are not mandates; rather, they serve as signposts that can furnish guidance and direction to one's program. Second, standards are not designed to stand apart from one another as discrete, unrelated entities. Their strength lies in their integration, just as a child's strength lies in her or his wholeness—the emotional, cognitive, social, spiritual, and physical dimensions of the self. Third, the emphasis placed on any given standard is related directly to the particular outdoor activity being implemented.

For the purposes of addressing each standard, we have selected two activities: orienteering, one of the most exciting and satisfying outdoor activities; and cycling in its various forms (e.g., touring, mountain biking). Orienteering is a relatively inexpensive sport requiring very little specialist equipment. Also, the school setting is an ideal starting point for introducing and developing orienteering techniques, then moving outdoors where most places have suitable orienteering terrain (e.g., school grounds, city parks). For those unfamiliar with orienteering, it is an activity that can be pursued at many levels, and appeals to both genders and all ages. Although a thriving and rapidly growing international sport, orienteering can begin with 2nd graders learning basic ideas indoors (a great opportunity to collaborate with the classroom teacher!), and then using newly acquired skills to navigate easy terrain such as school grounds and local parks before moving onto more challenging and unfamiliar fields, woods, and hills. The principle of orienteering is simple and familiar to anyone who has ever been on a scavenger hunt: using a map (and, sometimes, a compass), students seek out a series of checkpoints (sites marked with small flags), which must be visited in a specified order and in the shortest time possible. Blending navigational and physical skills, orienteering has great potential for inclusion in the physical education curriculum. (See References and Additional Resources for additional sources regarding orienteering and other outdoor activities.)

Another fun and popular outdoor activity is cycling. Cycling means different things to different people: from staying fit, to enjoying the feeling of a shared experience; from sightseeing around town and touring in the outdoors, to competitive road-cycling events, to riding off-pavement on all kinds of terrain. A good form of aerobic exercise, almost anyone can become a proficient rider with practice while, at the same time, building cardiorespiratory and muscular fitness. Although the price of bicycles varies widely, many youngsters already own one, and good used models can often be acquired at yard sales, through newspaper ads, from donations, and at police auctions. Consequently, cycling activities can be included in most school programs, especially when accompanied by a bicycle safety program designed to safeguard youngsters' everyday use of bicycles.

Therefore, using orienteering and cycling as our examples, the following comments provide some insight into how outdoor activities might address each of the standards.

Standard 1: Demonstrates competency in motor skills and movement patterns needed to perform a variety of physical activities. For orienteering, this standard would have a minor role. An important feature of orienteering is the mixture of mental and physical challenge, rather than acquiring or practicing new motor skills. For cycling, on the other hand, this standard would have a major role because proper technique is very important for safe, efficient cycling. And although there are different types of cycling (e.g., touring, mountain biking), some skills are basic to most types (e.g., ankling technique, proper pedaling cadence, changing gears).

Standard 2: Demonstrates understanding of movement concepts, principles, strategies, and tactics as they apply to the learning and performance of physical activities. Interpreted as cognitive understanding, this standard plays a major role in orienteering. Orienteering teaches students to have clear goals and to work hard and constructively to achieve those goals—concepts necessary for acquiring any motor skill, and applying it to varied situations. For cycling, this standard may play a more secondary role, although learning about bicycle maintenance and repairs, designing obstacle courses, planning routes, and learning local cycling rules or regulations can add a cognitive dimension to this activity. By including information about bicycle safety, history, rules, and maintenance, children can show large gains in their knowledge of bicycles.

Standard 3: Participates regularly in physical activity. This standard plays a minor role in orienteering and cycling, yet can be an important by-product for both. For example, in orienteering students often train harder and run further when they have the added interest of map reading. Also, because orienteering principles and skills can be used in a host of other outdoor activities (e.g., hiking, mountain biking, paddling), combining map reading and terrain following with these other outdoor activities can enhance the enjoyment and appeal of both. In other words, by combining orienteering with cycling and other outdoor activities, students may be more prone to participate.

For those so inclined, competitive orienteering emphasizes speed, fitness, and the thinking skills needed to use maps and compasses to find their way to the series of small flags—and to do it before anyone else. However, orienteering need not be grueling. Individuals can take part at their own pace, can choose appropriately simple treks, and then progress from there. Moreover, orienteering can become a family adventure. Many adults have become involved in orienteering because their children participate in the activity. Thus, unlike many other activities where a parent's role is limited to spectating or officiating, in orienteering the whole family can actively participate. In most European countries, orienteering is very much a family affair with entire families participating on different courses at the same event, or even participating as a family on a single course.

Standard 4: Achieves and maintains a health-enhancing level of physical fitness. Again, this standard is more a by-product of orienteering than an intention. Though it can easily be modified to accommodate the needs and aptitudes of different children, orienteering involves the ability to move fast, preferably at a run, requiring speed, agility, and strength. Healthy outcomes include cardiovascular endurance and general fitness. It is important to note that, although students may be physically exerting themselves, they still need to keep their minds clear in order to read the map, thus adding to the incentive to work on speed and fitness together with navigational skills.

As with orienteering, cycling often is not intended as a conditioning activity—but it can be. Cycling is one of the best forms of aerobic exercise. Anyone who cycles regularly can achieve health and fitness benefits. Many people of all ages choose cycling as their primary means for maintaining and improving physical conditioning.

Standard 5: Exhibits responsible personal and social behavior that respects self and others in physical activity settings. Depending on the instructional format, this can be either 1) a primary standard using orienteering or cycling as the means to promote responsibility, 2) a secondary intention, or 3) simply a by-product. (See Chapter 6: Personal and Social Responsibility for a more complete discussion of responsibility.) Students often start orienteering in small groups where they must learn to work with one another. The excitement of exploration, problem solving, challenge, and exercise is heightened when youngsters learn and participate together. Students must not only work together when interpreting information (usually from map to ground), making decisions, and progressively mastering new techniques, but also must be mindful that success and enjoyment will depend on respecting one another's interests and aptitudes.

Also, though not included in the physical education standards, students must exhibit responsibility toward their surroundings. As with all outdoor activities, the natural setting holds much more significance than for most other physical activities. Orienteering encourages an awareness and appreciation of the environment. It also requires an obligation to observe and apply appropriate standards of outdoor environmental ethics. Students should be able to discuss the consequences of individual and group behavior on the quality of the outdoor experience.

Cycling can support this standard in a similar fashion. Students must accept responsibility for themselves (e.g., watch for traffic and, if necessary, take evasive action; be prepared for weather conditions; avoid riding in the rain; stay in control; brake with back brakes first, then apply the front), for others (when in doubt, give anyone and anything the right of way; do not give others a ride, and do not pull them on skateboards, in-line skates, etc.), and the surroundings (work to keep bike paths open by being courteous and thoughtful; when zooming through forests, parks, and open spaces, respect both flora and fauna—that is, practice low-impact cycling; respect trail and road closures). Again, these may be aspects of a program that deliberately attempts to promote responsible behavior, or may purely be consequences of sensible cycling.

Standard 6: Values physical activity for health, enjoyment, challenge, self-expression, and/or social interaction. In orienteering, finding sites and objects through successful map reading leaves students with an authentic sense of achievement, fostering self-reliance and confidence. Students are responsible for making their own decisions about 1) which course to pursue (when arranged according to difficulty level); 2) which route to follow (trying to go straight up a hill may take longer than finding a path around it); 3) pace (minimal to high physical exertion); 4) competition (against others? with self? not at all?); and 5) whether to follow routes alone or with others, often as a team. These choices allow students to participate at their own level in the same event. Since cycling offers a wide range of options to a wide range of abilities and interests, cycling presents similar opportunities for health, enjoyment, challenge, and social interaction. It is important that students leave a cycling unit with a positive attitude, and a desire to take up more cycling activities.

Although not included in the physical education standards, orienteering, cycling, and other outdoor activities provide a wonderful opportunity for collaboration between the physical activity educator and the classroom teacher. In other words, outdoor activities lend themselves to working across the curriculum. To continue with our example of orienteering, cross-curricular links include: geography (using maps and interpreting contours, fieldwork techniques, cartography/designing maps, physical and environmental geography); mathematics (measuring and locating shapes in space, estimating distance, determining direction and scale, handling data); history (famous explorers, origin of the compass and its use in early navigation); language arts (creative writing, technical terms and symbols); and expressive arts (making your own orienteering equipment, making three-dimensional models from contour maps). Other outdoor activities offer similar possibilities. Linking the physical education curriculum to other school subject matter presents a wealth of opportunity (e.g., partnerships and projects with other teachers, community events and support, connections with families, increased perceptions by students of the relevance of school subjects) that is beyond the intent or scope of this chapter—yet may be worth considering.

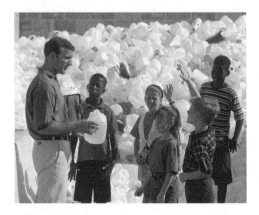

The previous remarks about decisions and choices warrant additional commentary and are particularly relevant and suitable to outdoor activities. Choice influences participation; choice accommodates individual differences; choice affects an individual's "buy in" or ownership. It is also indispensable for creating the conditions underlying any successful, positive learning climate (i.e., kids feel safe, capable, successful, motivated, and connected to others). Irrespective of whichever purposes, models, or standards are being emphasized, the success of any program will be shaped by its climate. A climate in which appropriate choices are presented in a thoughtful, deliberate manner is vital to ensuring that every student can gain the most from that program. Hence, we emphasize the holistic nature of outdoor programs, as well as the need to offer proper choices in those programs. With willingness and a little ingenuity, most outdoor programs and activities can be adjusted to provide choices that fit the needs and abilities of all students.

Examples of Programs

Some programs rely heavily on an outdoor component, often situated in a school that organizes much of its curriculum around outdoor pursuits. Examples include programs that incorporate the Wilderness Education Association (WEA) curriculum (Drury, Bonney, Berman, & Wagstaff, 2005), or Outward Bound's expeditionary learning principles (Voyageur Outward Bound School, 1993). In the latter, for example, true learning is considered an expedition into the unknown. Thus, students' education is organized into purposeful expeditions of inquiry, discovery, and action, designed to promote self-discovery and knowledge. Diversity and inclusion, the natural world, and responsibility for learning are some of the principles used in designing expeditionary learning curriculums.

A more far-reaching effort exists in England and Wales, where outdoor and "adventurous" activities are included in their National Curriculum for physical education. Organized on the basis of four key stages (Stage 1: ages 5–7; Stage 2: ages 7–11; Stage 3: ages 11–14; Stage 4: ages 14–16), physical education is included in all four stages, with outdoor activities included in Stages 2, 3, and 4. For each subject and each key stage, "programmes of study" set out what students should be taught (scope and sequence of activities), and "attainment targets" set out the expected standards of students' performance. To illustrate, in Stage 2, students are taught six areas of activity: games, gymnastic activities, dance, athletic activities, swimming, and outdoor and adventurous activities. Expectations in the latter include: 1) to perform outdoor and adventurous activities (e.g., orienteering exercises), in one or more different environments (e.g., playground, school grounds, parks, woodland, seashore); 2) challenges of a physical and problem-solving nature (e.g., negotiating obstacle courses), using suitable equipment while working individually and with others; and 3) the skills necessary for the activities undertaken.

Comprehensive outdoor programs such as those just mentioned are less common than are programs in which selected outdoor activities have been incorporated into a school's physical education curriculum. Though perhaps not yet as common as other models in this book, aspects of the outdoor model are being included in physical education programs at an increasing rate in both cities and rural areas. Seldom do we see a physical education activity program composed solely of backpacking, canoeing, cross-country skiing, cycling, kayaking, mountaineering, orienteering, rock climbing, sailing, scuba diving, snowboarding, snowshoeing, spelunking (caving), or winter backpacking and camping. Nor do we see programs that include all of these. Rather, after investigating which outdoor activities might best suit their needs, teachers proceed to add these to their existing physical education program. In addition to our earlier comments, and relative to the six standards, a teacher might ask:

1. What expectations are reasonable and achievable in my program, and would this outdoor activity promote those expectations?
2. What resources (e.g., budget, equipment and materials, transportation, insurance, space and site locations) do I need to begin and to maintain this activity?
3. What new skills may be needed, and how do I develop them (or gain the assistance of others who have those skills)?
4. What evaluative criteria and strategies will I need to fulfill my assessment obligations, as well as to provide me with direction?

The following is an example of one successful outdoor program where the physical education teacher examined and answered the above questions. The program, developed and implemented by Leo Malloy in Gunnison, Colorado, is but one aspect of his high school physical education program, which also includes adventure activities, as well as more traditional games and sports. For his outdoor component, activities selected by Leo are relevant to his location and skills, and they correspond to his budget allotment and needs. His offerings are also consistent with all six physical education content standards, due in part to his choice of activities, and his ability to present these activities successfully. Furthermore, he has developed an assessment component for each activity. Most students elect to take individual outdoor activities (e.g., kayaking, hiking), while some apply for a 16-week "block" designed for students in Grades 11 and 12. In the block situation, the class meets for 2½ hours, 4 times per week, plus 5 outings (two or three 1-day outings, one or two 2- to 4-day outings, and a culminating 10-day to 14-day outing). We will present an abbreviated version of

Leo's overall outdoor curriculum as follows: 1) general program content, 2) overall and content-specific goals, 3) sample assessment strategies.

I. **GENERAL PROGRAM CONTENT.** Content is separated into "hard" skills, "soft" skills, and interdisciplinary skills. Hard skills consist of the technical competencies necessary to perform the various activities (Standard 1). Examples in rock climbing include knots, rope care and management, belaying, **anchors,** proper use of equipment, and various techniques of climbing to include **rappelling.** Soft skills deal predominantly with the affective and cognitive domains to include communication, supporting others, cooperation, expressing feelings appropriately, respecting differences and commonalities, and trusting oneself and others (Standard 5). Interdisciplinary skills (Standard 2) for rock climbing may include life science (e.g., trees as anchors, animal ecology and habitats), physical science (e.g., boulders and rock formations, meteorology and lightning), and mathematics and physics (e.g., vector forces in various anchor configurations, pulley systems, forces generated by a fall). Leo identifies hard, soft, and interdisciplinary skills for each of his outdoor activities (which are admittedly broad in scope): rafting, river kayaking, rock climbing, mountain biking, map and compass, CPR and basic wilderness first aid, leave-no-trace minimum impact skills, winter skiing and camping, and backpacking.

II. **OVERALL AND CONTENT-SPECIFIC GOALS.** As a result of participating in some or all of Leo's outdoor offerings, students are expected to:

1. Understand the benefits of engaging in regularly scheduled physical activity.
2. Know where to seek further instruction and training in pursuing outdoor activities.
3. Demonstrate sound judgment and decision-making skills.
4. Identify personal strengths and limitations as they relate to outdoor activities.
5. Demonstrate competency in outdoor movement skills.
6. Recognize the benefits of interdisciplinary exploration and skills as taught in an outdoor environment.
7. Demonstrate responsible, considerate social behavior in all outdoor activities and settings.

In addition, Leo has developed specific expectations for each of the aforementioned content areas. For instance, upon completing the rock climbing sessions, students will possess the following skills and knowledge related to

anchors   Main protection points in a roped safety system.
rappelling   Descending a rope while controlling speed with friction.

movement and safety (and for those unversed in the terms used in rock climbing, you may notice that students also learn a new "language"):

1. Movement
    a) stretching and conditioning (for both training and for preparing to climb; Standard 3)
    b) **bouldering**: balance, friction, and weight transfer; traversing and downclimbing; resting to avoid fatigue
    c) intermediate movement: footwork (e.g., **edging, smearing**) and using hands (e.g., **positive pull**; **side pull**; **palming, push-off,** and **mantle**; types of grips)
    d) advanced movement: **opposition** (e.g., **stem, lieback, undercling**); **overhang** (e.g., **heel hook, deadpointing**); **crack climbing** (e.g., finger and fist **jam; off-width**)

bouldering   Climbing without ropes close to the ground.
edging   Pressing the edge and side of your climbing shoe into a hold and then standing on it.
smearing   Pressing as much of a shoe's rubber sole as possible into a rock to create friction.
positive pull   A handhold on which one can pull downward.
side pull   A hold that faces away from the climber (requires pulling sideways with fingers).
palming   Placing the entire hand over a rounded hold.
push-off   Pushing upward off of a hold.
mantle   Boosting into a hold or onto a ledge by locking the elbows and bringing the feet up.
opposition   Pushing in two different directions.
stem   Pressing both feet against opposite holds.
lieback   A move that involves pulling with the hands while pushing with the feet.
undercling   Grabbing the underside of a hold with the palm up.
overhang   A rock that is farther away at the top than at the base (requires tilting the head back to see the top of the wall or climb).
heel hook   Hanging by the heel.
deadpointing   When a climber makes a move for a handhold that appears out of reach, but he/she is able to complete the move with his/her feet still on holds (fully extended with four points of contact).
crack climbing   Involves jamming or torquing your limbs or body inside of a rock's natural crack systems.
jam   A cramming action that requires expanding a part of the body into a crack.
off-width   A crack that one can get his/her arms or legs into but not his/her entire body.

2. Safety
  a) spotting another climber (protecting a climber during short falls)
  b) selecting and appropriately using a harness and other equipment (e.g., helmet, climbing shoes)
  c) properly tying knots and using them correctly (e.g., tying in, connecting ropes or webbing)
  d) belaying (managing a climber's rope and catching falls), and communicating correctly using agreed-upon signals
  e) recognizing the elements of a correctly set up **top-rope** anchor system
  f) displaying and judging whether others in a top-rope climbing situation are adhering to requisite safety principles and procedures

Prior to introducing any specific outdoor activities, students begin with a class that emphasizes "ground rules," which are agreed-upon ways of behaving and interacting in any outdoor activity. Ground rules serve as the foundation and structure for how a group will function together during outdoor sessions. Students develop rules related to how they want to work together (e.g., cooperation, caring, abiding by rules for safety) and some of the negative things they want to avoid (i.e., unsupportive behaviors and language that will get in the way of a positive group experience such as put-downs, not listening, everyone talking at once, prejudice and stereotypes, and not involving everyone). Since the students generate these, and they are not just "another bunch of rules devised and enforced by the teacher," Leo finds that groups are much more likely to compliment one another on positive behaviors and attitudes, and to call each other on negative ones. These rules also provide a means to review a class session, to keep students focused on how they are treating each other, and to assist students in feeling safe, knowing what the expectations and consequences are for various behaviors. Finally, ground rules are flexible and may change over the course of a semester. But, whenever changes are made, there must be consensus among the class members for the changes to take place.

Next, students develop personal goals about what they want to accomplish in the program, followed by action plans for achieving those goals (Standard 6). The goals may relate to acquiring specific skills (e.g., paddling strokes) or adjusting behaviors or attitudes (e.g., managing fear of swift moving water). Additional suggestions for goals occur through adventure activities whereby Leo provides opportunities to explore and develop skills necessary for group unity. These skills typically include leading and following, listening, cooperating, expressing feelings appropriately, respecting one another's differences, trust,

top-rope   A belay that is above the climber (where the rope is attached to an anchor above the climber).

proper planning, importance of one's role in class or in a group, accepting ownership of behaviors and feelings (versus blaming others), and avoiding value judgments, among others.

Continuing with an example from Leo's program, Figure 9.1 is part of an outdoor climbing unit that focuses on snow rather than rock. Climbing on snow requires some different skills than does climbing on rock. Although footwork is again the foundation, distinct footwear (stiff-soled leather or plastic boots, sometimes with **crampons**, versus lightweight soft shoes with sticky rubber soles) and use of an ice ax are important differences between snow and rock climbing.

A Sample Lesson

Up to this point, we have given some indication of the wide assortment of activities comprising outdoor education. Some may be less practical in the typical physical education setting. For example, they may require special talents and experience from the teacher, or are relatively costly, necessitating ample resources and adequate outdoor facilities and sites. Others, such as orienteering, are more affordable and require fewer special teacher competencies and qualifications, while still addressing the physical education standards. Because orienteering allows for full participation by everyone at their own level of performance, and because it can be linked to other outdoor activities (e.g., ski orienteering, mountain bike orienteering, canoe orienteering, mountain and trail orienteering), we will close with a description of a session designed for middle-school youngsters. This session builds on students' skills in reading and using a map and compass. Assume that students are familiar with basic map symbols, can orient a map, and can take **bearings** of particular points of interest. This session is designed to enhance those skills, to involve students in decision making and problem solving, and to support them in sharing their learning in pairs and small groups.

Preparation: draw up a map of the area, including key features and locations of checkpoints (numbered tin can stakes).

Materials: one compass and map per team; numbered tin can stakes.

Description of activity: By participating in this team challenge, students practice skills they have already learned, and now must work with others in an event that involves speed and accuracy. Furthermore, each team must design a plan that takes into account each team member's fitness and navigational ability.

---

crampons   Steel-pointed attachments for mountain boots to help travel on steep snow and ice.

bearings   The direction one wants to travel.

Ice ax:

a) Parts: spike (plunge into softer snow, or use as balance point) connected by a ferrule to the shaft where, at the other end, there is the head of the ax consisting of a pick (for gaining purchase in hard snow and ice), an adze (for chopping), and a carabiner hole (for attaching a leash).

b) Carrying and using safely and effectively: how to carry when not in use; situations when leash offers advantage.

Techniques of snow climbing:

a) Principles: climb with feet (edging with boots), using ax for balance.

b) Self-arrest (to stop a slip or fall) sliding on belly: point toes and pick of ax into snow; feet shoulder width apart; bottom high in air (forces upper body weight onto ax head); securely hold ax in self-arrest position and pull spike high out of snow with other hand near ferrule.

c) Self-arrest sliding on back: roll toward ax head (ensures pick will hit snow first), and then continue as when sliding on belly.

d) Self-arrest sliding on back with head pointing downhill: plant pick near your hip; allow your hips and legs to rotate away; pull yourself into position as you slow, and then continue as when sliding on belly.

e) Techniques for ascending snow: walking, duckfoot, traversing, front-pointing.

    i. Walking. Feet flat on snow surface; ice ax held like a cane with one hand in self-arrest position. As slope steepens, carve steps by kicking with boot edge.

    ii. Duckfoot. Splay feet out and gain purchase on snow with inside edges of boots; use ice ax same as in walking, but if you feel insecure, plunge shaft into snow with each step (server as handhold in case of a slip); in steeper terrain, place both hands on ax's head.

    iii. Traversing. Another form of edging, keep ax in uphill hand; don't lean on ax, causing feet to slide out from under you if you slip. Each step gains same amount of elevation. Downhill foot must cross up and over uphill foot to kick a step, which is made by carving out an edge with the toe and then sliding the heel into place as the kick ends. Soles must be kept perpendicular to the fall line of the snow. After a kick, keep boot still for an instant before standing on the step (allows step to solidify). When uphill foot is in high step position, you are most balanced, and should move your ax. When downhill foot is crossed over the other and in the high step position, balance is more tenuous and you should not move your ax. Move ax with every other step, always from a balanced position.

    iv. Front-pointing. Used when slope is quite steep and traversing is difficult or insecure; kick toes of boots into snow, holding ax with both hands. To conserve energy (front-pointing is easy to learn, but tiring), combine this technique with duckfooting (i.e., one foot front-pointing, other duckfooting). Mix techniques as the terrain changes or as specific muscles tire.

f) Techniques for descending snow: (continuing with the preceding format, topics here include plunge step and glissades).

The above skills, especially self-arrest techniques, are demonstrated and practiced on moderately angled snow slopes that run out to a flat snow surface below (no rocks, tree stumps, or gullies). If students fall or cannot stop themselves, they will slide out to the flats and slow to a stop.

FIGURE 9.1 Skills developed during an ice climbing unit.

Points are awarded for the number of checkpoints located (e.g., some worth 50 points, others worth 200 points depending on their distance and difficulty) in a specified time (e.g., 50 minutes). The objective is for teams to achieve the highest score within a time limit, with points deducted for late return (e.g., two points deducted for every second beyond 50 minutes), for incorrect identification of checkpoints, or for incorrect answers to orienteering questions placed at each checkpoint. Questions at checkpoints may involve using a compass (e.g., What is located about 100 feet away on a 175-degree bearing? From where you are standing, what is the bearing to the water tower?), or may check students' understanding of orienteering principles (e.g., What are **contour lines**? What is a bearing? Draw the map symbol for a church).

Variations of this activity include:

1. Several questions at checkpoints, each varying in difficulty and worth different amount of points.
2. At some checkpoints, rather than answer a question, students can opt to copy and follow written bearings to another checkpoint; this option is worth more points, but presents a new challenge because it may disrupt the team's original plan.
3. Ensure wheelchair accessibility to most, if not all, checkpoints; "bonus" questions worth additional points are available only to groups in which at least one member is using a wheelchair (regardless of whether that person has a disability) or has a disability (e.g., visually impaired; blind-folded; breathing through a straw, thereby simulating asthma).
4. Extended or reduced time; difficulty of terrain; maps for some groups more detailed than for others; at each checkpoint, one player rolls a die to determine what exercise to perform (e.g., 1 = jumping jacks; 2 = push-ups; 6 = your choice), with a second roll determining the number of repetitions (e.g., 1 = five repetitions; 2 = 10 repetitions; 6 = your choice).

Assessing Student Progress

At the heart of standards-based education lies the principle that children learn better when they know what is expected of them. A primary goal for standards-based programs, therefore, is to set forth clear expectations for students' knowledge and skills (i.e., the six physical education standards), and benchmarks (points of reference) for measuring student progress toward achieving

contour lines   Lines on a map that connect points of equal elevation; each line indicates a constant elevation as it follows the shape of the landscape.

those content standards. Standards provide many ways for students to show their abilities, and strategies vary widely for showing student progress toward meeting standards. In outdoor education, as presented here, the student learning is predominantly centered around learning the psychomotor skills involved in outdoor activities, and the cognitive knowledge associated with the use of those skills. Assessment provides a mechanism for giving feedback to the students regarding their learning, as well as communicating how well learning goals have been achieved to the participants and others. Two sets of assessment examples are included here.

The Outdoor Education curriculum is replete with a multitude of psychomotor skills that must be mastered in order to participate safely and effectively in the activity. For example, in rock climbing, students must be able to belay correctly; in cross-country skiing they must be able to use a diagonal stride; and in canoeing they must be able to use a variety of strokes to maneuver the boat. Figure 9.2 represents an observational checklist that can be used to assess canoe strokes (such as **draw strokes, pry strokes,** and **J-strokes**) and the proper use of the stroke.

As with any content, the situation in which the canoeing assessment occurs is quite important. In the initial stages of learning, it would be important to simply ascertain if students were able to demonstrate the strokes correctly; therefore, the assessment might well be in calm, flat water. As students progress, it is not only the mechanics of the stroke that are important, but also the proper use of the stroke (such as knowing if students can properly **sweep**). In this situation, you may want to set up an obstacle course as included in Table 9.1, and assess paddling strokes in a more realistic situation. At this point, the scoring key could also be amended to include the correct use of the stroke to complete the task. Finally, Table 9.2 provides a more holistic canoe assessment that could be used on an extended trip.

Figure 9.2 provides an alternative assessment example for a hiking trip. Although hiking and walking are both psychomotor skills, the large majority of information needed for hiking is cognitive or affective. This assessment focuses on those aspects, not the psychomotor ones. Depending upon the group, the task can be completed with friends or on a class trip.

draw strokes   Stroke to move a canoe laterally.
pry strokes   Deep, powerful strokes used in whitewater to move the canoe away from the side of the paddler (also termed pryaways).
J-strokes   Forward-steering strokes that end with an outward hook.
sweep   Used for a major turn of the bow or for a complete pivot originating from the stern.

Student Name	Forward	Reverse	Draw	Pry	J-Stroke
Tim					
Christina					
Julie					
Gerald					

Key: ⊕ = Consistently performs stroke correctly using all cues
    + = Performs stroke correctly the majority of the time; at times has to think about cues
    − = Performs stroke incorrectly the majority of the time

FIGURE 9.2 Canoe stroke observation checklist.

Outdoor education is a curriculum arena which has long relied on its attractiveness and appeal to overshadow the need to document learning. In today's educational world, that is not acceptable. We, with everyone else, must be able to provide students with relevant feedback regarding their learning, and simultaneously be able to describe to others what students have learned.

TABLE 9.1

Paddling Obstacle Course

This is an open, flatwater tandem canoe assessment. Anchored buoys are placed in the shape of a square, each side at least 6 boat lengths long. The instructor anchors in the center of the square. Paddlers begin in corner one and do the following:
—Port turn circle around buoy 2 and continue to buoy 3.
—Starboard circle around buoy 3.
—Paddle backward to buoy 4.
—Stern to buoy, port pivot turn around buoy 4.
—Paddle in to the instructor's boat and perpendicular dock.
—Leave dock and paddle to buoy 1; bow to buoy starboard pivot turn until bow returns to buoy 1.

Note: Paddlers must not change paddling sides during the assessment.

Source: Adapted for canoeing from Steffen, J., & Grosse, S. (2003). *Assessment in outdoor adventure physical education.* Reston, VA: NASPE.

TABLE 9.2

Canoe Trip Scoring—Outdoor Education Practicum

5: We'll Take You Anywhere . . . if, you are able to maneuver a canoe efficiently through the proper choice and effective use of the forward, backward, pry, draw, "J," and sweep strokes while paddling on the trip. You can control the canoe seemingly effortlessly without having to think about what you are doing. Your strokes appear automatic. You don't have to switch paddling sides unless tired. It is clear that you control the canoe, rather than the canoe controlling you.

4: You'll Get There . . . if, you are able to paddle a canoe properly while on the trip using the forward, backward, pry, draw, "J," and sweep strokes. Yet, the strokes and the maneuvering of the canoe might not be as efficient or effective as possible, e.g., paddler persists in the execution of strokes, yet at the same time the canoe may zigzag. Essentially, timing is a little off.

3: The Rudder . . . if, on the trip, you demonstrate the correct motion of the forward, backward, pry, and draw, but are unable or unwilling to move beyond continual ruddering as the means of steering. When not ruddering, the canoe forward motion is erratic through ineffective steering strokes or extreme over-correction. The canoe zigzags well beyond a straight line.

2: The Lilly Dipper . . . if, when on the trip, you use only forward and backward strokes, and/or paddle only in the bow or stern. It seems you are passively going through the motions; the paddle is at least a 90° angle to the water. There is little power and little effort. You may be able to control the direction of the canoe, but when applying effective power, control is off.

1: Get Out of My Boat . . . if, when on the trip, you use only forward and backward strokes poorly (incorrectly), and/or only paddle in the bow or stern. You may switch sides constantly to control the direction of the canoe, and/or paddle on the same side as your partner. Speed is the only way to make a turn.

Source: Developed and adapted from Parker, M., Young, A, & Ramsey, T. (2008). *Outdoor education staff manual.* Cortland, NY: Department of Recreation and Leisure Studies, State University of New York at Cortland.

Just yesterday we were asked twice what students learn on a two-week canoe/hike/climbing trip to the Colorado Canyonlands. And so our responses included: safety and judgement, expedition behavior, leadership skills, travel skills, camping skills, environmental awareness, physical conditioning, and technical skills. We needed, and need to be able, to answer that question honestly and accurately. Appropriate assessments will allow us to do so.

Task and Directions
As we finish the hiking aspect of the class, your task is to document that you have gained the necessary knowledge to safely hike with friends. To do this, you will have the opportunity to develop a hiking portfolio while on a day hike. The following hiking aspects need to be included in your portfolio.

Portfolio Format and Contents
Format. Typed, except for any hand-written reflections or sketches, and in the order presented below.

Contents
1. Goal(s)
2. Hike itinerary to include:
    a) Leader and partner(s) names
    b) Date
    c) Map (with hiking route highlighted)
    d) Starting and anticipated ending times
    e) Emergency contacts (leader/partner friends; your cell phone number, if appropriate) and name(s) of everyone who has copy of hike itinerary (including instructor)
    f) Brief (single-page) reflection about the experience.
3. Photos of the following:
    a) Your essentials (with labels)
    b) You and trailhead sign (and relevant regulations/cautions, if any)
    c) You at bridge that crosses Big Thompson River (approx. 1.5 miles from start)
    d) You at Fern Falls (another 1.2 miles beyond the bridge)
    e) You at Fern Lake (another 1.1 miles beyond the falls)
    f) Two photos of anything interesting or unusual (e.g., arch rocks about a mile from the start, hanging garden at the falls, scat/droppings, trash, critters, tracks)
    g) Two photos of anything of your choice (e.g., cloud formations, wet huddled hikers, ghastly blister, celebrity hiker spotted along the way)

Hike

Location: Rocky Mountain National Park (RMNP)
Activity: Day hike
Travel time: From Greeley, 1:30 hrs. (approx. 55 miles)
Starting point: Fern Lake Trailhead
Ending point: Fern Lake Trailhead

Directions: Travel west on Hwy 34 to Estes Park, turning southwest on Hwy 36 to Park Headquarters (7840'). Proceed through Beaver Meadows Entrance ($15 per car fee). Follow signs to Club Lake trail, but go one (1) mile beyond to Fern Lake Trailhead (8155'). Park in designated lot.

    Hike 2.5 miles to Fern Falls (645' elevation gain), proceeding to hike another 1.3 miles to Fern Lake (730' additional elevation gain).
    Difficulty = *moderate* (*easy* = 0'–1,000' elevation gain or 0–3 miles 1-way distance; *moderate* = 1,000'–2,500' gain or 3–6 miles 1-way distance; *difficult* = more than 2,500' gain or more than 6 miles 1-way distance)

Total hike time: Approximately 6 hours

Hazards/   Dangers related to automobile travel. While hiking, possibility of high
obstacles: altitude illnesses (e.g., increased chance of dehydration, hypothermia, severe sunburn, mountain sickness); giardiasis; animal/insect bites; route finding; loose rocks; mountain weather (e.g., thunderstorms, lightning, early snowstorms); streams, lakes, and waterfalls; human error.

Emergency   RMNP Headquarters: 970-586-1399
contacts: UNC Campus Police: 970-351-2245
    Estes Park Police: 970-586-4000
    Note: 911 is operational in this area.

FIGURE 9.3 Hiking portfolio assessment.

Summary

Including outdoor activities in any physical education program can be immensely rewarding for the many youngsters who enjoy excitement, challenge, and sometimes a degree of risk (both real and perceived). The challenges of nature demand special skills and knowledge, individual responsibilities, and social interactions that may not occur in more traditional physical activity settings. Although many outdoor activities demand certain instructor competencies that exceed the skills and experience expected of most physical educators, some outdoor activities require neither extensive training nor undue funds, equipment, or organization. Moreover, each of the six physical education standards can be incorporated as either a primary or secondary standard, or as a by-product of participating in outdoor activities.

References

Dougherty, N. J., IV. (Ed.). (1998). *Outdoor recreation safety*. Champaign, IL: Human Kinetics.

Drury, J., Bonney, B., Berman, D., & Wagstaff, M. (2005). *The backcountry classroom* (2nd ed.). Merrillville, IN: ICS Books.

Parker, M., Young, A, & Ramsey, T. (2008). *Outdoor education staff manual*. Cortland, NY: Department of Recreation and Leisure Studies, State University of New York at Cortland.

Steffen, J., & Grosse, S. (2003*). Assessment in outdoor adventure physical education*. Reston, VA: NASPE.

Stiehl, J. (2000). Outdoor and adventure programs. In D. Hellison, N. Cutforth, J. Kallusky, T. Martinek, M. Parker, & J. Stiehl (Eds.), *Youth development and physical activity: linking universities and communities* (pp. 67–85). Champaign, IL: Human Kinetics.

Voyageur Outward Bound School. (1993). *Manual for expeditionary learning*. Minneapolis, MN: VOBS.

Ziegler, E. F. (2003). Names should reflect what we do! *Chronicle of Physical Education in Higher Education, 14*(3), 3–4.

Additional Resources

Bates, T., McLaughlin, T., Ewert, A., & Gilbertson, K. (2005). *Outdoor education: methods and strategies*. Champaign, IL: Human Kinetics.

Bunting, C. (2005). *Interdisciplinary teaching through outdoor education*. Champaign, IL: Human Kinetics.

Hammerman, D., Hammerman, W., & Hammerman, E. (2000). *Teaching in the outdoors* (5th ed.). Englewood Cliffs, NJ: Prentice-Hall.

Kosseff, A. (2003). *AMC guide to outdoor leadership*. Boston, MA: Appalachian Mountain Club Books.

Ladigin, D. (2005). *Lighten up!: a complete handbook for light and ultralight backpacking*. Helena, MT: Falcon Books.

O'Bannon, A., & Clelland, M. (2001). *Allen and Mike's really cool backpackin' book*. Helena, MT: Falcon Books.

Smith, J., Carlson, R., Donaldson, G., & Masters, H. (1972). *Outdoor education* (2nd ed.). Englewood Cliffs, NJ: Prentice-Hall.

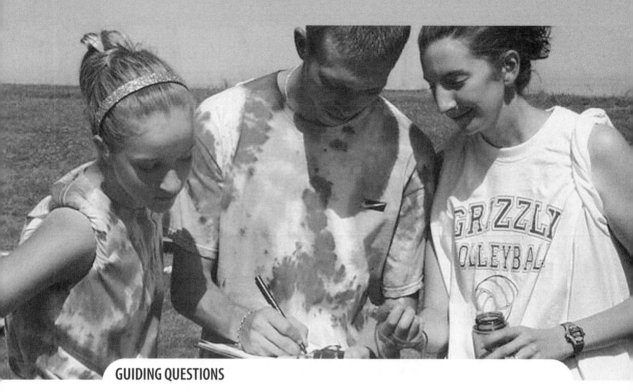

GUIDING QUESTIONS

1. How is Teaching Games for Understanding (TGFU) different from traditional games teaching?
2. Why was TGFU developed?
3. What are tactics?
4. What are the four categories of games in the TGFU classification system? Can you name and define them?
5. How can you sequence content in TGFU/TGM?
6. How is game play assessed?
7. Which of the NASPE content standards does this curriculum model best support?
8. Why might there be an interest in this curriculum model for contemporary youth?
9. How might this curriculum model be incorporated into the physical education curriculum?
10. Describe assessment within this curriculum model.

Teaching Games for Understanding

Steve Mitchell, Kent State University
Judy Oslin, Kent State University

Rationale and Development of the Model

From a glance at a typical school district, county, or state physical education curriculum guide, it is clear that games teaching is a prominent part of what goes on in the name of physical education. Games teaching often begins at about the 2nd grade level, following instruction in fundamental locomotor and manipulative skills, and continues throughout elementary, middle, and high school. Games have traditionally been taught from a skill-based perspective, with units and lessons planned around the skills required for students to be successful. Teachers who use this traditional approach often teach games lessons that include little or no game play, instead providing a diet of skill drills with the goal of improving students' technical performance. Complete lessons of drills might be followed by complete lessons of game play, based on the assumption that, at some point in time, practiced skills will transfer to game play.

Initial criticisms of skill-based games teaching were voiced by David Bunker and Rod Thorpe, two teacher educators at Loughborough University in England, who noted the problems their pre-service teachers had first in motivating students for games instruction, and second in improving student game performance (Bunker & Thorpe, 1982). They identified several specific concerns with skill-based games teaching, including the lack of motivation students in schools showed for participation in skill practices, the inability of students to make appropriate decisions when they did have the opportunity to play in game situations, and the inability of students to implement learned skills within game play.

After much observation and discussion, Bunker and Thorpe determined the need for an alternative approach to games teaching, an approach that would focus student attention on the problems posed by game situations and the solutions to those problems. The resulting instructional model, termed Teaching Games for Understanding (TGFU), was developed primarily for secondary school physical education, and the secondary emphasis was retained in instructional materials developed by Griffin, Mitchell, and Oslin (1997). In recent years the model has been further developed and refined for use at the elementary level (Mitchell, Oslin, & Griffin, 2003).

The original TGFU model of Bunker and Thorpe is presented in Figure 10.1. The model represents a format for games teaching, and presents the games lesson with the learner at its center in problem-solving situations presented by the game being taught. The model has six stages, and rather than repetitive skill practices, a lesson begins with game play (Stage 1). This initial game takes a different form than the full version, by virtue of modifications made to present problems to students. Such modifications might include changes to rules that involve alternative equipment, team size, and playing areas. Students begin to appreciate that it is the game rules, modified to present problems, that dictate the way the game must be played (Stage 2), and students become aware that they must employ certain **tactics** (decisions about what to do in response to problems arising during a game) to play the game successfully (Stage 3). This requires students to think about decisions regarding what to do and how to do it when problems arise during game play (Stage 4). At this point, skill practice makes sense because solutions to tactical (what to do) problems are usually found in the form of game skills and/or movements (Stage 5). Having practiced the required skills, for which students now see the need, a lesson might close with game play to determine the degree to which performance is improved as a result of skill practice (Stage 6).

In our own later work (Mitchell et al., 2003), we have sought to make the model somewhat more user friendly, resulting in a lesson plan outline such as that presented in Table 10.1. This planning guide presents major components of a lesson plan in bold print, with points for the teacher to consider in *italics*. For some teachers the unusual feature of this planning format is that a lesson begins with game play. In fact, we are often asked why this is the case. The initial game sets up the problem to be solved and, in doing so, helps the learner to see the need for particular skills and/or movements as solutions to the problem, and to appreciate the value of practicing these skills. Perhaps it might best be thought of in this way: The game sets the problem; the skill practice solves (or provides solutions to) the problem. By logical extension then, the closing game is where the learner finds out the extent to which the solutions (skills or movements) work to solve the problem during game play.

> **tactics** Decisions about what to do in response to problems that arise during a game.

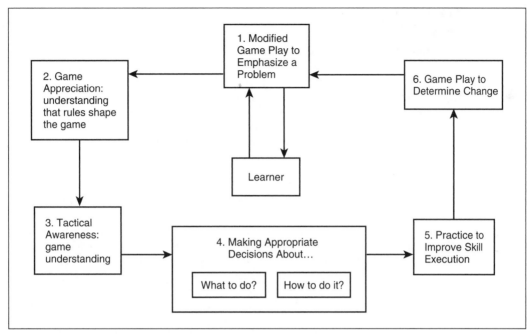

FIGURE 10.1 Original teaching games for understanding model.
Source: Adapted from Bunker, D., & Thorpe, R. (1982). A model for the teaching of games in secondary schools. *Bulletin of Physical Education, 18*(1), 5–8.

Experienced teachers who have used the model cite several observable benefits for both themselves and their students. First, increased time spent in game play provides a more enjoyable and motivational experience for students. They will not need to ask the all too common question, "When are we going to play a game?" Second, the approach enables students to see the link between the skills they practice and the application of those skills to game situations. Third, in any given lesson students learn to appreciate the value of skill practice, first through early game play and discussion, which demonstrate the need for skill practice, and second through later game play, which allows the application and performance of learned skills in the game. This makes for a more motivational environment during skill practice. Fourth, learning the tactical components of one game can help students learn another tactically similar game. A teacher gave us this example during the early stages of a 2nd grade invasion games unit in which students were playing a modified game of team handball. When a girl, whose play indicated a good understanding of supporting movements, was asked by the teacher, "How did you know that was a good place to move to?" she replied simply, "I play soccer!" Other middle and high school teachers have reported strong transfer between net games such as badminton, pickleball, and tennis, in terms of students understanding court dimensions and use of (and defense of) space to successfully win points.

TABLE 10.1

Planning Outline for a TGFU Lesson

Game _____   Lesson # _____   Grade Level _____

Tactical problem:	*What is the tactical problem being addressed during the lesson?*
Lesson focus:	*What is the focus of the lesson—how will the tactical problem be solved?*
Objective:	*What are the major cognitive and psychomotor learning objectives for the lesson?*

1. Game	*What is the modified game being played?*
Conditions	*What conditions will you put on the game to ensure that students have to address the tactical problem?*
Goal	*What performance goal will you give to the students for the game?*
Questions	*After this initial game play, what are the questions you might need to ask (and what answers do you anticipate) to help students focus on the tactical problem and its solution?*

2. Practice task	*What skill practice is appropriate to help students develop a solution to the tactical problem when they return to game play?*
Goal	*What performance goal will you give to the students for the skill practice?*
Cues	*What teaching cues will you use to help the learner focus on critical elements of execution?*
Extension	*How might you extend the skill practice to make it more challenging, or easier, for students of varying abilities?*

3. Game	*What is an appropriate modified game to help students apply newly learned skills, so you and the students can determine improvement?*
Conditions	*What conditions will you put on the game to ensure that students use the skills learned to address the tactical problem?*
Goal	*What performance goal will you give to the students for the game?*

4. Closure	*What are the critical points for discussion and/or demonstration when you close the lesson?*

Source: Adapted from Mitchell, S. A., Oslin, J. L., & Griffin, L. L. (2003). *Sport foundations for elementary physical education: a tactical games approach.* Champaign, IL: Human Kinetics.

The issue of transfer described above is important because many games have common tactical elements. By this we mean that seemingly different games have common problems to be solved, though solutions to these problems might be different by virtue of different skill requirements. The concept of transfer is the basis for the games classification system originally developed by Almond (1986) and presented, in modified form, in Table 10.2. Perhaps the best example is the similarities between the invasion games of soccer and field hockey,

TABLE 10.2

A Games Classification System

Invasion	Net/Wall	Striking/Fielding	Target
Basketball (FT)	*Net*	Baseball	Golf
Netball (FT)	Badminton (I)	Softball	Croquet
Team Handball (FT)	Tennis (I)	Kickball	Bowling
Soccer (FT)	Table Tennis (I)	Rounders	Lawn Bowls
Field/Ice/Floor	Pickleball (I)	Cricket	Pool
Hockey (FT)	Volleyball (H)		Billiards
Lacrosse (FT)			Snooker
Water Polo (FT)	*Wall*		Shuffleboard
	Racquetball (I)		
Speedball (FT/OET)	Squash (I)		
	Handball (H)		
Rugby (OET)			
Football (OET)			
Ultimate (OET)			

FT = Fixed Target   I = Implement
OET = Open End Target   H = Hand

Source: Adapted from Almond, L. (1986). Reflecting on themes: A games classification. In Thorpe, R., Bunker, D., & Almond, L. (Eds.), *Rethinking games teaching* (pp. 71–72). Loughborough: University of Technology.

two essentially identical games when considered from the viewpoint of what must be done effectively to score and prevent an opponent from scoring. In both soccer and hockey, the main tactical concerns for the novice related to scoring are keeping possession of the ball and attacking the goal, while defensively, teams must defend space and defend a goal in order to prevent the opponent from scoring. Badminton, tennis, and racquetball are also similar tactically, and so they are classified as net/wall games. The other categories of games with similar rules, and hence tactics, are striking/fielding games and target games. Brief descriptions of each game category follow.

Invasion Games

The fundamental problems to be addressed in any game are scoring and prevention of scoring. In invasion games, teams score by moving a ball (or other projectile) into another team's territory, and either shooting into a fixed target (a goal or basket) or moving the projectile across an open-ended target (i.e., across a line). To prevent scoring, one team must stop the other from bringing the ball into its territory and creating scoring attempts. Solving these offensive and defensive problems will require similar tactics (similar things that have to be done), even though many of the skills to be used will be quite different. For example, while players must understand the need to shoot if they are to score in both floor hockey and team handball, the striking and throwing skills used to shoot in these two games are very different.

Net/Wall Games

In net/wall games, teams or individual players score by hitting a ball into a court space with sufficient accuracy and/or power that opponents cannot hit it back before it bounces once (as in badminton or volleyball) or twice (as in tennis or racquetball). To prevent scoring, players and teams must return the ball before it bounces once or twice.

Striking/Fielding Games

In striking/fielding games, players on the batting team must strike or kick a ball with sufficient accuracy and/or power that it will elude players on the fielding team, and give time for the hitter to run between two or more points (bases or wickets). To prevent scoring in striking/fielding games, members of the fielding team must position themselves in such a way that they are able to gather a hit ball and throw it to the base or wicket (to which the hitter is running) before the hitter reaches this base or wicket.

Target Games

In target games, players score by reaching a target with a ball, either by throwing or striking the ball. Some target games are unopposed (e.g., golf, ten-pin bowling), whereas others are opposed (e.g., bocce, lawn bowling, croquet), in which one participant is allowed to block or hit the opponent's ball. In opposed target games, players seek to prevent scoring by hitting the opponent's ball to place it in a disadvantageous position relative to the target.

Similarities and the Oppositional Relationship Among Games

TGFU has become something of a worldwide movement, with proponents developing variations on the theme with different nomenclatures. An Australian conception of TGFU, known as Game Sense, was developed in the 1990s and was the first approach to address the use of TGFU as a coaching methodology at varying levels of youth sport development. Early efforts to publicize and educate coaches in Game Sense were cosponsored by the Australian Sport Commission, the Australian Coaching Council, and Aussie Sport. Game Sense stays very close to the original TGFU model with its focus on conditioned game play, modifying and exaggerating game conditions to place players in problem-solving situations as the means for players to learn (and only teaching technique when necessary), but it places specific emphasis on using questions and challenges to promote learning and problem solving (Den Duyn, 1997). Much is made of setting challenges and designing questions, emphasizing that these things are difficult pedagogical skills. In particular, Game Sense focuses on questions related to time (when will you . . . ?), space (where is . . . ?), and risk (which option . . . ?). Again, the nature of these types of questions provides a focus on decision making and problem solving.

In his discussion of using Game Sense in coaching, Light (2005) describes several strengths that Australian coaches have identified across different sports. These strengths include developing players' ability to work off the ball; transfer of training to the game by ". . . placing all learning in game-like environments structured by the coach to develop particular skills and tactics" (p. 171); developing independent players who can think and make decisions without coach input; motivating players in training by keeping practice activities close to the game and allowing players to set their own challenges; and the applicability of game sense training to performers of varied abilities, particularly because of the decreased emphasis on technique, which is to the benefit of the less technically gifted player. Certainly these facets were all deemed important by Bunker and Thorpe (1982) and were also emphasized by Mitchell et al, (2003, 2006). In particular, the latter authors placed considerable emphasis on off-the-ball movement, given the large amounts of time players spend without the ball (or other projectile) in most games. However, whereas Games Sense places all learning within modified games (Chen & Light, 2006), the Tactical Games Model (Mitchell et al., 2003, 2006) accepts that isolated technical development might be necessary in some cases, particularly for players with very poor technical ability, so that novice players' decision making is not completely constricted by an inability to execute once decisions are made.

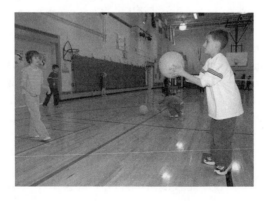

Also developed in Australia and with a youth sport coaching emphasis, Play Practice (Launder, 2001) holds true to many of the tenets of TGFU, particularly the emphasis on the development of player understanding as a critical component of learning and performance improvement, and the use of conditioned game play as a means of diagnosing performance problems before practice takes place. According to Launder, three questions drive the concept of Play Practice:

1. What do young people want from a sport experience?
2. Under what conditions do young people best learn?
3. What competencies do young people need to participate effectively and enjoyably in a sport?

In his explanation of Play Practice theory, Launder provides answers to these questions, some of which indicate strong alignment to the intentions of TGFU. Among other things, Launder suggests that young people prefer to play games rather than to practice, want to be challenged, and see practice as a means to an end not an end itself. Hence Bunker and Thorpe's idea of only practicing technique or skill execution as warranted by game performance is evident here. Responding to the second question, Launder suggests that children learn best when they understand the relationship between the practice and its application, and when they are quickly able to apply what they have learned in practice in what they view as real situations. This brings to mind Stages 4–6 of the original TGFU model in which any necessary technique or skill practice is followed by the opportunity to perform in a game setting. Launder answers the third question above by focusing primarily on notions of "effective participation," affective outcomes such as fun and enjoyment, and perseverance when faced with a challenging environment. This speaks to the motivational intent of Play Practice and also TGFU and, indeed, the latter was intended as a motivational model through its emphasis on players seeing the value and necessity of practice through participation in game play.

A French model of game play analysis, the Tactical Decision Learning Model (TDLM), also has roots, in part, in TGFU. This model was developed by Grehaigne and his colleagues during the 1990s (Grehaigne & Godbout, 1995; Grehaigne, Godbout, & Bouthier, 1997, 1999, 2001) and later formally presented in textbook format (Grehaigne, Richard, & Griffin, 2005). TDLM focuses specifically on team sports and makes a very thorough analysis of the complexities of team play, particularly in invasion games. Again, TDLM has decision making and problem solving as core components, in particular problems related to space, time, information, and organization. However, this model also emphasizes the interdependent nature of tactics, technique, and "athletic potential," meaning conditioning or fitness in this case.

Grehaigne et al. (2005) suggest that TDLM is a systemic model in that it seeks to ". . . explain game play from the oppositional relationship that constantly exists between opposing teams" (p. 9). Hence TDLM views as critical the *force ratio*, positions of advantage or disadvantage that are subject to momentary change, between opponents if game play performance is to be understood in its entirety, and uses the concept of *tactical intelligence* to distinguish a performer's ability (or lack thereof) to understand the reciprocal relationships between the movements of both teams within game play situations. As with all TGFU perspectives, decision making is central in TDLM, in terms of both initial decisions and adjustments made during the course of game play. Decision making is seen as related to and influenced by factors such as a player's motivations, concentration, conditioning, and ability to execute whatever action is decided most appropriate.

Somewhat similar to the frameworks developed by Mitchell et al. (2003, 2006), Grehaigne and Godbout (1995) formulated the notion of *action rules* to provide a potential breakdown of possible tactical decisions within game situations, though the latter authors also emphasize the momentary nature of action rules as solutions to tactical problems arising instantaneously during game play. And again similar to Mitchell et al. (2003, 2006), Grehaigne et al. (2005) suggest that action rules might be used as a tool in curriculum planning for the teaching and learning of team sports. Offensive action rules include keeping the ball, playing in movement (movement of the ball in a forward direction), exploiting and creating available space, and creating uncertainty. Defensive action rules include defending the target, regaining possession of the ball, and challenging the opponent's progression.

Clearly these components of game play apply across invasion games, and the identification of similarities across games has clear implications for curriculum development, in terms of content selection and sequencing. The process of developing the TGFU curriculum is discussed in the next section of the chapter.

Curriculum Development in TGFU

The Tactical Games Model

More recent work in TGFU has focused on moving the model from the stage of being an alternative lesson format to being a means of selecting and sequencing content in the curriculum. In our own work we have developed what we call the Tactical Games Model (Mitchell et al., 2003), based on the original TGFU model of Bunker and Thorpe (1982), and the games classification system of Almond (1986). In our formulation of the Tactical Games Model (TGM), we suggest that games can be taught using a tactical approach, rather than a skill-based approach, beginning at about age 8, or 2nd grade. At the elementary level, a thematic approach would have teachers select several games from within the same category, for example, soccer, floor hockey, and team handball, to emphasize game similarities (Mitchell et al., 2003). At the secondary level, content selection and instruction might be more game specific, with a focus solely on one game (Griffin et al., 1997) to allow for greater tactical and skill complexity.

SCOPE AND SEQUENCE IN TGM. Regardless of whether teachers opt to plan content across games or teach a specific game, TGM advocates the development of **tactical frameworks**, and identification of game complexity levels to facilitate the planning of scope and sequence. Table 10.3 provides an example of a tactical framework, illustrating the possible tactical breakdown of invasion games for instruction at the elementary level, by identifying tactical problems and solutions to these problems. Solutions are in the form of decisions to be made, on-the-ball skills, and off-the-ball movements, and these solutions represent the content of games instruction at the elementary level. This framework provides the "scope" of content for teaching invasion games at the elementary level by breaking down invasion games according to the problems associated with scoring, preventing scoring, and starting/restarting play.

The levels of "game complexity" provided in Table 10.4 provide an appropriate "sequence" for this content. Taken together, the framework and levels of game complexity provide developmentally appropriate scope and sequence of invasion games content for elementary children. Ideally, game play should occur between teams no larger than 3v3 at first, progressing to a maximum of 6v6 in games such as soccer and hockey.

The *sequence* of learning suggested in Table 10.4 is designed to make games instruction developmentally appropriate. We recommend identifying levels of game complexity for each games category. These levels include the learning of concepts and skills across a variety of games. So, at Level I, teachers might teach students to keep possession of a ball by passing, receiving, and supporting in soccer, hockey, and basketball. Depending on the length of time spent on invasion games, Level I might also include the learning of shooting techniques in these games. Table 10.4 presents three possible levels of game complexity, upon which the development of unit and lesson plans can be based, if teaching invasion games at the elementary level. Notice that we advocate beginning invasion games play with no more than three players per team. This allows for some **decision making** (should I pass to player A or player B?), but does not force a vast range of possibilities. We have even found 2v2 games to be effective because this would only force players to make pass/shoot/dribble decisions. This represents decreased complexity in the early stages of invasion games learning. Note in

---

tactical frameworks   Ways of thinking about games based on the problems that need to be solved in order to be successful.

decision making   The process of deciding what to do, particularly when selecting and executing skills during game play.

TABLE 10.3

A Framework for Invasion Games Content in Elementary Physical Education

Tactical Problems	Decisions and Movements	Skills
Offense/Scoring		
Keeping possession of the ball	Supporting the ball carrier / When to pass (timing the pass to beat a defender)	Passing and receiving the ball skillfully
Penetrating the defense and attacking the goal	Using a target forward or post player / When to shoot and dribble	Moving with the ball (usually dribbling with hand, feet, or stick) / Shooting for power and accuracy
Transition: defense to offense	Moving to space after a shot or save	Quick passing
Defense/Preventing Scoring		
Defending space	Marking/guarding / Footwork: stance and sliding the feet / Pressuring the ball carrier	Clearing the ball away from goal / Quick outlet passes
Defending the goal	Goalkeeping: positioning, angle play (cutting down angles) / Rebounding: boxing out	Goalkeeping: stopping and distributing the ball to teammates / Rebounding: catching the ball
Winning the ball		Tackling and stealing the ball
Starting/Restarting Play		
Beginning the game	Positioning	Initiating play
Restarting from the sideline	Supporting positions	Putting the ball in play
Restarting from the endline	Supporting positions	Putting the ball in play
Restarting from violations	Supporting positions	Putting the ball in play

Source: Adapted from Mitchell, S. A., Oslin, J. L., & Griffin, L. L. (2003). *Sport foundations for elementary physical education: a tactical games approach.* Champaign, IL: Human Kinetics.

Table 10.4 that game complexity increases as students progress through Levels II and III. For example, transition is a more complex tactical problem, and is addressed only at Level III.

Similar frameworks and game complexity levels might be developed for other game categories at the elementary level (Mitchell et al., 2003) or for specific games at the secondary level (see Griffin et al., 1997, for examples).

TABLE 10.4

Levels of Game Complexity for Invasion Games in Elementary Physical Education

Tactical Problems/Concepts	Game Complexity Level I 3-a-Side Maximum	Game Complexity Level II 4-a-Side Maximum	Game Complexity Level III 6-a-Side Maximum
Offense/Scoring			
Keeping possession	Pass, receive, footwork	Pass, receive, footwork	
	When to pass— timing the pass	Support	
Penetration/attack	Shooting, moving with the ball (dribbling)	Shooting for power, feinting	Using a target or post forward
	When to dribble and shoot		Shooting for accuracy, change of speed, moving with the ball (dribble)
Transition			Moving to space, quick passing
Defense/Preventing Scoring			
Defending space		Marking/guarding, pressure	Clearing the ball, quick outlet pass
		Stance/footwork	
Defending the goal		Goalkeeper: positioning, angle play	Goalkeeper: shot stopping and distribution
			Rebounding
Winning the ball			Tackling and stealing the ball
Starting/Restarting Play			
Beginning the game	Initiating play	Positioning in a triangle	
Restarting from side and end line	Putting ball in play	Positioning	Quick restarts
Restarting from violations	Putting ball in play	Positioning	Quick restarts

Source: Adapted from Mitchell, S. A., Oslin, J. L., & Griffin, L. L. (2003). *Sport foundations for elementary physical education: a tactical games approach.* Champaign, IL: Human Kinetics.

Relationship of TGFU/TGM to the National (NASPE) K–12 Content Standards

The National K–12 Content Standards (National Association for Sport and Physical Education [NASPE], 2004) described in Chapter 1 of this book provide a comprehensive definition of a physically educated individual. That said, most curriculum models will not address all standards equally, and TGFU is no exception. The standards table in the introductory chapter of this book indicates that TGFU places greater emphasis on Standard 1 (competency in several forms), Standard 2 (application of movement principles), and Standard 6 (enjoyment of movement), with a minor emphasis on Standard 3 (maintenance of an active lifestyle).

TGFU was originally conceived as a more effective model of games instruction, particularly in secondary physical education, and more recently developed relative to elementary physical education. The model has a clear focus on Standard 1. A thematic approach to content selection advocated by ourselves (Mitchell et al., 2003), together with a more sport-specific approach at the secondary level (Bunker & Thorpe, 1982; Griffin et al., 1997; Thorpe & Bunker, 1982), can clearly enable students to develop competence in several games. A thematic approach at the elementary level, where teachers emphasize and have students experience the commonalities between different games within the same games category (i.e., invasion, net/wall, striking/fielding, target), is intended to develop more knowledgeable and adaptable games players who can take a broad understanding and apply it to specific games in the pursuit of competence.

Although TGFU concentrates on games content, the cognitive focus of TGFU also suggests a strong emphasis on NASPE Standard 2. TGFU addresses games content through a problem-solving approach in which students are placed in game situations that have been designed by the teacher to present particular problems. For example, one school program that uses TGFU extensively is Nordonia Middle School in Macedonia, Ohio. In the badminton class the teachers emphasize the problem of court space by having students play singles on a long, narrow court, perhaps using just half of the full court. With only very limited width to the court, students are limited in their attacking options, and must focus on playing a "long and short" game in which they attempt to set up attacks by pushing opponents to the back of the court with overhead and underhand clears, before exploiting the space created in the front of the court by using drop shots. In TGFU, students are first placed in game play in which they must solve this problem. They must apply the principle of space creation and use of space to their game play, practicing relevant shots when they see the need to use these shots, before returning to game play to determine game performance improvement.

For many people, game playing is an enjoyable activity, and indeed, a lifetime activity, hence the focus on Standard 6 and also Standard 3. The movements and skills performed during game play are kinesthetically pleasing when performed successfully, and challenging when performance is less than successful. The element of appropriate competition (Siedentop, 1998) in game playing adds a layer of excitement and intensity to the physical education environment, and is a component that most students find engaging and stimulating.

The presence of competition, particularly in the case of elementary students, does present a concern for some physical educators. It will be necessary to train students to play small-sided games in an organized and fair manner, because it is likely that most lessons will involve the use of multiple small-sided games being played simultaneously. With reference to NASPE Standard 5, it will also be necessary to foster respect, responsibility, and appropriate behavior by teaching rules and routines for equipment management, entry and exit to and from the gymnasium, and starting and restarting game play (Mitchell et al., 2003).

Examples of TGFU/TGM in the Curriculum

Many teachers now use TGFU/TGM as their preferred approach to games teaching. It is beyond the scope of this chapter to present examples covering all levels and all games categories, so we give you a sample unit used by one of our local teachers, Linda Clemens at Davey Elementary School in Kent, Ohio, to introduce net/wall games to her 2nd grade students. Having been introduced to the principles of net games play at an early stage, it would be an easy transition for students to move on to learn games such as pickleball and badminton, games in which the same principles of play apply, in upper elementary and secondary physical education.

In this short unit (six lessons only), instruction focuses on the problems of space creation and defense (Figure 10.2). Notice that Linda spent time in the first lesson to familiarize students with the playing areas and procedures to set up

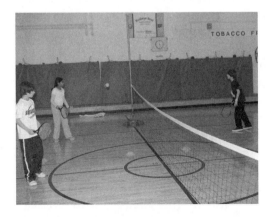

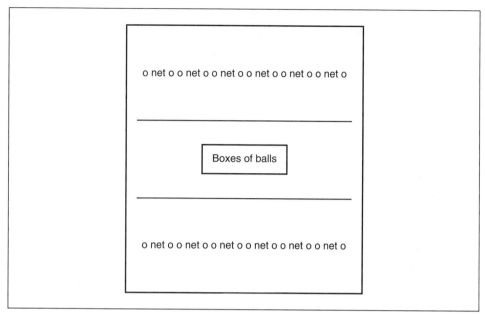

Figure 10.2 Explanation of court spaces.

these areas. Also interesting is the link made between net and wall games—at the point where students were able to play a simple, but competitive, throw and catch net game, Linda then modified the game so students played off a wall. The positive transfer of understanding from the net game to the wall game was substantial in these 2nd grade students. The following lessons, designed for approximately 35 minutes' duration, use the planning format previously presented in Table 10.1.

An Introductory Net/Wall Game Unit

Lesson 1. Tactical problem: Maintaining a rally.

    Game: Throw tennis (singles—student's own choice of ball). Mini courts set up on volleyball court.

    Lesson focus: Court spaces, etiquette, and the cooperative game.

    Objectives: Students will learn to recognize court spaces and play a cooperative game keeping the ball in their own court.

    1. Selection of partners. Selection of ball. Throw/catch warm-up; play with different balls (one bounce).

    2. Explanation of court spaces. Cones (red or yellow) mark the "net" of each court.

3. Game. Throw and catch over the "net."
Conditions. All throws must be underhand.
Throw over the net; ball must bounce only once on the other side of the net.
Ball cannot bounce on your own side of the net.
Goal. Rallies of 10 throws, keeping ball in court (discuss width of court—in line with cones—and depth of court).
4. Closure. Set up and take down practice.

Lesson 2. Tactical problem: Maintaining a rally.
Game: Throw tennis (singles).
Lesson focus: Court spaces, etiquette, and the cooperative game.
Objective: Students will play a cooperative game keeping the ball within the defined court.

1. Game. Throw and catch over the "net."
Conditions. All throws must be underhand.
Throw over the net; ball must bounce only once on the other side of the net.
Ball cannot bounce on your own side of the net.
Goal. Rallies of 10 throws, keeping ball in court (discuss width of court—in line with cones—and depth of court).
Questions:
Q. What makes it easier to keep the ball in court when you are throwing?
What should your throw look like? (Perhaps present some options here: one hand, two hand, feet still, stepping, etc.)
A. One or two hands (depending on the ball they have chosen). Step as you throw (step with opposite foot).
Q. What makes it easier to catch the ball? Where should you be?
A. After it bounces, let it come up and then down so it is falling when you catch it (this makes it easier to catch and encourages them to move their feet).
2. Practice task. Partner throw/catch over the net.
Goal. Rallies of 10 throws, keeping ball in court.
Cues: Throwing—step with the opposite foot (to the throwing hand).
Swing through to your target.
Catching—let the ball drop after the bounce.
3. Game. Same as game 1.
4. Closure. Where would you throw the ball if you wanted to make it harder for your partner to get it before it bounced twice?

Lesson 3. Tactical problem: Playing a competitive game and setting up to attack.
Game: Throw tennis (singles).

Lesson focus: Game rules and use of court spaces.

Objective: Students will play a competitive game, with appropriate rules, and try to move their opponent to the back of the court.

1. Game. Throw and catch over the "net."

Conditions. All throws must be underhand.

Throw over the net; ball must bounce only once on the other side of the net.

Ball cannot bounce on your own side of the net.

Goal. Try to make your opponent move around the court.

Questions (interjected during game play):

Q. What spaces are there on the court for you to throw the ball into?

A. Front and back.

Q. Is it hardest to make a good throw from the front or the back?

A. Back.

Q. So, where should you try to make your opponent move to (front or back)?

A. Back. Try to get the ball to bounce close to the back line.

Continue game play.

Q. When you have gotten your opponent to move back, where is the space now?

A. In the front.

Q. So, to make it hard for your opponent, where should you throw to now?

A. The front.

Q. Should you throw quickly or should you wait to throw? Why?

A. Quickly. Because your opponent will be further away.

Continue game play.

Q. When should you stop and restart a rally?

A. Restart a rally if:

- ball bounces twice on opponent's side.
- opponent throws the ball out of court.
- opponent makes the ball bounce on his/her own side.
- opponent throws overhand.
- opponent catches the ball before it bounces.

Note: Set up demonstrations of these scoring rules.

Continue game play.

2. Closure. Review restart rules.

Lesson 4. Tactical problem: Defending space.

Game: Throw tennis (singles).

Lesson focus: Recovering to a base position.

Objective: Students will play a competitive game, with appropriate rules, and try to defend their own space by moving back to the center of the baseline between throws.

1. Game. Throw and catch over the "net."
   Conditions. All throws must be underhand.

   Throw over the net; ball must bounce only once on the other side of the net.

   Ball cannot bounce on your own side of the net.

   Goal. Try to make your opponent move around the court.
   Questions (interjected during game play):

   Q. If your opponent is moving you around your court, where should you move to in between your own throws?
   A. The middle of your court. At the baseline.
   Q. Why?
   A. So you can move up or back easily.

   Continue game play.
   Cue: Move back to the line between throws.

2. Game. Three-minute games against rotating opponents.
   Conditions. Alternate underhand serve.

   Follow rules and score the game according to the restart rules.

   Score a point if:
   - ball bounces twice on opponent's side.
   - opponent throws the ball out of court.
   - opponent makes the ball bounce on his/her own side.
   - opponent throws overhand.
   - opponent catches the ball before it bounces.

   Goal. Move your opponent, recover, and score the game.

3. Closure. Review court spaces, recovery, and scoring.

Lesson 5. Tactical problem: Setting up an attack.
   Game: One wall handball (singles throw and catch).
   Lesson focus: Court spaces.
   Objective: Students will play a cooperative and competitive game of one wall handball, trying to move their opponent around the court.

1. Game. Throw and catch against the wall.
   Conditions. All throws must be underhand.

   Ball must bounce once after hitting the wall.

   Ball must bounce inside the boundary (cones).

   Goal. 20-throw rally (cooperative game to introduce shift to wall game).

Try to make your opponent move around the court (competitive game).

Questions (interjected during game play):

Q. Where should you try to make the ball bounce to make it hard for your opponent?

A. Near the back.

Q. Where on the wall do you need to aim to do this (high or low)?

A. High up.

Continue game play.

Q. When you have gotten your opponent to move back, where is the space now?

A. In the front.

Q. So, to make it hard for your opponent, where should you throw to now?

A. The front.

Q. Where on the wall should you aim (high or low)?

A. Low.

Continue game play.

Q. When should you score a point?

A. Score a point if:

- ball bounces twice in court.
- ball bounces outside the court lines.
- ball bounces before it hits the wall.
- opponent throws overhand.
- opponent catches the ball before it bounces.

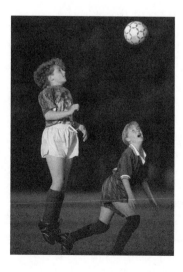

Note: Set up demonstrations of these scoring rules.

Continue game play.

2. Closure. Review restart rules.

Lesson 6. Tactical problem: Defending space.

Game: One wall handball (singles throw and catch).

Lesson focus: Recovering to a base position.

Objective: Students will play a competitive game, with appropriate rules, and try to defend their own space by moving back to the center of the court between throws.

1. Game. One wall handball.

Conditions. All throws must be underhand.

Ball must bounce once after hitting the wall.

Ball must bounce inside the boundary (cones).

Goal. Try to make your opponent move around the court (competitive game).

Questions (interjected during game play):

Q. If your opponent is moving you around your court, where should you move to in between your own throws?

A. The middle of your court.

Q. Why?

A. So you can move up or back easily.

Continue game play.

Cue: Move back to the center between throws.

2. Game. Three-minute games against rotating opponents.

Conditions. Alternate underhand serve.

Follow rules and score the game according to the restart rules.

Score a point if:

- ball bounces twice in court.
- ball bounces outside the court lines.
- ball bounces before it hits the wall.
- opponent throws overhand.
- opponent catches the ball before it bounces.

Note: Set up demonstrations of these scoring rules.

Continue game play.

3. Closure. Review recovery. Center of court.

Assessment of Student Learning

An integral part of the elementary net/wall games unit was assessment of student performance. This was done on an ongoing basis, by recording performance levels of a few students in each lesson, and again during the final lesson when all were looked at as they played. There are few instruments available for assessing **game performance**, largely because of the difficulty in determining student intent during game play situations. Although skill performance (i.e., execution) is easily observed, it is more difficult to observe and measure critical components of game performance, such as *decision making*, when choosing actions or positional play when movement is required. One available instrument is the Game Performance Assessment Instrument (GPAI; Griffin et al., 1997; Mitchell & Oslin, 1999). The GPAI enables teachers to assess game performance relative to important components, including:

1. *Use of a base position*: The performer appropriately returns to a recovery (base) position between skill attempts.

2. *Decision making when in possession of the ball*: Performers must make appropriate decisions about what to do with the ball (or projectile) during a game.

3. *Skill execution*: Performers must then execute the selected skills.

4. *Support for teammates in possession of the ball*: Performers should provide appropriate support for a teammate with the ball by being in position to receive a pass.

5. *Marking or guarding opponents*: Performers should defend space by appropriate guarding or "marking" of an opponent who may or may not have the ball.

6. *Covering for teammates who are defending against opponents*: Players should provide appropriate defensive cover, help, or backup for a player making a challenge for the ball.

7. *Adjusting to the flow of a game*: Players should move, adjusting position either offensively or defensively as necessitated by the flow of the game.

It is important to note that not all components relate strongly to all games. For example, although supporting, decision making, skill execution, and guarding are all critical to good invasion game performance, the same is not necessarily true of the component of base position. On the other hand, support is not relevant to most net games, particularly in singles play in a racket game. The elementary net/wall games unit only focused on three of the above components of game performance, numbers 1–3. Although the decision-making component clearly speaks to NASPE Standard 1, the components of base position and decision making have a cognitive emphasis related to NASPE Standard 2. Using the GPAI, the teacher defines criteria for the components in terms of what he or she

game performance   A student's ability to play in game situations.

TABLE 10.5

Game Performance Assessment Instrument for Elementary Net/Wall Games

Game Performance Assessment Instrument

Class: _____   Evaluator: _____   Game: Net/Wall

Observation Dates: ___ / / ___   ___ / / ___   ___ / / ___   ___ / / ___

Scoring Key: 5 = Always does this
4 = Usually does this
3 = Sometimes does this
2 = Rarely does this
1 = Never does this

Components/Criteria:
1. Base: Return to appropriate position at mid-court between skill attempts.
2. Decision making: Makes appropriate choices about which skills to use—deep throw if opponent is at mid-court or front, short throw if opponent is deep.
3. Skill execution: Executes chosen skills proficiently—deep throw lands close to the baseline, short throw lands close to the net.

Recording Procedures: Observe the selected player(s) for 5–10 minutes, observing only performance related to the above criteria. After the observation period give each player a score from 1–5 on each component.

Name	Base	Decision Making	Skill Execution

expects to see, and records student performance based on the defined criteria. A sample observation form is presented in Table 10.5 (an elementary example). For other assessment ideas addressing other standards, see Mitchell, Oslin, and Griffin (2003).

Summary

Whether considered an instructional approach or a curriculum model, TGFU has provided a viable alternative approach for games teaching. Teachers cite numerous benefits, including their own teaching pleasure, increased student motivation, and improved student game performance. We conclude with the remarks of a teacher who, having changed her approach to games teaching, reflected on the efficacy of TGFU:

> There have been a number of positive outcomes using this approach. If my goal was to have students play the game more effectively, then letting them play the game was critical. Because my students have had increasingly more opportunities to play games and solve tactical problems, they seem to have a better understanding of games in general. Technical skill work still occurs but never in isolation, always as it would in the game and mostly as a means to accomplish the tactical problems. Students come in excited, positive, and ready to go because they know they are going to get to play a game of some form. I no longer hear, "are we going to play a game today?" (Berkowitz, 1996).

References

Almond, L. (1986). Reflecting on themes: a games classification. In R. Thorpe, D. Bunker, & L. Almond (Eds.), *Rethinking games teaching* (pp. 71–72). Loughborough: University of Technology.

Berkowitz, R. J. (1996). A practitioner's journey from skill to tactics. *Journal of Physical Education, Recreation and Dance, 67*(4), 44–45.

Bunker, D., & Thorpe, R. (1982). A model for the teaching of games in secondary schools. *Bulletin of Physical Education, 18*(1), 5–8.

Chen, Q., & Light, R. (2006). Encouraging positive attitudes toward sport through game sense pedagogy in an Australian primary school. In Liu, R., Chung, L., & Cruz, A. (Eds.), *Teaching games for understanding in the Asia-Pacific region* (pp. 47–58). Hong Kong: Hong Kong Institute of Education.

Den Duyn, N. (1997). *Game sense: developing thinking players*. Belconnen, Australia: Australian Sports Commission.

Grehaigne, J-F., & Godbout, P. (1995). Tactical knowledge in team sports from a constructivist and cognitivist perspective. *Quest, 47*, 490–505.

Grehaigne, J-F., Godbout, P., & Bouthier, D. (1997). Performance assessment in team sports. *Journal of Teaching in Physical Education, 16*, 500–516.

Grehaigne, J-F., Godbout, P., & Bouthier, D. (1999). The foundations of tactics and strategy in team sports. *Journal of Teaching in Physical Education, 18*, 159–174.

Grehaigne, J-F., Godbout, P., & Bouthier, D. (2001). The teaching and learning of decision making in team sports. *Quest, 53*, 59–76.

Grehaigne, J-F., Richard, J-F., & Griffin, L. (2005). *Teaching and learning team sports and games*. New York: RoutledgeFalmer.

Griffin, L. L., Mitchell, S. A., & Oslin, J. L. (1997). *Teaching sport concepts and skills: a tactical games approach*. Champaign, IL: Human Kinetics.

Launder, A. G. (2001). *Play Practice: the games approach to teaching and coaching sports*. Champaign, IL: Human Kinetics.

Light, R. (2005). Making sense of games sense: Australian coaches talk about games sense. In Griffin, L., & Butler, J. (Eds.), *Teaching games for understanding: theory, research and practice* (pp. 169–181). Champaign, IL: Human Kinetics.

Mitchell, S. A., & Oslin, J. L. (1999). *Assessment in games teaching: assessment series for K–12 physical education*. Reston, VA: National Association for Sport and Physical Education.

Mitchell, S. A., Oslin, J. L., & Griffin, L. L. (2003). *Sport foundations for elementary physical education: a tactical games approach*. Champaign, IL: Human Kinetics.

Mitchell, S. A., Oslin, J. L., & Griffin, L. L. (2006). *Teaching sport concepts and skills: a tactical games approach* (2nd ed.). Champaign, IL: Human Kinetics.

National Association for Sport and Physical Education. (2004). *Moving into the future: national standards for physical education*. Reston, VA: National Association for Sport and Physical Education.

Siedentop, D. (1998). *Introduction to physical education, fitness and sport*. Mountain View, CA: Mayfield.

Thorpe, R., & Bunker, D. (1982). From theory to practice: two examples of an "understanding approach" to the teaching of games. *Bulletin of Physical Education*, 18(1), 9–15.

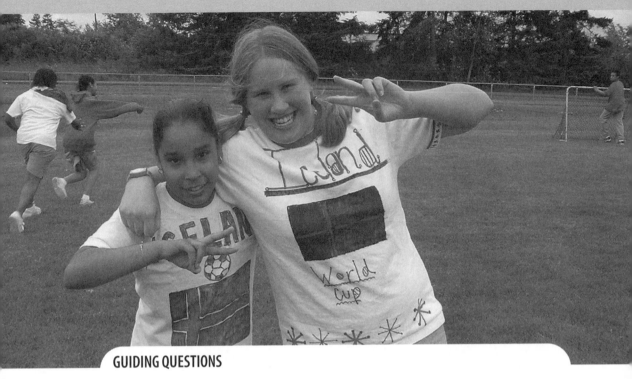

GUIDING QUESTIONS

1 Describe the underlying goal of Sport Education.

2 What constitutes a competent sportsperson? A literate sportsperson? An enthusiastic sportsperson?

3 Discuss the purpose of the 10 short-term objectives.

4 Link Sport Education to each of the NASPE standards.

5 Why does Sport Education suggest not using the parent game version of sports?

6 What is the purpose of the non-playing roles that students learn to play? Describe several of these roles, and the aligned responsibilities.

7 Describe the role of fair play in a Sport Education season.

8 What is meant by the rituals and conventions that make sports unique?

9 Describe what is meant by a more complete and authentic sport experience.

10 Describe the primary features of Sport Education that are typically seen in authentic sport.

11 How does sport differ from Sport Education?

12 How does the role of the teacher and the student change in physical education when implementing Sport Education?

13 Develop a set of authentic assessment tools to match the 10 Sport Education objectives.

14 Outline your own Sport Education season.

Sport Education: Authentic Sport Experiences

Hans van der Mars, Arizona State University
Deborah Tannehill, University of Limerick

Physical education professionals generally agree that instruction in sport continues to be the dominant feature of many secondary school physical education programs in the United States. At the elementary level, it is also common to see students being introduced to basic sport techniques as early as 3rd grade. In recent years, this dominance has faced frequent criticism, based on a growing body of research (e.g., Carlson, 1995; Ennis, 1996, 1999) that points to 1) frequent marginalization of lower-skilled students and girls by higher-skilled students (and at times teachers themselves); and 2) sport being perceived by students as something to be tolerated at best, and irrelevant at worst.

Across the country, many physical education programs are characterized by multi-activity, exposure-oriented approaches to physical education programming, where sports/activities form the bulk of the program's menu. Generally, teachers introduce basic techniques in isolated drill practice conditions, and then place students in games that largely mirror the official parent game structure; units are short (generally no more than 10–12 lessons). It is quite typical for students to experience three weeks of volleyball, followed by three weeks of basketball, and so on. With such short units, students' opportunity to demonstrate any type of mastery that can be attributed to the experiences in the unit is limited. Students will likely experience a similar sequence of activities across grade levels. During these units, much of class time is devoted to learning and practicing isolated sport skills. Toward the end of the short unit, teams are organized to play games, but the team membership changes frequently. The techniques practiced in drill-oriented conditions do not find their way into the more complex game conditions. The higher-skilled players take charge of the action, while lesser-skilled players often find ways to look involved without actually contributing. Research on the physical education experiences of youth points to the inescapable conclusion that for many students (especially girls), physical activity becomes something to be avoided at all cost (e.g., Hastie, 2003; Siedentop & Tannehill, 2000). If the standards-based movement increases its hold on daily education practices, programs that continue to offer the type of physical activity programming described above will be exposed, and will be completely indefensible.

At the same time, the world of sport continues to offer our profession many reasons to become more and increasingly disenchanted, and to seek other forms of physical activity that can be promoted. As dissatisfaction with team sport–only curricula increases and public health concerns mount, other curriculum models such as Outdoor Education (Stiehl & Parker, Chapter 9) and Fitness Education (e.g., Corbin & Lindsey, 1997, 2005; McConnell, Chapter 13) are emerging as powerful alternatives. Yet, two important developments offer hope for sport as viable and legitimate content in today's school-based programs, including the in-roads being made by the Teaching Games for Understanding (TGFU) approach (Mitchell & Oslin, Chapter 10) and the emergence of Sport Education. At the instructional level, the TGFU approach forms a radical departure from traditional designs of instruction, aimed at getting students to develop a better understanding of the tactical dimensions of games. At the curricular level, Siedentop (1994) proposed a more authentic approach to teaching sport in the context of school physical education. This chapter will provide an overview of the Sport Education model, considerations for its use across grade levels, its alignments with the latest National Association for Sport and Physical Education (NASPE) Content Standards (NASPE, 2004), several examples of how teachers might formally assess their students' learning, as well as its benefits and limitations.

Sport Education was developed in the early 1980s in the United States by Daryl Siedentop as a result of his view that sport as it was being taught in physical education focused on isolated skills decontextualized from their authentic role in sport and games (Siedentop, 1984). He set out to design a model that would develop young people as competent, literate, and enthusiastic sport persons who are able to take responsibility for their own sport experiences (Siedentop, 1998). Sport Education and research on its design and implementation has spread internationally from New Zealand (Grant, 1992) and Australia (Alexander & Luckman, 2001; Alexander, Taggert, & Luckman, 1998) to Ireland (Kinchin, MacPhail, & Ni Chroinin, 2009) and the United Kingdom (Almond, 1997; MacPhail, Kinchin, & Kirk, 2003) and from Russia (Sinelnikov & Hastie, 2008) to Korea (Kim, Penney, & Cho, 2006). Although the initial focus and a continuing theme in Sport Education is around games, there are numerous examples of Sport Education being applied to other contexts such as dance

(Graves & Townsend, 2000), fitness (Sweeney, Tannehill, & Teeters, 1992), and gymnastics (Bell, 1994) and at both the elementary (Strikwerda-Brown & Taggart, 2001) and secondary levels (Kinchin, Penney, & Clarke, 2001). We have read about efforts to deliver Sport Education seasons to both low-skilled (Carlson, 1995) and high-skilled students (Kinchin, 2001), as well as those labeled "at risk" for learning (Hastie & Sharpe, 1999) or who have shown little to no interest in physical education (Curnow & Macdonald, 1995; Hastie, 1998). There are reports of Sport Education being the framework for collegiate physical activity programs (Bennet & Hastie, 1997) and the focus of research in the education of prospective physical education teachers (Collier, 1998; McMahon & MacPhail, 2007). In the last decade, interest in research on Sport Education has grown as well. Although this is not the place for a full review of literature on Sport Education, we direct you to the following sources: 1) The 2005 edited text by Penney, Clarke, Quill, and Kinchin titled *Sport Education in Physical Education: Research Based Practice*; 2) Wallhead and O'Sullivan's (2005) review of research on Sport Education in *Physical Education and Sport Pedagogy*; and 3) the 2006 Kinchin review chapter on Sport Education in the *Handbook of Physical Education* edited by Kirk, Macdonald, and O'Sullivan. However, there is extensive evidence that lower-skilled students as well as those who typically do not participate are afforded increased opportunities to learn and come to view the physical education experience more positively. For example, in their review of over 20 research studies, Wallhead and O'Sullivan (2005) found that the extensive focus on persistent team memberships was a key contributor to creating more equitable learning experiences and improved cooperation and responsibility among students.

Sport Education Model: An Overview

Sport Education's Long-Term Goals

Sport Education has three central long-term goals for students supported by 10 specific objectives, aimed at providing students more complete and authentic sport experiences. Sport Education aims to have students learn to become players in the fullest sense, and have them develop into competent, literate, and enthusiastic sportspersons (Siedentop, Hastie, & van der Mars, 2004).

COMPETENCY IN SPORT. **Competent sportspersons** are those who have sufficient command of the techniques to participate in games and activities with satisfaction. They recognize, understand, and are able to execute strategies and tactics

competent sportspersons People with sufficient skills to 1) participate in games at a satisfactory level, 2) be knowledgeable players, and 3) execute strategies appropriate to their levels and the complexity of the game.

appropriate to the complexity of the activity, and are knowledgeable participants. Sufficient command refers to a level where persons would feel comfortable and confident to participate in a community sport league (such as a city volleyball league).

LITERACY IN SPORT. Truly **literate sportspersons** understand and appreciate the rules, rituals, and traditions that surround sport activities. They can distinguish between good and bad sport practices at the various levels. As well, they are more discerning sport consumers, whether as spectator or fan. This literacy is vital because it helps ensure that sport and activity programs are educationally sound and contribute to a safer, more positive, and saner sport and activity culture.

ENTHUSIASTIC IN SPORT. **Enthusiastic sportspersons** value and find meaning in their sport experiences, and pursue other venues in which to participate. They tend to put more effort into every sport season, take their role in sport seriously, and demonstrate high levels of peer support within their teams. These individuals are eager to share their positive attitude about sport with others in a variety of settings, from working with youth to organizing sport experiences in the community.

Sport Education's Short-Term Objectives

The long-term goals of competency, literacy, and enthusiasm are sought by pursuing 10 short-term objectives during each Sport Education season. As shown in Table 11.1, these objectives align well with NASPE's Content Standards (2004). Recognition of this link is essential when teachers move to standards-based instruction in their program. Good programs stand for something, and clearly articulated goals are a major component of these programs. It is not unusual for teachers to think that because there are new content standards and a push for standards-based programs, they need to develop completely new content to guide their program. In fact, what is needed is a more clear articulation of the relationship among program goals, assessment, and learning experiences.

1. DEVELOP TECHNIQUES AND FITNESS SPECIFIC TO PARTICULAR SPORTS (NASPE STANDARDS 1 & 3). For people to learn to play tennis well, they have to reach some mastery in using serves, drop shots, forehand passing shots, and lobs.

---

literate sportspersons People who understand and appreciate the rules, rituals, and traditions that surround sport and are able to distinguish between good and bad sport practices.

enthusiastic sportspersons People who find additional outlets (outside of class) to participate in that provide meaning to sport experiences and actively support the sport culture.

TABLE 11.1

Relationship of Sport Education's Goals and Objectives with NASPE's Latest National Content Standards

Sport Education's Central Goals	Sport Education's Objectives	NASPE's National Content Standards
Competency	1. Develop Techniques, Tactics, and Fitness Specific to Particular Sports	Standard 1: Demonstrates competency in motor skills and movement patterns needed to perform a variety of physical acivities
	2. Appreciate and Be Able to Execute Strategic Play Specific to Particular Sports	
	3. Participate in Game Contexts Appropriate to Their Stage of Development	Standard 2: Demonstrates understanding of movement concepts, principles, strategies, and tactics as they apply to the learning and performance of physical activities
	4. Work Effectively Within a Group Toward Common Goals	
Literacy	5. Develop and Apply Knowledge About Officiating/Refereeing and Scorekeeping	Standard 3: Participates regularly in physical activity
	6. Provide Responsible Leadership	
	7. Develop the Capacity to Make Reasoned Decisions About Sport Issues	Standard 4: Achieves and maintains a health-enhancing level of physical fitness
	8. Share in the Planning and Administration of Sport Experiences	Standard 5: Exhibits responsible personal and social behavior that respects self and others in physical activity settings
Enthusiasm	9. Understand/Appreciate the Rituals and Conventions That Give Sports Their Unique Meanings	
	10. Decide to Voluntarily Become Involved in Sport Beyond School	Standard 6: Values physical activity for health, enjoyment, challenge, self-expression, and/or social interaction

Alan Launder (2002) refers to these as "techniques." Being able to control and handle an implement in sport is a necessary (though not sufficient) prerequisite to experience success in playing. In addition, players need to be able to move quickly and adjust position on the field or court during most games. Developing good trunk and shoulder flexibility is critical when learning to play golf—not only from an injury prevention perspective, but also for more sound swing execution. The physical conditioning needs differ across sports, as well.

When programs can demonstrate that their students have learned to use the sport techniques and fitness activities unique to that sport, NASPE Content Standard 1 is met. In addition, one can argue that Content Standard 3 is addressed indirectly during physical education classes.

2. Appreciate and Be Able to Execute Strategic Play Specific to Particular Sports (NASPE Standards 1 & 2). Volleying a tennis ball successfully, or trapping a soccer ball during a technique drill, is a level of mastery that will not ensure success in actual game play. Picking the right time to approach the net, and finishing the rally with a well-placed volley in tennis is an example of what Launder (2002) refers to as "skillful play." This lies well beyond isolated technique execution. Recognition of what to do and where to move or position oneself on the field or court during game play requires a higher level of understanding by learners. Hence, this objective directly targets NASPE Content Standard 2.

Moving students to better understanding the games' tactical dimensions can be accomplished by employing the TGFU and Play Practice approaches to instruction (e.g., Griffin, Mitchell, & Oslin, 1997; Launder, 2002; Mitchell, Oslin, & Griffin, 2003). Players using the right techniques and tactics at the right time reflect more advanced levels of decision making (i.e., understanding). Instruction in Sport Education should strike a balance between emphasizing technique and understanding/applying tactics. Both are needed for more skillful play to emerge, and require the teacher to actively instruct during both technique practice and game play.

3. Participate in Game Contexts Appropriate to Their Stage of Development (NASPE Standards 1 & 3). Successful game play can be enhanced if the game structure is appropriately matched to the students' developmental level. Thus, teachers' decision making on what game structure to employ (i.e., via graded competition and/or progressive competition) is critical. Use of small-sided games allows for more active participation by more students in game conditions that are less complex and less overwhelming, especially from a tactical perspective. Hence, quality Sport Education seasons should not include parent game versions.

Modifications such as softer or lighter balls, shorter equipment, nearer or lower targets, larger goals, and playing 3v3 all offer ways to reduce the game's complexity. Such game modifications align well with TGFU and Play Practice approaches, and allow teachers to directly target Content Standards 1 and 3.

4. WORK EFFECTIVELY WITHIN A GROUP TOWARD COMMON GOALS (NASPE STANDARD 5). Sport Education depends largely on getting small heterogeneous groups of students to learn to work together toward common goals in the context of sport. Students are always part of teams (even in the case of "individual" activities), and these teams remain together throughout the entire season. In addition, each team member has additional non-playing **roles** and responsibilities. Team success is very much dependent on each member making contributions and learning to recognize and respect each other. This objective directly targets NASPE Content Standard 5.

A common goal for teams is to finish first in the season's competition. However, in Sport Education, the teams' standing in the league depends not only on games won or lost. Effectively performing non-playing roles and exhibiting fair play at all times are of equal importance. If these aspects of sport are actively taught, and teams recognize how their performance influences the team standings, teammates learn what it means to work together.

5. DEVELOP AND APPLY KNOWLEDGE ABOUT OFFICIATING/REFEREEING AND SCOREKEEPING (NASPE STANDARDS 2 & 5). With few exceptions (e.g., ultimate), sport events rely on the use of game officials to ensure that teams play within the rules of the game. All students will referee/judge and keep score at some point during each season. Opportunities to learn these roles must be built into each season. Through explanation, modeling by the teacher, and most importantly, extensive practice of scorekeeping and refereeing during between-team scrimmages, students can develop these critical skills.

This Sport Education objective directly addresses the completeness and authenticity in students' sport experiences. Thus, it links directly with the cognitively focused Content Standard 2, and by successfully fulfilling their non-playing roles, students also demonstrate responsible and respectful behavior (Content Standard 5).

6. PROVIDE RESPONSIBLE LEADERSHIP (NASPE STANDARD 5). The success of Sport Education seasons is dependent on students learning to take on more responsibilities to ensure the seasons' authenticity. Ideally, high school–level students will seek to have more input into how seasons are designed, how competition is structured, additional student roles that can be included, how **culminating events** can be organized, and so on. This active involvement should

roles   Help students gain a more complete understanding of sport by assigning students to experience roles beyond that of just a participant.
culminating events   Festive, exciting, and appropriate conclusions to sport seasons, which involve all participants.

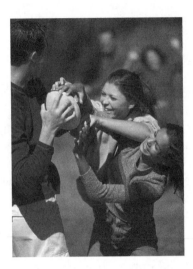

be fostered in elementary and middle school programs, and teachers should gauge which tasks and responsibilities are within the students' grasp.

The role of team coach offers excellent leadership opportunities. Coaches work with their teams to plan practice sessions and choose player positions for games. As students gain more experience over multiple seasons, team coaches (in conjunction with team scouts, perhaps) can design game strategy for upcoming games. A team's fitness trainer is responsible for team conditioning, leading warm-ups, and designing physical conditioning routines for the team geared specifically to the particular sport. The process of infusing leadership roles occurs gradually over multiple seasons. This objective links particularly well with Content Standard 5, as students learn that by taking on leadership roles they can contribute to a more positive sport experience (at the individual, team, and class levels).

7. DEVELOP THE CAPACITY TO MAKE REASONED DECISIONS ABOUT SPORT ISSUES (NASPE STANDARD 5). The responsibilities that students have in Sport Education each requires decision making within and among the teams. As seasons progress and teams compete, tensions and conflicts will often arise, and these need to be resolved in a constructive manner. Because **fair play** is an integral part of Sport Education, issues of what is fair and what is appropriate conduct arise throughout a season. These become critical "teachable moments," where students can be confronted with issues that pertain to their own sport experience. Students can learn to resolve those conflicts with teacher guidance. Such conflicts can serve as springboards to discuss controversial issues in sport be-

fair play   Behaving in positive and cooperative ways so that all participants can enjoy the sport experience.

yond the physical education program. This process can help students become more informed (i.e., literate) about sport practices in various sport settings.

8. SHARE IN THE PLANNING AND ADMINISTRATION OF SPORT EXPERIENCES (NASPE STANDARD 5). In many physical education programs, the only responsibility students have is to follow class rules and do exactly what instructors tell them to do. This is hardly a context within which one would expect people to develop into independent, responsible, and informed players, let alone become leaders in sport and physical activity. As noted earlier, in Sport Education, other key sport roles are learned as well, including that of coach, captain, manager, game official, statistician, conditioning trainer, or member of a sports council. With experience, students can and should become actively involved in the planning and administration of sport seasons. This will allow them to take ownership, and view the total experience in the program as more meaningful, which, according to Ennis (1996, 1999), is often absent. For example, forming even teams for more balanced competition requires students to recognize and respect differences among peers.

9. APPRECIATE THE RITUALS AND CONVENTIONS THAT GIVE SPORTS THEIR UNIQUE MEANINGS (NASPE STANDARD 6). This objective with its strong affective focus relates directly to Content Standard 6. Sport Education aims to take learners beyond learning the techniques and tactics of sport. The development of a deeper appreciation for sport is vital to ensuring what Siedentop et al. (2004) call a more sane **sport culture**. Students should learn not only the appropriate post-game behavior of players, such as thanking the opponents and game officials, but also what it means to truly respect one's opponents, the officials, and the play experience itself. Students should learn about the fundamentals of fair play and playing by the rules (and act accordingly). Such content is central to Sport Education, because we should not assume that students come to us knowing such rituals and conventions of behavior.

10. DECIDE TO VOLUNTARILY BECOME INVOLVED IN SPORT BEYOND SCHOOL (NASPE STANDARD 6). Rarely has the promotion of physical activity behavior beyond the walls of a physical education program been emphasized more than in recent years. If school physical education experience turns students away from physical activity, then even the best opportunities in the community may not draw them in. Students who have learned about sport in a well-taught Sport Education–based program may be more inclined to continue participation, and seek and accept volunteer roles as coaches and/or officials in local community-based sport programs. It is here that, according to Siedentop et al. (2004), Sport Education can help assure that a healthy sport culture is maintained. NASPE's Content Standard 6 targets enjoyment and valuing of physical activity. Sport Education

sport culture The collective beliefs, customs, practices, and behaviors of people in the context of sport; a healthy sport culture contributes to a healthy society.

aims to contribute to this standard, at the individual level and beyond, to ensure that future generations look at sport as an important aspect of the culture.

Sport Education: Its Main Features

As noted, Sport Education is aimed at youth ages 9–18, with the overriding goal to provide them with **authentic (more complete) sport experiences** through the design of developmentally appropriate competition. The following italicized words form key differences with how sport has typically been taught in schools. Sport in society (e.g., community, youth, interscholastic, intercollegiate, and professional) is characterized by enthusiasm, excitement, and passion by participants, spectators, parents, and the surrounding community. Games matter in the context of formal competition; team practices have a purpose, and being on a team means something special. In other words, the sport experience is authentic. Figure 11.1 illustrates the primary features of Sport Education that typically reflect institutional forms of sport. They include seasons, affiliation, formal competition, record keeping, culminating event, and festivity. These features give sport meaning, and make it uniquely different from other types of physical activity and what we typically see in physical education sport.

SEASONS. Sport is done in **seasons**. Seasons are long enough so students have a chance to learn something. Seasons include time for both team practices and formal competition schedules that are central to the success of the season. The length of a season is dependent on various contextual factors. Generally, a complete season in a secondary school program will take approximately 25 class sessions of 50 minutes, or between 12 and 15 lessons in the case of schools with block periods.

A key reason for longer seasons is the need for students to learn to perform essential roles beyond that of a player. That is, students are responsible for learning to keep score, officiate, coach a team, lead conditioning sessions, and so forth. Learning to perform these roles well takes time. As will be shown later, in a longer season with more content to teach, having more time available is crucial both from an instructional perspective and for teachers' assessment efforts.

AFFILIATION. Students are members of teams, and retain membership for the duration of a season. Teams that participate in a season of competition are essentially working toward a set of common goals. Much of what it means to be an athlete, and a significant part of one's personal growth as an athlete, is related to being affiliated with a team. In Sport Education, team success is defined not only by how many games are won, but also by how the various roles were

authentic (more complete) sports experiences Experiences that reflect all of the key characteristics generally seen in institutional versions of sport.
seasons Length of time a sport is played; in sport education, seasons are longer than what is typical in physical education.

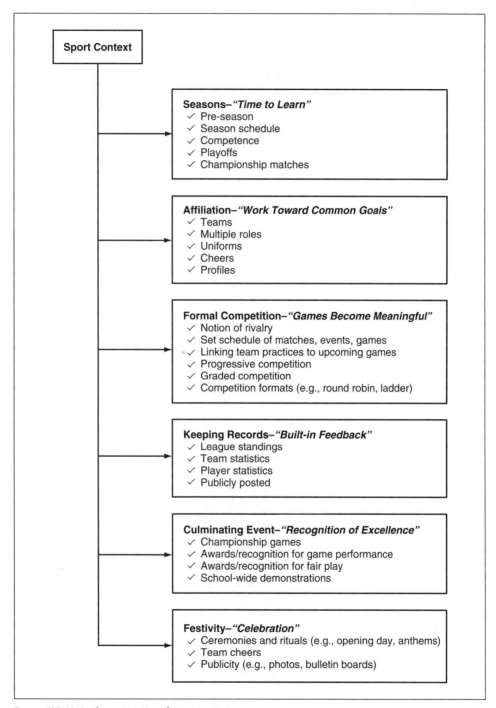

FIGURE 11.1 Main characteristics of sport context.

performed and the level of fair play exhibited. That is, if individual students recognize that their individual efforts across the various non-player roles will contribute to the total team's results, they are more inclined to contribute, thus building a stronger sense of **affiliation**. Teams creating a name, choosing a team color, developing a team cheer, and/or creating a team mascot also serve to strengthen the sense of affiliation.

FORMAL COMPETITION. Sport seasons are defined by a schedule of games or meets around which teams hold team practices. On "Opening Day," all teams know whom they play on which day so they can prepare appropriately. Thus, team practices become more meaningful, because they serve as preparation for scheduled **formal competitions**. Also, the games and contests themselves become more meaningful because they are part of a full schedule that ultimately leads to a season champion. With a longer season, students/teams learn to recognize areas of improvement, and areas of technical and tactical weakness that they must work on to compete equitably in subsequent games.

Competition formats in Sport Education vary from dual meets to round robin, compass, ladder, or event meets with a heavy emphasis on using modified games in order to accommodate students' developmental levels. This is accomplished by using either "progressive" and/or "graded" competition formats. In **"progressive" competition**, a season may start off with a series of 1v1 games that are followed by 2v2 and 4v4 games (depending on how students progress in their game play). Even with teams of 8, the results of each 1v1 game are totaled. **"Graded" competition** includes games at three different skill levels. For example, there might be novice, minor league, and major league divisions. Teams themselves choose which players will compete at which level. And again, the game results from each level are pooled and contribute to each team's position in the league standings.

KEEPING RECORDS. Sport performance **records** come in many different forms. They might include shot attempts, free throw percentage, assists, kills, time, distance, and points per game, shooting averages, or rebounds. Player and

> **affiliation**   Being a member of a team; in sports, this can come out in team names, uniforms, mascots, and working together to achieve a common goal.
> **formal competitions**   Reflected by a schedule that lays out all of the competitions that will make up the season.
> **"progressive" competition**   Becomes more complex as the season progresses, from 1v1 to 3v3 to 4v4, depending on how the game performance develops.
> **"graded" competition**   Based on levels of performance—novice or advanced, minor leagues or major league, and recreational or competitive.
> **records**   Provide feedback to players, can be used as an assessment for the teacher, or can help as a goal setting tool for players; tracking student performance can vary from shots on goal to gymnastics event scores.

team records offer important feedback for teams to help recognize where team and individual performance has taken place, set goals for further improvements, and plan for team practices. For example, a soccer team that reduces turnovers and can increase possession time increases its chances of success. A sprinter in track and field who reduces his or her time on the 60-meter sprint race has improved. In activities such as dance and gymnastics, the results would consist of judged performances.

Siedentop et al. (2004) points to the importance of keeping (and publicizing!) records because they serve to define standards of performance, and can become an important part of the tradition of a sport. It is here that the important roles of scorekeepers, team statisticians, and team publicists become clear. Team statisticians become responsible for maintaining, updating, and making public the team's performance records. At the same time, these same records provide teachers with authentic forms of student assessment.

CULMINATING EVENT. It is inherent in sport to identify which individuals and teams perform the best in a particular season. In collegiate and professional sport in the United States, events such as the NCAA finals in basketball, American football's Super Bowl, and baseball's World Series have become events of national importance. Internationally, the summer and winter Olympics and soccer's World Cup serve a similar function. Though on a smaller scale, culminating events in Sport Education can create similar excitement within a class, and sometimes even for an entire school.

Culminating events can be structured in a variety of ways. They may include a two-day track and field competition, a 3v3 volleyball competition, or a skills challenge competition. However, the culminating event need not always be a game-related event. For example, a frequently used culminating event has been the awards banquet, during which team, individual, and league awards are presented. It might also take the form of having a well-known guest speaker attend and give a talk on the sport being played.

FESTIVITY. The *festive* nature that surrounds sport can be seen everywhere in the world and at every level of sport, from the state championship to the local Friday night high school game, from the pageantry of the Olympic Games to the state track and field finals, from the World Cup in soccer to the Saturday afternoon youth soccer games on a community field. The festive nature of sport provides excitement and meaning for the participants, and adds an essential social element to the experience. In Sport Education, **festivity** is created in many

festivity   A celebration that is present in sport of all levels; Sport Education encourages making sport festive by building the team spirit, publicizing records, creating team cheers, taking pictures, and holding culminating events that are meaningful to all learners.

ways, including the use of team names, colors, and pictures; publicizing team and individual performances; "Opening Day" ceremonies; celebrating fair play; and creating publicity within the school for the Sport Education seasons.

Sport and Sport Education: Not the Same Game

As noted by Siedentop et al. (2004), Sport Education differs in three essential ways from how sport is practiced in community, high school, and collegiate, international, and professional settings. They include:

PARTICIPATION REQUIREMENTS. The rule is simple: **Everybody plays**—no exceptions. Regardless of the players' skill level, the time of season, level of competition—everyone plays. This can be accomplished by designing the competition around small-sided games, thus preventing domination by higher-skilled players. In addition, season tournaments are never structured so that teams get eliminated.

DEVELOPMENTALLY APPROPRIATE GAME FORMATS. For most beginners, the adult version of a game is overly complex, and likely reduces the chance for success in the early stage of learning. In Sport Education, the games used for competition should match the developmental level and needs of the players.

ROLES BEYOND THAT OF A PLAYER. As noted, students learn to perform the many other roles and responsibilities that surround sport. Learning to be a coach, trainer, official, scorekeeper, and/or statistician contributes to making the experience more complete and more authentic. If participation by all, modified game structures, and/or diversity in student roles are absent, the curriculum loses its central educational focus.

The types of roles vary by the sport/activity that is the focus of the season, the number of students and their age, the students' previous experience in sport and particularly Sport Education, and the ideas that both the teacher and the students can identify. Identifying role responsibilities, designing materials to assist students in performing these roles, and determining how students will learn to perform these roles can be time consuming. However, once you have begun to develop these and begin to see the result of students taking responsibility for their teams and their sport experiences, it becomes worthwhile. We encourage you not to try to start your first season with all of these roles because it may be a bit overwhelming for both you and the students. Start small, select the roles that might provide you with the most assistance and that the students might be

everybody plays   A playing requirement of Sport Education where everyone is a participant; in Sport Education, sport should be developmentally appropriate so all players can take part and feel valued.

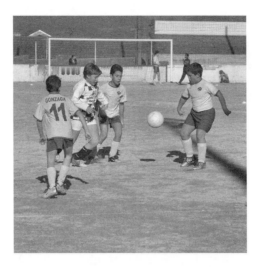

most familiar with, and then build from there. Roles generally fall within four different categories:

- *Player:* Every student is a player and is expected to participate on this level throughout the season.
- *Duty team/flights:* This role is actually one that all students must be able to perform on competition days and might include referee, scorekeeper, event director, or judge. It may be that you have a "lead" team member in charge of each of these roles who takes responsibility for ensuring that all team members are prepared to meet the expectations of the role on a given day.
- *Team roles:* These are those roles that assist in the smooth running of a season and the cooperative nature within a team. For instance, the team trainer might be in charge of the warm-up and cool-down component of class while the team manager is charged with ensuring the team space is set up and all equipment is available and in good working condition. The team captain would be responsible for the "nuts and bolts" of daily organization as well as arrangements for team entries in competitions while the team coach plans for and directs team practice sessions and oversees team performance on a daily basis as well as during competition. A sport journalist (Figure 11.2) or sport photographer is a role that can add an additional element of festivity and reality to the season.
- *Specialist roles:* These roles relate specifically to the activity or sport that is guiding the season. For example, you might have a choreographer in dance, a field events coordinator or place judge in track and field, a timekeeper in cross country, a lane judge in swimming, or a spotter in weight training. These specialist roles may not have duties to perform on a daily basis, yet they are none the less important to team cohesion.

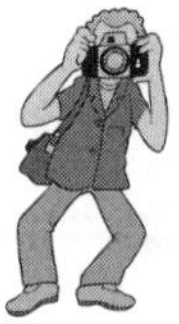

I, _____ , agree to take
responsibility for the following tasks throughout the season:

1. Take team photos for sports board and newsletter.

2. Develop a weekly story that highlights one of the teams.

3. Design, print, and distribute an end-of-season newsletter.

Signature _____

FIGURE 11.2 Sport journalist contract.

Sport Education's Philosophy

At the curricular level, Sport Education seeks to create learning conditions that 1) offer students opportunities to learn the subject matter (sport) more authentically, 2) increase the chances of students learning the subject matter more completely, and 3) make the experiences more important and relevant for all students. This can be accomplished only if students are given sufficient time, and are provided with content that reflects the full nature of the sport experience.

At the instructional level, Sport Education changes daily life for both teachers and students. Instead of teachers being in charge of everything and students simply doing as they are told, Sport Education is a more student-centered model (Alexander et al., 1998) where students become increasingly more invested in the experience by helping and learning from each other. This gradual shift toward making the program more student-centered occurs over multiple seasons and across grade levels. Teachers need to carefully gauge what types of roles and responsibilities students can handle. The initial research on teachers and students' responses to employing Sport Education suggests that if the model is implemented faithfully, the product sells itself.

Teachers who wish to implement Sport Education need to recognize two critical changes that have to occur if Sport Education is to flourish. The first occurs in the role that teachers play. Teachers who have traditionally been the sole source of information and have served as "traffic cops" will, in fact, have more opportunity to actively instruct students as the season progresses. Thorough planning and preparation by the teacher will allow for many of the managerial tasks to be handled by students. Once the tasks and responsibilities of the various student roles have been practiced and learned, and once students recognize that the team's standing in the league competition is based on games won, fair play, and performance in non-playing roles, much of the general class management will become more seamless. That is, teams know where they are supposed to be for practices and for games; non-playing teams know that they are responsible for serving as referees, scorekeepers, and so on. Consequently, teachers find they have an increased opportunity to cover more content and actively instruct students throughout the season.

The second change is one of increased student ownership in the design and management of the Sport Education seasons. In traditional physical education classes, students mostly follow teachers' directions and become involved in the sport only as players. In contrast, within Sport Education they become actively involved in tasks such as selecting teams, becoming a member of the sport board, or learning to be a game official, scorekeeper, team captain, or publicist. As students gain experience in doing Sport Education, the number and sophistication of students' roles increase.

Planning a Sport Education season involves issues that revolve around the framework for the season: organization, sequencing and progressions, and management. On a second level, teachers must plan for and design student learning experiences that relate to the specific sport or activity around which the season is framed. Within this planning phase there must be room for student involvement as they begin to take charge of their own learning experiences under the guidance of a knowledgeable and informed teacher. Table 11.2 provides a worksheet to take you through the design of a Sport Education season on an outline level to guide your development/selection of materials, learning experiences, and assessment tools.

Assessment Within Sport Education

If Sport Education intends to provide children and youth with authentic and realistic sport experiences, then it is only appropriate that assessment strategies be designed to determine how well this goal is achieved. This will also allow teachers to determine how instruction might better be designed to facilitate student success and provide students with a means of documenting their progress. Questions the teacher might ask include: Are students able to demonstrate skills and tactics in "real" game situations that are in line with their individual development? Do we see strategic play that is appropriate for the sport in which students are participating? Are teams able to work cooperatively toward a season goal, which they set and define? During game play, are student officials making appropriate calls and enforcing correct consequences? When serving as team captains, do we observe students using positive and effective leadership skills to

TABLE 11.2

Sport Education Season Design

This outline plans for the design and implementation of a sport education season. Once the plan is complete, use it to guide development of tools and materials to facilitate implementation of the season. Be innovative, personalizing the season to reflect you and what you deem important.

1. **Context for season**	
a. Age group (Elem 4–6, MS, HS)	
b. Sport	
2. **Content standard(s)/outcome(s) to be assessed**	
a. Competency	
b. Literacy	
c. Enthusiasm	
3. **Assessment tool(s) to be used**	
a. Play performance	
b. Duty team	
c. Fair play	
4. **Teams**	
a. Number of teams	
b. Team size	
c. Team selection process	
d. Building affiliation (team name, color, mascot, cheer, team space)	
5. **Roles**	
a. Determining roles	
b. Defining roles	
c. Students selecting roles	
d. Strategies for teaching roles	
6. **Class management**	
a. Fair play agreement	
b. Routines (link to teams and student roles)	
7. **Festivity**	
a. Awards	
b. Recognition	
c. Rituals and traditions	

Continued

TABLE 11.2	
Sport Education Season Design—Cont'd	
8. Season design	
a. Daily practice	
b. Practice and game play connections	
c. Competitive schedule	
d. Culminating event	
9. Record keeping	
a. Daily records	
b. Statistics	
c. Portfolio	
10. Extra touches	
a. Newsletter	
b. Handbook	
c. Creative options	
11. Sport/activity focus	
a. Concept map	
b. Learning outcomes	
c. Learning experiences	
d. Instructional strategies	
e. Student task cards	
12. **Final season plan** (developing materials to implement above plans)	

guide their peers? When given the opportunity, do students choose to become involved in sport experiences outside of physical education as participants, coaches of younger youth, or in some other capacity? As spectators in after school or community sport, are students able and willing to stand up for what is "right," when fair play comes into question? As noted in Table 11.1, these are the types of skills, knowledge, and behaviors we would expect students to demonstrate as a result of participating in a Sport Education season, and tend to integrate the standards in a holistic way.

With seasons longer than the traditional physical education unit, teachers have more time in which to assess student performance. In addition, having students working together in a team context allows them to be involved more easily in peer assessment. Assessments that are authentic serve to motivate youth, and are more meaningful because they provide realistic and applied knowledge on "how am I doing?" What might these authentic assessments look like, how are they implemented, and what tools are necessary? It is important to keep in mind that assessments are also learning tools for students to improve performance. As in sport, games are the best assessment there is because they let the player know if he or she is developing the skills necessary to be successful.

As we know, when designing assessment measures it is critical to ask, what was the intended outcome for student performance? If these goals were the intended learning and guided instruction, then the assessment tasks should match the goals. For Sport Education, this suggests that if we chose competency, literacy, or enthusiasm, and the aligned objectives to guide our instruction, then we should design assessment tools that would let us know if students reached those goals. Referring back to Table 11.1 will provide a framework to guide this discussion.

One Sport Education goal aligned with NASPE Standard 1 is development of skills, tactics, and strategic play in a game-like setting. Instruction would include what these skills look like, when they are used, how they are performed, and students practicing them during game play. Assessment, therefore, should take place during games to give students the opportunity to demonstrate that they can perform the skills, tactics, and strategies successfully at a level appropriate to their development. For example, if a teacher chooses to focus on students' development relative to transition play in basketball, Figure 11.3 provides a tool the teacher can use to analyze this aspect during the games played as part of a basketball season. Team players can also be invited to self-assess their game performance/improvement using the tool presented in Figure 11.4.

Because a basketball season is longer in Sport Education than the typical unit seen in more traditional physical education, students will have increased opportunities to engage in more authentic learning (i.e., basketball matches). Coupled with the increased involvement in managing the season by students, the teacher can actually devote time to ongoing formative (and formal) assessment of students across the intended outcomes. For example, for each lesson teachers might select three to four students who would be the "students of the day" for the purpose of actually observing and recording assessment data. Such assessments can focus on game play performance, students' knowledge, and/or fair play. Regular season games are not to be considered "testing" days (as in traditional end-of-unit skill tests or written tests). Thus, teachers can and should use the information they gather and inform students about their performance/development.

As the season progresses, teachers can always return to re-assessing students who they formally assessed earlier in the season. Thus, the assessment of student learning not only becomes more authentic, but also is more fair because students will have multiple opportunities throughout the season to demonstrate their progress toward competency (i.e., meeting the standard), as opposed to the one-shot opportunity on an end-of-unit skill or written test.

Select the term that best matches the player or players' performance for the observed skill/tactics(s).

Skill/Level	EXCEEDS (Mastery/Competence) (3)	MEETS (Emerging/Coping) (2)	DEVELOPING (Struggling/Surviving) (1)
Off-the-ball play Transition play	**Switches quickly** between offense and defense Able to **double team at right time**, looking to force a turnover by opponent Adjusts to the position/direction of ball and teammates in both offense and defense **Initiates fast breaks quickly**, looking to counterattack opponents	Does respond to changes in possession, but at times still slowly, thus delaying contribution **Recovers** back behind the ball on defense **slowly** Is **reactive to counterattack** opportunities, therefore limiting fast break opportunities **At times still lingers with ball**, thus missing fast break opportunites	Only **watches the ball** Waits around for other team-mates to regain ball possession OR **Does not move with team** when it regains ball possession

Observed Students' Names:	Rating (1–3):
1.	
2.	
3.	
4.	
5.	
6.	
7.	
8.	
9.	
10.	

Observer Name: _____   Date: _____

FIGURE 11.3 Analyzing transition play in basketball.

Source: Adapted from Siedentop, D., Hastie, P. A., & van der Mars, H. (2004). *Complete Guide to Sport Education*. Champaign, IL: Human Kinetics.

Name _____

On- and off-the-ball skills/movements

Strong player   Adequate player   Getting better

Improved during season

3 = a great deal   2 = somewhat   1 = a little

During the season I was able to . . .	On- and off-the ball-skills/movements			Improved during season
	Getting better	Adequate player	Strong player	1, 2, or 3
Successfully serve using the overhead floater serve				
Forearm pass to the setter				
Open up and set to the hitter				
Transition off the net to set up for an attack				
Perform a hit to win the point				
Communicate with my teammates by consistently calling for the ball				
Set up and play cooperatively as a member of my team				
Improve my overall game play				
Help defend court space				

FIGURE 11.4 Volleyball game play self-assessment.

Student ability to apply knowledge of officiating or scorekeeping is a goal guiding instruction in Sport Education that fits into NASPE Standard 2. There are several ways in which this type of knowledge can be assessed. For example, teachers can employ the assessment tool in Figure 11.5, which reflects students' ability to use the knowledge of basketball's most basic game rules "in action." Students can be asked to self-assess their officiating performance following each turn at serving as the game's referee. An initial written scenario quiz, given prior to the opening day of the season, would allow the teacher to determine who is ready to tackle officiating a contest (e.g., we have heard of teachers using the successful passing of such pre-season quizzes as a qualifier for subsequent seeding in the season's tournament). The use of peer feedback on how well an official monitored and directed game play would also provide useful information for students as they learn this role and demonstrate achievement of this standard. During pre-season scrimmages, the assessment tool shown in Figure 11.5 can be used by students to determine if they can recognize when their peers are breaking rules during a game of basketball. Once they have done this, they might be ready to demonstrate knowledge by passing an officiating exam for a given sport and be assigned to an officiating role based on their score (lead official, apprentice, or assistant).

NASPE Standard 3 focuses on students participating regularly in physical activity, and is a key element of Sport Education. The instructional aspect of this model encourages small-sided games to allow students to have more opportunity to be active in a game-like context. Asking students to respond to a reflective journal focused on their activity involvement would provide a self-report measure of activity level, as would a team activity participation log kept by the trainer or an event task card that records activity responses for each student. Obviously, game play statistics would show the students' participation level, as would the wearing of a pedometer throughout the season. The latter tool would allow teachers to accumulate important data on the degree to which students are meeting the recommended levels of physical activity for Physical Education as reflected in the United States' national health objectives and guidelines for physical activity (e.g., U.S. Department of Health and Human Services, 2000, 2008).

Although achievement and maintenance of fitness is not a primary focus of Sport Education, it is certainly an excellent opportunity for students to learn about the types of fitness activities appropriate to improve sport performance, and assist them in meeting the physical conditioning demands of a selected sport. An indirect fitness assessment for Sport Education is students having the stamina to complete an entire competition, the flexibility to meet the demands of a given sport with maximal performance and without injury, and the agility to successfully move in response to game play. These are informal assessments because they are measured by student accomplishment and teacher observa-

Select the term that best matches the player or players' performance for the observed skill/tactics(s).

Skill/Level	EXCEEDS (Mastery/Competence) (3)	MEETS (Emerging/Coping) (2)	DEVELOPING (Struggling/Surviving) (1)
Knowledge of rules	*Few, if any, basic rule violations* (e.g., steps out-of-bounds) *Restarts games appropriately* (i.e., passes ball in play) *Acceptable physical contract* with opponents (eg., going for ball)	*Double dribble* and *travel violations occur infrequently* *Restarts game appropriately* (i.e., passes ball in play) *Sporadic physical contact* with opponents Appears *aware of violation(s)*	Regularly *double dribbles* and/or *travels* Runs with ball *Restarts game inappropriately* (e.g., starts to dribble off and out-of-bounds) *Uncontrolled and perhaps excessive physical contact* with opponents Appears *unaware of violation(s)*

Observed Students' Names:	Rating (1–3):
1.	
2.	
3.	
4.	
5.	
6.	
7.	
8.	
9.	
10.	

Observer Name:	Date:

FIGURE 11.5 Knowledge of rules in basketball.

Source: Adapted from Siedentop, D., Hastie, P. A., & van der Mars, H. (2004). *Complete Guide to Sport Education.* Champaign, IL: Human Kinetics.

tion, yet they address the intent of NASPE Standard 4—achieving and maintaining a health-enhancing level of physical fitness. Having students maintain a journal reflecting on their fitness development during game play would be useful for goal setting and its measurement.

Sport Education can also target physical fitness directly. Just like "nontraditional" activities such as dance and orienteering, Sport Education allows for the design of a fitness conditioning season (Sweeney et al., 1992). Teams train together and compete by engaging in cardiovascular and muscular strength/endurance activities on alternating days throughout the season, with competitions designed using various formats.

Standard 5, students exhibiting responsible personal and social behavior that respects self and others in physical activity settings, is a huge focus of Sport Education. A number of useful instruments can be designed to assess personal decision making, fair play behaviors demonstrated during game play, leadership demonstrated as part of a given role, and how well students achieved as a cooperative member of a team. One such tool, displayed in Figure 11.6, asks students to assess the type of team player they are each week during a season; a record of this can be maintained in a season portfolio. Siedentop et al. (2004) also included several assessment tools specifically geared for assessing students' fair play behavior. Self-assessing role performance of a captain, trainer, or publicist might involve a checklist, criteria rubric, or reflective journal. This same student could receive feedback from a peer or each member of his or her team through a roles and responsibilities checklist. In another instance, being a "good" team member is demonstrated daily by being on time to practice, dressed in uniform, supporting all teammates regardless of ability level, contributing to all team efforts (portfolio, competition, team poster), and performing the assigned role completely. Each of these assessments demonstrates student achievement of NASPE Standard 5; an example can be viewed in Figure 11.7 where captains are asked to assess their performance as team captain in a badminton season.

Each day when we observe students reporting quickly to their team court to begin warming up, acknowledging a well-played point by an opponent, or challenging themselves to strive toward higher goals, we are observing them work toward achieving NASPE Standard 6 (i.e., values physical activity for health, enjoyment, challenge, self-expression, and/or social interaction). These all demonstrate informal assessments of this standard. Completing an investigative assignment that requires identification of community outlets, costs, and requirements for participation in golf, or defining traditions, rituals, or conventions unique to soccer would be a more formal measure of this standard.

A number of well-designed, effective, and easy-to-use assessment strategies have been developed for use in Sport Education (Siedentop et al., 2004; Townsend, Mohr, Rairigh, & Bulger, 2003, 2006). The National Council for

Your Task: At the close of each week, self-assess your participation as a team player in the gymnastics season by sharing at least one thing you did in the category. Keep this assessment in your season portfolio.

Active and Fair Player
- Followed Fair Play Agreement and prompted others to do so
- Frequently shared ideas with team
- Provided support to team and individual players
- Played an active and substantive role as a team member
- Helped to build a festive and enjoyable season
- Served as a leader by taking on my individual team/duty role
- Interacted with peers and the teacher in a positive way.

Helpful Player
- Occasionally shared ideas with team
- Occasionally provided support to team and individual players
- Played a role as a team member
- Played a role in team/class activities
- Served as a member of class learning experiences, occasionally leading
- Interacted with peers and the instructor in a positive yet non-specific way

Less than Adequate Player
- Did not share ideas with team
- Did not support team or individual players
- Did only what was necessary in team/class activities
- Did only what was necessary as a team member
- Server as a reluctant member of class in team learning experiences
- Interacted with peers and the teacher only when necessary

FIGURE 11.6 Assess your team player behavior.

Curriculum and Assessment (NCCA), in conjunction with the Junior Cycle Physical Education Support Services in Ireland, has developed a set of assessment tools that both teachers and students have found helpful in determining progress toward learning goals (MacPhail & Halbert, 2009). One of these tools, the assessment wheel displayed in Figure 11.8, provides the opportunity for students to assess their own performance for given learning outcomes by shadowing in their level of achievement on the wheel and then commenting on that performance in the student space provided. The teacher is then able to review the student's self-assessment and provide his or her view on student performance by marking a solid line around the boundary of the wheel where he or she feels the student is

Coach/Captain

Reflect upon your performance in the role you selected. Review the criteria outlined below for which you agreed to be responsible. Assess your performance of these responsibilities as we progress through the season.

3 = strong   2 = adequate   1 = need improvement

3	2	1	
			Checked season board daily and shared new and important information with team
			Reported team attendance, uniforms, and timeliness to season board
			Led practice sessions on team court following warm-up with trainer
			Submitted practice plans, as assigned, to the teacher at beginning of week
			Led team in determining flights for practice and competition
			Monitored safety in practice and games
			Hustled team when transitioning
			Took the initiative to determine how else my role might take responsibility
			Resolved any disputes that surfaced within team
			Submitted reflection of practice session

Identify what you *will* do to strengthen your role performance.
1.

2.

3.

Comments

FIGURE 11.7 Badminton season assessment of role.

performing. This type of formative assessment could prove useful in Sport Education by providing an overall picture of how the student and teacher perceive student achievement and where further instruction or practice might be useful, and could be repeated at various points during the season (pre-season, competition, and culminating).

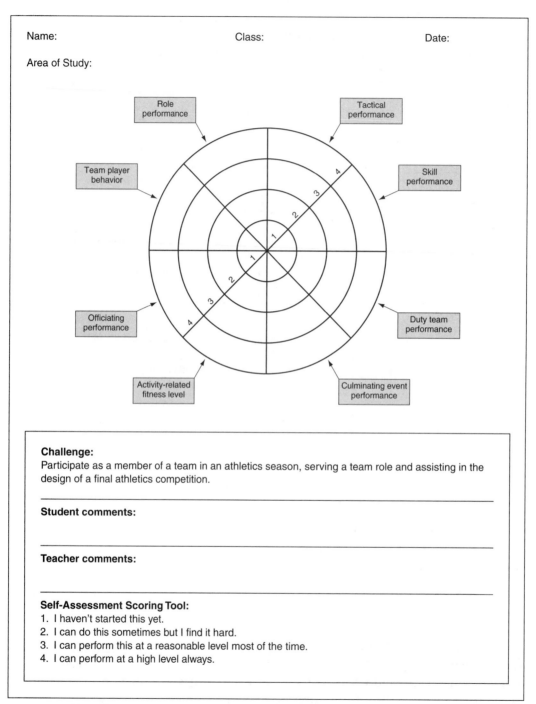

Name: Class: Date:

Area of Study:

Challenge:
Participate as a member of a team in an athletics season, serving a team role and assisting in the design of a final athletics competition.

Student comments:

Teacher comments:

Self-Assessment Scoring Tool:
1. I haven't started this yet.
2. I can do this sometimes but I find it hard.
3. I can perform this at a reasonable level most of the time.
4. I can perform at a high level always.

FIGURE 11.8 Athletics season student's record of learning.

Source: Adapted from Junior Cycle Physical Education. *Guidelines for teachers.* Ireland: National Council for Curriculum Assessment.

Sport Education in Action: Tahoma Middle and High School

What does Sport Education look like in practice? Numerous sources provide examples of how Sport Education is applied and adapted to the learning context, the sport, and the students participating (Bechtel, O'Sullivan, & Oliver, 2001; Siedentop et al., 2004; Sweeney et al., 1992). Teachers in two secondary schools in Maple Valley, Washington, have committed themselves to designing and delivering Sport Education seasons for all sports they offer across the 7–12 curriculum. Seasons at the middle school level include soccer, basketball, badminton, lacrosse, pickleball, volleyball, and weight training. The high school program includes and extends Sport Education beyond these activities to softball, flag football, dance, aerobics, and outdoor adventure. When they first began, the teachers worked in pairs to develop the learning goals and design the block plan, learning experiences, and instructional/assessment materials necessary to deliver an effective Sport Education season to meet the stated goals. They consulted the literature and those knowledgeable about the model, yet have learned from their students and each other on a daily basis about what works and what needs to be adapted for their settings. The overall response of these teachers is that Sport Education does make a difference, to both the students and the teachers. They find that students who in the past were unwilling to dress or take part are now excited and eager to participate in all aspects of class. Peer pressure to be a contributing member of the team has had a huge impact on student effort and team camaraderie. With students taking more responsibility for their own sport experience, the teachers find they have more time to interact with and teach students in a one-on-one fashion.

In both the middle school and high school setting, classes are 100 minutes every other day, with the first 30 minutes focused on fitness. Classes are run independently, jointly (team taught), or in a combination format for competitions. Table 11.3 provides the outline teachers used to guide initial season planning, and highlights student roles, the competition format, festivity and affiliation strategies, and an outline of assessment measures. Once these key points are determined, teachers move on to designing a season block plan such as that shown in Table 11.4.

Teachers are quickly learning that students do not know how to take responsibility for their sport experience and different roles, which Sport Education encourages. Teaching these skills and behaviors is like teaching anything else; it requires guidance, modeling, practice, and feedback. Development of teaching tools to guide team members in the learning process is fundamental to teaching with this model, and is admittedly time consuming initially. Examples of Sport Education materials and tools used in this setting, as well as others, are provided in the ancillary materials accompanying this text.

TABLE 11.3

Initial Planning for Tahoma High School Volleyball Season

Season Goals:
- For learners to gain enough skill and tactical knowledge to successfully partici-pate in a volleyball season
- For learners to work together to successfully perform as a team that shows fair play and respect
- For learners to develop leadership skills and/or respect for those peers who are performing leadership roles

Length of Season:	12 lessons (100 minutes every other day with first 30 minutes focused on fitness)
Class Size:	40 students
Number of Teams:	6
Roles:	Captain, coach, referee

Nature of Competition:
- Round Robin Tournament to determine seeding for championship tournament. Round Robin games are played to 15 points.
- Championship Tournament consists of the best of 3 games each played to 15 points.

Assessment:	Skill and tactical play assessment conducted by coaches to inform practice plans, and guided by a teacher-developed checklist.

Festivity & Affiliation Strategies

Team			Awards	Culminating Event	
Team Name	Team Banner	Individual	Fair Play Points	Championship Game	Awards Day
Team Chant	Team Photos	Team	Certificates	Banquet	

Sport Education: Its Benefits, Limitations, and Cautions

Developing a coherent K–12 physical education program is a daunting task re-gardless of the primary focus. Building a program using Sport Education as the guiding model is no different. In this chapter, we have tried to demonstrate how teachers implementing Sport Education, with authentic and meaningful approaches to student assessment, can show how NASPE's Content Standards can be targeted. We believe that Sport Education, when faithfully implemented, brings with it several benefits, but we would be remiss if we didn't offer several limitations and cautions for teachers.

TABLE 11.4

Tahoma High School Volleyball Block Plan

Days	Instructional Focus		Application Context (i.e., type of game)	Sport Education Focus
	Technique (Skill)	Strategy/Tactic		
1			3v3 Practice Games	Selection of Captains and Teams
2	Skill evaluation by coach		3v3 Practice Games with New Teams	Selection of Coach Coaching Clinic
3	Passing	Forearm pass to target (setter) with/without movement to ball	Team Practice (coach-led) Practice Game	Selection of Team Officials Rules Clinic
4	Passing	Overhead pass (set) to target (hitter) with/without movement to ball	Team Practice (coach-led) Practice Game	
5	Digging	Hard toss Out of net	Team Practice (coach-led) Begin Round Robin Tourney	
6	Serving	Overhead and underhand for accuracy	Team Practice (coach-led) Round Robin	
7	Hitting/Blocking	Drills for technique and accuracy	Team Practice (coach-led) Round Robin	
8	To be determined by coach evaluation	As specified by practice plan (coach)	Team Practice (coach-led) Complete Round Robin	Coach's Skill Evaluations and Practice Plans Due
9			Begin Championship Tournament	Team Posters, Chant, and Warm-up
10			Continue Championship Tournament	Team Posters, Chant, and Warm-up
11			Complete Championship Tournament	Team Posters, Chant, and Warm-up
12				Awards Banquet

BENEFITS. The Sport Education model offers teachers the following benefits:

1. A clear focus that aligns well with current trends in education, both in terms of its goals and objectives, and the instructional approaches.
2. Aims to include all students, not just the privileged or gifted.
3. Allows teachers to spend more time actively instructing the subject matter and assessing students' progress.
4. Students experience more authentic and complete learning experiences that reflect the context of sport as experienced beyond school; that is, they learn to be more than just players.
5. Sport Education can be applied to "non-traditional" activities as well, including dance, orienteering, and fitness/conditioning courses. As noted earlier, a fitness conditioning season could be designed around alternating days of muscular strength/endurance activities and cardiovascular activities. Assessment can revolve around teams' improvement of process indicators (e.g., total miles traveled by a team) and/or product indicators (e.g., performance on fitness test components).
6. If assessment is employed well, teachers can demonstrate program impact across the three learning domains.
7. The research base on Sport Education shows quite consistently that when implemented faithfully, teachers and students like it.

LIMITATIONS AND CAUTIONS. The following do not necessarily apply only to Sport Education, but are important to note:

1. *Overcoming the inertia to begin:* Implementing Sport Education demands extensive planning and forethought on the part of teachers. The model calls for new roles and responsibilities for both teachers and students. However, especially in secondary school programs, the more active involvement by students in designing seasons can foster a greater sense of ownership.
2. *Needed class management skills:* It does not matter that Sport Education looks great on paper. Successful implementation will not occur unless teachers employ the class management skills known to be associated with effective teaching.
3. *Teacher content knowledge:* Teachers will find that as seasons progress, students will seek assistance in performing better as a team, because the competition is more meaningful. Increasingly, the instructional focus will shift toward the tactical dimensions of sports and games.
4. *Start small and build on the previous seasons:* Teachers are strongly encouraged to try Sport Education with sports and activities with which they are more knowledgeable. Initial seasons need only include basic, non-playing roles (e.g., referees/judges, scorekeepers, publicists, statisticians, and coaches). As these roles become more "routine," and students

understand the associated responsibilities, additional roles can be added (e.g., sport boards, team scout, broadcasters).

Summary

Historically, the type of passion and enthusiasm surrounding sport has been largely absent in physical education classes. Many students find their sport experiences in physical education classes to lack relevance and meaning. The Sport Education model seeks to reverse this negative trend. It aims to foster competency, literacy, and enthusiasm in sport by creating more authentic and complete learning experiences for students. The latter are matched with the students' developmental levels. Sport's authenticity is maintained by ensuring that the central features of sport (e.g., affiliation, season, formal competition) are present. Learning experiences are more complete by having students learn to perform roles beyond that of player/performer. Such roles include coach, scorekeeper, game official, and publicist. The intent is for students to take an active part in the organization and design of the season, in which teams that are evenly matched compete with each other. Consequently, Sport Education shifts the roles of both teachers and students.

The season champions are determined not only by the number of events or games won, but also by how teams performed other roles and exhibited fair play behavior. For programs employing Sport Education to demonstrate impact, teachers need to assess students on all three dimensions of competency, literacy, and enthusiasm. Assessments related to NASPE Content Standards should occur throughout the entire season. Assessments aimed at demonstrating competence in technical and tactical aspects of game play should occur during games/events that are part of the formal competition, in order to maintain their authenticity.

References

Alexander, K., Taggart, A., & Luckman, J. (1998). The Sport Education crusade down under. *Journal of Physical Education, Recreation and Dance, 69*(4), 21–23.

Alexander, K., & Luckman, J. (2001). Australian teachers' perceptions and uses of the sport education curriculum model. *European Physical Education Review, 7*(3), 243–267.

Almond, L. (1977). *Physical education in schools.* London: Kogan Page.

Bechtel, P. A., O'Sullivan, M., & Oliver, R. M. (2001). Implementing Sport Education: staying sane when making change. *Strategies, 15,* 19–24.

Bell, C. (1998). Sport education in elementary school. *Journal of Physical Education, Recreation, and Dance, 69*(3), 36–48.

Bennet, G., & Hastie, P. (1997). A Sport Education curriculum model for a collegiate physical activity course. *Journal of Physical Education, Recreation and Dance, 68*(1), 39–44.

Carlson, T. B. (1995). "We hate gym": student alienation from physical education. *Journal of Teaching in Physical Education, 14*, 467–477.

Collier, C. (1998). Sport Education and preservice education. *Journal of Physical Education, Recreation and Dance, 69*(5), 44–45.

Corbin, C. B., & Lindsey, R. (1997). *Fitness for life teacher's edition* (4th ed.). Glenview, IL: Scott Foresman.

Corbin, C. B., & Lindsey, R. (2005). *Fitness for life* (5th ed.). Champaign, IL: Human Kinetics.

Curnow, J., & MacDonald, D. (1995). Can sport education be gender inclusive: a case study in upper primary school. *The ACHPER Health Lifestyles Journal, 42*(4), 911.

Ennis, C. D. (1996). Students' experiences in sport-based physical education: (more than) apologies are necessary. *Quest, 48*, 453–456.

Ennis, C. D. (1999). Creating a culturally relevant curriculum for disengaged girls. *Sport, Education and Society, 4*, 31–49.

Grant, B. C. (1992). Integrating sport into the physical education curriculum in New Zealand secondary schools. *Quest, 44*, 304–316.

Graves, M. A., & Townsend, J. S. (2000.) Applying the Sport Education curriculum model to dance. *Journal of Physical Education, Recreation and Dance, 71*(8), 50–54.

Griffin, L. L., Mitchell, S. A., & Oslin, J. L. (1997). *Teaching sports concepts and skills: a tactical games approach*. Champaign, IL: Human Kinetics.

Hastie, P. (1998). The participation and perception of girls within a unit of sport education. *Journal of Teaching in Physical Education, 17*(4), 151–171.

Hastie, P., & Sharpe, T. (1999). Effects of sport education curriculum on the positive social behavior of at-risk rural adolescent boys. *Journal of Education for Students Placed At Risk, 4*(4), 417–430.

Hastie, P. A. (2003). Sport education. In A. Laker (Ed.), *The future of physical education: building a new pedagogy* (pp. 121–135). New York: Routledge, Taylor, & Francis.

Kim, J., Penney, D., & Cho, M. (2006). "Not business as usual": Sport Education pedagogy in practice. *European Physical Education Review, 12*(3), 361–379.

Kinchin, G. (2001). A high skilled pupil's experiences with Sport Education. *ACHPER Healthy Lifestyles Journal, 48*, 5–9.

Kinchin, G., MacPhail, A., & Ni Chroinin, D. (2009). Pupils' and teachers' perceptions of a culminating festival within a Sport Education season in Irish primary schools. *Physical Education and Sport Pedagogy*, in press.

Kinchin, G., Penney, D., & Clarke, G. (2001). Teaching the national curriculum physical education: try Sport Education. *British Journal of Teaching Physical Education, 32*(2), 41–44.

Launder, A. (2002). *Play practice: the games approach to teaching and coaching sports*. Champaign, IL: Human Kinetics.

MacPhail, A., & Halbert, J. (2009). "We had to do intelligent thinking during recent PE": students' and teachers' experiences of assessment for learning in post-primary physical education. *Assessment in Education*.

MacPail, A., Kinchin, G., & Kirk, D. (2003). Students' conceptions of sport and Sport Education. *European Physical Education Review, 9*(3), 285–299.

McMahon, E., & MacPhail, A. (2007). Learning to teach Sport Education: the experience of a pre-service teacher. *European Physical Education Review, 13*(2), 229–246.

Mitchell, S. A., Oslin, J. L., & Griffin, L. L. (2003). *Sport foundations for elementary physical education: a tactical games approach*. Champaign, IL: Human Kinetics.

National Association for Sport and Physical Education. (2004). *Moving into the future: national standards for physical education* (2nd ed.). Reston, VA: Author.

Penney, D., Clarke, G., Quill, M., & Kinchin, G. (Eds.). (2005). *Sport Education in physical education: research based practice*. New York: Routledge, Taylor, & Francis.

Siedentop, D. (1994). *Sport education: quality PE through positive sport experiences*. Champaign, IL: Human Kinetics.

Siedentop, D. (1998). What is Sport Education and how does it work? *Journal of Physical Education, Recreation and Dance, 69*(4), 18–20.

Siedentop, D., Hastie, P. A., & van der Mars, H. (2004). *Complete guide to Sport Education*. Champaign, IL: Human Kinetics.

Siedentop, D., & Tannehill, D. (2000). *Developing teaching skills in physical education* (4th ed.). Palo Alto, CA: Mayfield.

Sinelnikov, O., & Hastie, P. (2008). Teaching Sport Education to Russian students: an ecological analysis. *European Physical Education Review, 14*(2), 203–222.

Strikwerda-Brown, J., & Taggart, A. (2001). No longer voiceless and exhausted: Sport Education and the primary generalist. *ACHPER Healthy Lifestyles Journal, 48*, 14–17.

Sweeney, J., Tannehill, D., & Teeters, L. (1992). Teaming up for fitness: a Sport Education model approach to fitness instruction. *Strategies, 5*(6), 20–23.

Townsend, J. S., Mohr, D. J., Rairigh, R. M., & Bulger, S. M. (2003). *Assessing student outcomes in Sport Education: a pedagogical approach*. Reston, VA: NASPE.

U.S. Department of Health and Human Services. (2000). *Healthy people 2010*. Washington, DC: U.S. Government Printing Office.

U.S Department of Health and Human Services. (2008). *2008 physical activity guidelines for Americans: be active, healthy, and happy*! Washington, DC: U.S. Government Printing Office.

Wallhead, T., & O'Sullivan, M. (2005). Sport Education: physical education for the new millennium? *Physical Education and Sport Pedagogy, 10*(2), 181–210.

Additional Resource

Mohr, D. J., Townsend, J. S., & Bulger, S. M. (2002). Maintaining the PASE: a day in the life of Sport Education. *Journal of Physical Education, Recreation and Dance, 73*, 36–44.

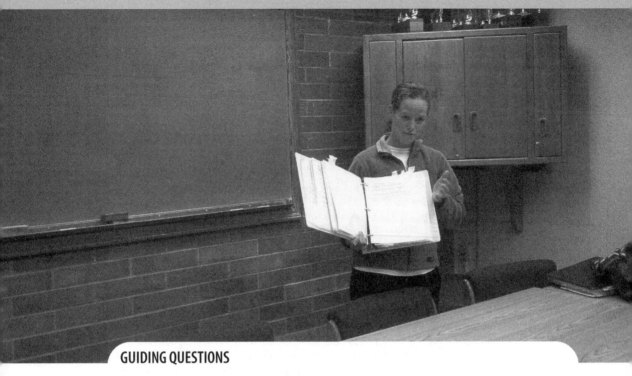

GUIDING QUESTIONS

1 What is a major goal of the Cultural Studies model?

2 What does it mean to be a critical consumer of sport?

3 There is a practical and a cognitive component to the model. What are the three major strands of the model?

4 Which of the NASPE Content Standards (2004) does this curriculum best support?

5 In what ways are the literate sportsperson in the Cultural Studies model similar to and different from the literate sportsperson in Sport Education?

6 Why might there be an interest in the Cultural Studies curriculum approach to physical education among contemporary youth?

7 What are some different types of assessments to be used in a Cultural Studies model?

8 The Cultural Studies model requires a significant shift in thinking about and planning of a physical education curriculum. What arguments could you make in support of such a shift of focus in the curriculum?

9 Describe one assessment that would align with each of the three strands of the model.

10 Debate the following statement: Physically educated students should be critical consumers of sport.

11 How is Cultural Studies different from Sport Education? In what ways are they similar?

Cultural Studies Curriculum in Physical Activity and Sport

Mary O'Sullivan, The University of Limerick
Gary Kinchin, University of Southampton

Overview of the Model

It has been exciting in recent years to see the positive and enthusiastic development of and experimentation with different K–12 curricular models in physical education. The co-editors of this textbook realized correctly that major curricular initiatives have gained the attention of physical education teachers and teacher educators who are looking for curricular models that better reflect and address contemporary American life, and the needs and interests of adolescents educated in a diversity of school contexts. These exciting curriculum models are described in other chapters in this textbook and include Sport Education, Adventure Based Education, and Outdoor Education, among others.

In the models presented in this textbook, there has been little consideration of physical education as a place for young people to develop as literate and critical consumers of sport, physical activity, and the **movement culture**. The **Cultural Studies (CS) curriculum** model described in this

> **movement culture** The infrastructure, norms, practices, policies, and values associated with sport, recreation, and physical activity at the local, national, and international levels.
> **Cultural Studies (CS) curriculum** Involves the practical and cognitive involvement of students in learning not only how to participate in sport and physical activity but also in learning how sport and physical activity contributes positively and negatively to individual well-being and to group, community, and national cultures.

chapter is quite different from the curricular experiences of most U.S. physical education teachers, and the other models presented in this textbook. As one effort to reflect the local regional needs and interests of children and youth from a range of backgrounds and populations, the CS approach to curriculum in physical education attempts to encompass an integration of practical and cognitive student involvement in sport and physical activity.

A key prerequisite of the CS approach is the use of a physical activity component in conjunction with a critical investigation of physical activity and sport in society. To this end, our work to date has employed Sport Education for this purpose (Siedentop, Hastie, & van der Mars, 2004), but other curricular approaches might also be considered, such as a Sport for Peace unit (Ennis et al., 1999), a Sport Education/Teaching Games for Understanding hybrid unit (Hastie & Curtner-Smith, 2006), or the approach to physical education taken at senior level in syllabi in Australia (Queensland Board of Senior Secondary School Studies, 1998), New Zealand (New Zealand Ministry of Education, 1999), and the United Kingdom (Oxford Cambridge and RSA [OCR], 2008).

The CS curriculum approach (Kinchin & O'Sullivan, 1999) is to develop students as literate and critical consumers of sport, physical activity, and the movement culture. A key goal of CS is the development of student-as-critical-consumer. We want students who are informed, watchful, and have the knowledge, skills, and confidence to critique physical activity provision and presentation on local and national levels.

We want students who can question and challenge the status quo related to access and influence of the physical activity and sport infrastructure. We want students who can unravel the hidden agendas and complexities and make known/public who is potentially being oppressed and silenced in the physical activity, sport, and movement culture. We want students to see themselves as part of diverse cultures and to be able to both connect school-to-home learning and reflect critically upon this learning. We also hope for students to be **Cultural Studies connoisseurs** (Eisner, 1985) of local and national physical activity and sport infrastructure and cultures. These are huge challenges requiring "risk-taking" students who will also *act*. Several learning experiences enable students to present, defend, and act where appropriate on their ideas related to issues of social justice in sport and physical activity. The learning experiences include journal writing, student presentations, in-class discussions, and action

Cultural Studies connoisseurs   Students who have heightened awareness or educated perceptions of the nuances; educated perceptions allow students to illuminate, interpret, and appraise physical activity, sport infrastructure, and sport cultures.

research projects or community mapping. The CS materials shared here have been designed, implemented, and revised by four teachers in three school districts in Ohio, when the lead author and two of her graduate students at the time approached some high school teachers with these ideas. This approach has also been implemented with adolescent girls in an Irish secondary school (Enright, 2007; Enright & O'Sullivan, in press). Early experiences with implementation of the curriculum have been shared at an American Association For Health, Physical Education, Recreational and Dance (AAHPERD) national convention (O'Sullivan, Kinchin, Kellum, Dunaway, & Dixon, 1996) and more recent experiences shared at the British Educational Research Conference (Enright). Although the curricular model has been designed for and delivered to high school students, it has potential application, with modifications, for middle school programs and students. Indeed, some work by Kim Oliver and her colleagues (Oliver, 2001; Oliver, Hamzeh, & McCaughtry, in press; Oliver & Lalik, 2001, 2004) with middle school students in the southern United States and with high school students (Knop, Tannehill, & O'Sullivan, 2001) aligns well with the goals and objectives of this curricular approach. This curriculum model is a work in progress. It is a response to changing cultural and social circumstances of our times where cultural diversity and identity are becoming increasingly significant. Teachers may not believe it is their responsibility to shape the curriculum to address serious social and ethical issues in sport and health. Curriculum development specialists may not view physical education as a place for discussion and critique of the public health agenda for the nation (such as trends in overweight and obesity and the principles of personal responsibility for one's health and wellness) or of the role of sport in contemporary culture, but as we shall shortly set out, some settings have included this content within their schemes of work/syllabi.

The above may be reasons enough for physical education teachers, curriculum developers, and teacher educators to reject the ideas described in these pages. However, we hope some readers will find the ideas exciting and thought provoking and will want to experiment with some of these ideas in their physical education classes and programs. In New Zealand and Australia, such a sociocultural perspective "now underpins most syllabuses . . . and may include classroom based lessons where students explicitly learn about physical activity, exercise and sport" (Wright, 2004, p. 10). Hopefully, U.S. teachers who experiment with these ideas will provide us with feedback on their efforts. The second author of this chapter focused his doctoral dissertation on implementing the Cultural Studies approach within an urban high school physical education program. The research focused specifically upon the perceptions of students and the extent to which students could engage with issues of gender, the body, and media influences in sport during a Cultural Studies unit (Kinchin, 1998; Kinchin & O'Sullivan, 1999, 2003). Data from the study indicate that the

Cultural Studies unit offered a very relevant and meaningful examination of sport in society for some students (Kinchin & O'Sullivan, 2003).

Enright and O'Sullivan (2007, 2008) carried out a 2-year participatory action research (PAR) project with disengaged students in an urban post-primary school in Ireland. The aim of the project was to work with the students to understand and transform barriers to their physical education engagement and physical activity participation. The PAR project was initially focused on the engagement of one class of teenage girls as physical education curriculum designers and evaluators (Enright & O'Sullivan, 2007). The project extended to a further two classes and to the design and evaluation of an after-school physical education club in the second year (Enright & O'Sullivan, 2008), thereby challenging formal physical education learning boundaries.

Traditional physical education programs in the United States have tended to focus on the development of fundamental skills, sport skills, and tactical development of game play, with a growing interest currently in health-related physical activity. American high school physical education programs in the past have focused almost exclusively on competitive team sports and fitness activities that are described in most school district courses of study as lifelong leisure activities. There has been a focus in recent years on student engagement in moderate to vigorous levels of physical activity, with a broadening of curricular offerings moving us away from a program dominated by games and teacher interests and expertise. The newer curricular models described elsewhere in this text expand upon the goals of physical education in positive and important ways. However, the perspective that physical education's role is also in developing critical and literate **consumers of sport and physical activity** in the local (school and community) and national cultures has never been considered an important task of American schooling. This seems particularly curious to us given the prominent role of sport and fitness/wellness in multiple facets of contemporary American society such as the media, schooling, economics, politics, and public health. The ideas presented here are different from how physical education teachers experienced physical education in school, or during their teacher preparation programs. Hence, we suspect this CS approach to physical education curriculum planning will be most challenging to physical education teachers. The basic contexts to understanding or appreciating this approach to the subject matter has probably not been a part of their experience or professional preparation.

consumers of sport and physical activity   Students are educated not only to appreciate the intrinsic benefits of participation in health-enhancing physical activity but also to exercise critical judgment when evaluating the role and function of sport and physical activity in their lives.

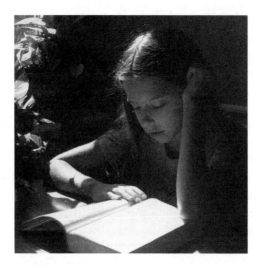

A CS approach to a physical education curriculum encourages students to consider and question their experiences in school physical education classes. It also allows for the opportunity to review their involvement (or lack of involvement) in physical activity outside of school and question taken-for-granted assumptions about sport, fitness, health, and physical education in their school, community, and today's society (e.g., the so-called obesity epidemic). Such assumptions have received significant attention globally (Kirk & Tinning, 1990; Wright, Macdonald, & Burrows, 2004). Such a curriculum approach offers a potentially exciting complement to the practice of physical education in American high schools for some teachers and students.

For many adolescents (more boys than girls), sport and physical activity play a central role in their lives, yet all too many students (more girls than boys) are disenfranchised from the joys and benefits of physical activity. The CS approach to high school physical education attempts to offer physical educators an opportunity to help students appreciate and critique the role of physical activity and sport in their own lives, and the life of their schools, their community, and the wider society. The curriculum attempts to make meaningful connections between what occurs in the name of physical education in school, and the access to or engagement with sport and physical activity, or lack thereof, in students' lives and the lives of members of other communities.

Characteristics of the Model and Unique Contributions

A CS unit includes a practical and academic component. It attempts to encompass an integrated and sustained practical and academic engagement with sport and physical activity, and examines what these physical activity experiences mean to young people, their school, and their community. The first component of the CS curriculum includes a focus on a specific physical activity. Teachers choose specific physical activities (games, track, aquatics, outdoor pursuits) as the foundational content of the curriculum. For the purposes of this chapter, this practical component of our model utilizes Sport Education to structure and deliver the content, but as we have indicated other models of learning and teaching may be equally suitable, particularly given a number of Sport Education variants do exist within the literature. The Sport Education model provides students with opportunities to engage in the practice of sport (see Chapter 11 by van der Mars and Tannehill), and the model complements several of the curriculum goals of the Cultural Studies model. The second component (a classroom-based component) engages students in a discussion and critique of several contemporary social issues in sport, health, and physical activity, through public presentations, private journals, class discussions, and group projects. Students can undertake some of this classroom-based work in their sport education "teams," which enables the established group structure to be retained and developed in contexts outside the physical activity setting (thus enabling affiliation and membership to be further enhanced). The goals of this component are for students to recognize the role and meaning of sport and physical activity in their lives, and in the wider community in which they live. It also allows for a space to discuss who has access to physical activity and sport cultures, and who benefits from opportunities and access provided to physical activity experiences. The CS approach aligns with some of the key objectives of the sport education experience: students should develop as both literate and critical sportspersons. A literate sportsperson would be "a more discerning consumer whether fan or spectator" (Siedentop, 1994, p. 4). Classroom experiences are designed to help students become aware of factors that support or inhibit their own and others' access and interest in physical activity and sport. The classroom-based activities provide students with chances to critically question the place of sport and physical activity in their lives and in the wider society.

In addition to following a season of sport education, students gain an appreciation of sport and physical activity from social and cultural perspectives (Kinchin, 1997). In schools where we experimented with the model, the teacher presented the historical and geographical roots of a specific sport. The students had opportunities to consider the role of sport (in our case, the sport of volleyball) in their lives and the lives of their family, friends, school, and local community. Students researched possibilities for sport and physical activity in their school and community, and considered that what influenced access to and interest in sport for themselves, their friends, and neighbors was a function of their gender, race, or class, or other family circumstances. Students discussed the availability of sport at their school, and debated the appropriateness of a school serving a small percentage of the school population by their use of school facilities during non-instructional time for physical activity (i.e., full court basketball played during open gym). They engaged in discussions on gender and body image associated with the role of sport in society, and how sport and physical activities are used at times to both support and oppress different groups of males and females (Kinchin, 1997). Physical education provides a suitable backdrop to debate many issues (issues of gender, body image, access to physical activity and sport facilities, and instruction), especially when discrimination in wider aspects of sport, as perceived by students, mirrored that in other contexts such as the school or community. These issues were appreciated by some students as topics for discussion during physical education curriculum time. The following provides an example of where students could see a connection between access to opportunities for physical activity in and out of school (referring to lunchtime "open gym" basketball):

> *Jaimee: Right now there are probably all guys out there [in the gym] playing basketball.*
> *Teresa: If there is a girl out there, she is probably having a hard time trying to play.*
> *Jaimee: If she [points to Keesha] was out there . . . I mean you should see the way she dribbles.*
> *Keesha: If I do play with the boys, they say 'pass it to the girl.' Why can I not be just another player instead of being 'the girl.' I don't like that.*

Philosophy of the Model

Some scholars have lamented the lack of substantive change between today's curriculum offerings and practices in physical education (particularly at the secondary level), and those of previous decades (Steinhardt, 1992). Although scholars concur on the need for radical and extensive change to high school programs (Capel & Blair, 2009; Kirk, 2005; Locke, 1992; Rink, 1993; Siedentop, 1994; Tinning & Fitzclarence, 1992), until recently, few have engaged in researching the process of and/or impact of curriculum change on school programs, teachers, or students (Ennis et al., 1997; Glasby & MacDonald, 2004; Jewett & Bain, 1987; Oliver, Hamzeh, & McCaughtry, in press; Sparkes, 1988).

The Cultural Studies model is similar in many ways to the content that is described in physical education[1] syllabi for senior high school students in Australia, New Zealand, and more recently in Ontario, Canada. New Zealand scholar, Lissette Burrows (2004) recently noted that:

---

[1] We are using physical education here in its broad sense. In Ontario, the courses we are referring to are labeled Sport Science and Recreation and Physically Active Lifestyle.

Curricular frameworks, at least in Australia, New Zealand, and the UK, are increasingly acknowledging that physical education must contribute to students' understanding of the diverse meanings and practices attached to physical culture . . . concepts like critical thinking, critical inquiry and problem-solving feature prominently in syllabus documentation, reflecting the now widespread educational interest in fostering students' capacity to learn how to learn and to engage with the proliferation of uncertain knowledge. . . . (p. 105)

In New Zealand, students of health and physical education[2] explore:

. . . how sporting experiences influence the development of people's physical and social lives. They investigate and critically appraise the educative value of sport and consider the effects of sport from social, cultural, and scientific perspectives. (New Zealand Ministry of Education, 1999, p. 44)

In Queensland, Australia, senior physical education involves the study of physical activity and:

. . . engages students as intelligent performers, learning in, about, and through physical activity . . . and engages students not only as performers but as analysts, planners, and critics in, about and through physical activity. (Queensland Board of Senior Secondary School Studies, 1998, p. 1)

In England, Anthony Laker (2002) and David Kirk (1997) have argued that physical education programs must better reflect and contribute to the popular physical culture. The current **standardized examination courses** in physical education in England are made available to pupils ages 16 to 18 years. These courses offer specific content that focus on sociocultural aspects of physical education and sport. For example, the Oxford Cambridge and RSA Examinations (OCR) is one of the major awarding bodies involved in the development of these courses, which are studied at advanced level in English schools.

Physical Education is one such course that students can elect to follow (OCR, 2008). A review of the physical education syllabus in England makes

> **standardized examination courses**   Rigorous tests that analyze students' practical and cognitive knowledge of sport, health, and fitness as well as the natural sciences (e.g., physiology, anatomy, biomechanics) and the social sciences (e.g., psychology, sociology).

---

[2] Health and physical education are regarded as one subject in New Zealand, and teachers are certified to teach both areas. In recent years in the United States, we have seen a number of states discussing or implementing legislation that combines health and physical education teacher certification as one combined subject in schools.

explicit within its aims that students become "... informed and discerning decision makers" (p. 7). This syllabus includes a significant sociocultural element where learners are encouraged to critically evaluate contemporary key influences that might limit or promote young people's involvement in physical activity (such as gender, race, age, or disability). In addition, this element stresses a critical appraisal of "... current product and consumer-focused influences" (p. 7) that might affect young people's ability to become involved in physical activity pursuits. Summative assessment involves the external grading of two written papers that may require the student to interpret visual material, including photographs and diagrams.

The CS unit described in this chapter is about developing students' intellectual curiosity about sport and physical activity on both a local and national scale. With the goals of the CS unit in mind, the extracts from students who have engaged in a unit of CS suggest many are able to talk about these aspects of our subject matter in quite thoughtful and encouraging ways. A Cultural Studies (CS) approach to physical education has not gained much attention or consideration in the United States. Some exceptions are Fernandez-Balboa (1997), Kinchin and O'Sullivan (1999, 2003), Oliver (2001), and perhaps Siedentop (2002). Siedentop alludes to critical literacy as a potential outcome of Sport Education, though other aspects of the model, rather than the literate sportsperson, are emphasized in his text and articles written about the model by other scholars.

We suggest that the inclusion of a CS component in the physical education curriculum could be divided into major content strands over the course of a school year or several years. Each strand could be tied directly to one or more physical activities. The first strand might focus on the Personal Dimension of Physical Activity and Sport. This strand provides opportunities for students to develop their personal biographies focused around physical activity, physical education, and sport since childhood, and examines the role of family, friends, and community in enhancing or inhibiting their levels of physical activity participation. In this chapter, we have provided examples of assignments that align with this objective. One of the culminating activities for this strand could be a poster display where students invite family, school, and community members to discuss their physical activity biographies. Such an exercise would indeed be relevant to the contemporary debates about obesity, youth physical activity levels, and childhood diabetes. It would also be an opportunity to learn how the adults spent their lives as children, and their physical activity levels as children. This strand is in alignment, for the most part, with Standard 5, though it sees personal choice and responsibility as just one factor in explaining interest and participation by children and young adults in regular physical activity.

A second strand of the curriculum could focus on sport and physical activity in the school and local community. What activities are available at the

TABLE 12.1

Sport Coverage Assignment

Purpose of assignment	Role of physical activity/sport in school culture.
Materials needed	Yearbook, student newspaper, or school bulletins.
Procedure to complete task	Review the last 10 (or more) years of the school yearbook and/or the last 10 issues of the school newsletter/newspaper to determine what physical activities are most promoted and supported at the school. Discuss your findings with your small group. What physical activities are given most coverage in text and in photos? What did you notice about how physical activity coverage changed over time in terms of type of activity, space allocation in the text, photos, gender, ability, and race/ethnicity? Prepare a summary of your findings for the class and your conclusions/recommendations related to equitable access to physical activity over time.

school and local levels, and who is recruited and attracted to these activities? Table 12.1 describes an assignment that provides students an opportunity to review sport and physical activity in their school and how it has changed over time. Students discuss what efforts are made to encourage all students to be active. One of our colleagues, an urban elementary physical education teacher working with the Columbus PEP grant, has addressed these kinds of issues in a creative way with his elementary students. He had his 3rd and 4th grade elementary students interview members of their family about their physical activity patterns as children and how the neighborhood supported such activity after school. The children learned that the two urban local parks, where the adults played after school as children, were now apartment blocks and a business plaza. They heard about how much easier it had been for these adults to walk to school and stay out in the evening playing on the street, something these children are not allowed to do because of parental safety issues. This strand is somewhat aligned to Standard 5 of the NASPE content standards in that the students are learning about their personal responsibility for physical activity, but it goes further in helping them see how changes in the environment around them impacts the potential choices they can make.

A third focus of the curriculum could be to look at physical activity and sport in the wider society. Many of these issues will intersect with school and community issues, looking at sport and the media, sport and drug use, and sport and violence, as well as physical activity, health, and its intersections with race, ethnicity, and social class. Table 12.2 describes an assignment where

TABLE 12.2

Percentage of Children Ages 9–13 Years Who Reported Participation in Organized and Free-Time Physical Activity During the Preceding 7 Days, by Selected Characteristics (Youth Media Campaign Longitudinal Survey, United States, 2002)

Characteristic	Participated in Organized Physical Activity During Preceding 7 Days %	(95% CI*)	Participated in Free-Time Physical Activity During Preceding 7 Days %	(95% CI)
Sex				
Female	38.6	(±2.5)	74.1†	(±2.0)
Male	38.3	(±2.9)	80.5†	(±1.7)
Age (years)				
9	36.1	(±4.0)	75.8	(±3.1)
10	37.5	(±4.0)	77.0	(±2.7)
11	43.1	(±3.6)	78.9	(±3.0)
12	37.7	(±4.1)	77.5	(±3.5)
13	38.1	(±4.2)	78.0	(±4.0)
Race/Ethnicity§				
Black, non-Hispanic	24.1†	(±3.8)	74.7	(±4.6)
Hispanic	25.9†	(±4.0)	74.6	(±3.9)
White, non-Hispanic	46.6†	(±3.0)	79.3	(±1.7)
Parental education				
<High school	19.4†	(±4.8)	75.3	(±5.7)
High school	28.3†	(±3.4)	75.4	(±2.9)
>High school	46.8†	(±2.5)	78.7	(±2.0)
Parental income				
≤$25,000	23.5†	(±3.7)	74.1	(±3.1)
$25,001–$50,000	32.8†	(±3.4)	78.6	(±2.5)
>$50,000	49.1†	(±2.6)	78.3	(±2.0)
Total	38.5	(±2.0)	77.4	(±1.2)

* Confidence interval.
† Statistically significant difference ($p < 0.05$).
§ Numbers for other racial/ethnic populations were too small for meaningful analysis.
Source: Centers for Disease Control and Prevention. (2003). Physical activity levels among children Aged 9–13 Years—United States, 2002. *Morbidity and Mortality Weekly Report, 52*(33), 785–788. Retrieved February 25, 2004, from http://www.cdc.gov/mmwr/preview/mmwrhtml/mm5233a1.htm

students review the barriers to participation in physical activity, and what actions could be recommended to improve physical activity levels in their school or community. In the work at our high schools, we found a portion of the student body eager and enthusiastic to engage in discussions of these issues. They are issues that are central to the health of the nation and the quality of sporting experiences at school, college, and professional levels. The intent of this strand includes many of the elements of Standard 6 (values physical activity for health, enjoyment, challenge, self-expression, and/or social interaction). It also demands students ask questions about the local, national, and economic factors that impact differential equity of access to and benefits from engagement in physical activity over the lifespan.

Relationship of NASPE Content Standards to Cultural Studies Curriculum

The Cultural Studies curriculum prioritizes Standards 3, 5 and 6 (see Table 12.3).

Standard 2, "Demonstrates understanding of movement concepts, principles, strategies, and tactics as they apply to the learning and performance of physical activities," considers the application of knowledge to the learning and performance of motor skills. The CS curriculum probably stretches the NASPE standards in ways not envisaged by those who helped to write and revise the standards. We suspect some will see this as a problem of the curriculum model. Our view is that there are gaps in the standards that this model highlights that should be addressed

---

TABLE 12.3

NASPE Content Standards for Physical Education (NASPE, 2004) and Alignment with Cultural Studies Curriculum

Alignment	National K–12 Content Standards
M	*Standard 1.* Demonstrates competency in motor skills and movement patterns needed to perform a variety of physical activities.
M	*Standard 2.* Demonstrates understanding movement concepts, principles, strategies, and tactics as they apply to the learning and performance of physical activities.
X	*Standard 3.* Participates regularly in physical activity.
M	*Standard 4.* Achieves and maintains a health enhancing level of physical fitness.
X	*Standard 5.* Exhibits responsible personal and social behavior that respects self and others in physical activity settings.
X	*Standard 6.* Values physical activity for health, enjoyment, challenge, self-expression, and/or social interaction.

M = moderate alignment; X = strong alignment.

in a contemporary physical education program for reasons we described earlier. In the NASPE standards as interpreted to date, there is little to no "curricular space" for consideration of the role of sport and physical activity in students' lives, or how individual, community, and societal factors enhance or inhibit personal and sustained commitments to lifelong healthy lifestyles. The CS model focuses on this aspect of physical education with the intent that such connections among school, home, and community life will encourage more active participation in physical activity. The model also recognizes aspects of school and community life that limit such participation, as well as discussion of action steps to resolve these issues. Such a goal is not easily aligned with the NASPE content standards. Using Sport Education as the format and structure for the delivery of physical activity, there is an alignment with Standards 3, 5, and 6, with some consideration to Standards 1 and 2 in helping students learn how to play, referee, and coach physical activities in the physical education program. The larger goal of understanding how society impacts the scope and nature of participation in physical activity is not a focus of any of the current NASPE standards. Perhaps discussions about this chapter may plant some seeds for further revision of the standards, or at least beg the question as to whether this should be a priority for physical education programs in American schools.

Benefits and Limitations of the Model

There are at least three major benefits for teachers and students with a CS approach as part of a physical education program at the middle or high school level. First, many physical education teachers will see the relevance of "foundation courses" such as sociology, philosophy, psychology, and exercise physiology in their undergraduate major, and many will find teaching about the sociocultural dimensions of physical activity intellectually stimulating. Second, activities and discussions that allow students to connect their interests and involvement in physical activity outside of school will make for more meaningful physical education lessons. The following quote from the transcripts of Kinchin's (1997) research describes an additional student perspective on the relevance of the CS assignments and class-based discussions during physical education to his life outside of his class and his high school.

> *There is always going to be discrimination and there is always going to be problems arising . . . it is just when we were talking about the conflicts like the funding [of school sport] and the discrimination issues, sexual discrimination, racial discrimination [in sport] . . . I mean we also touched on sexuality. I mean these are problems that you deal with in everyday life. When you turn on the TV and there they are not just in sports but in the workplace. (High school student interview)*

Third, this curriculum has the potential to engage students in new ways with and about physical activity, and help them become more informed (i.e., literate) and critical consumers of physical activity and sport in their own lives, and become aware of the significance of sport in their community and society at large. This could provide those alienated from physical education with a chance to understand why, and perhaps get reconnected in other ways.

We would suggest there are three substantive limitations to the model given our experience with it, current realities of the American public school, and conversations with teachers who have pondered the relevance of the model for their physical education programs. The first limitation relates to allocated time for physical education in the American public school. Allocated time for physical education in middle and high schools has decreased in recent years. Daily enrollment in physical education classes dropped from 42% to 25% among high school students between 1991 and 1995 (Centers for Disease Control and Prevention, 2004). Consequently, there is increased pressure on teachers to maximize students' class time engaged in moderate and vigorous activity. Taking class time to discuss the role of sport in students' lives, and in the life of their school and community, may not be a priority for teachers. We suggest that time spent in such discussions may lead to a better understanding by students of the role of sport and physical activity in developing their own and others' healthy lifestyles. However, like many claims for physical education, we don't have any solid evidence to support this position. At this time, our claims are a leap of faith. The second limitation with implementing the model is teacher expertise. Although prospective teacher candidates take courses on the sociological, psychological, and biological dimensions of sport and exercise, there is little, if any, discussion in these college classes of the relevance of this content for K–12 students and programs. Because this model actually demonstrates an application of some of this coursework, and represents a link between theory and practice, it would be appropriate for physical education faculty to introduce this curricular model as a way of helping teacher candidates better see the relevance and application of this coursework. There are few, if any, opportunities in American schools to learn how to teach adolescents about these dimensions of physical activity. Discussion of concepts of health-related fitness, such as the fitness-based education curriculum as discussed in Chapter 13 would be an exception. Many physical education teachers who don't teach health have little to no experience teaching "academic" content in a classroom setting. A third limitation is access to classroom space. Schools in many districts lack adequate space to teach traditional physical education programs, and finding an alternate classroom space to accommodate debates, group projects, lectures, and classroom work would be quite challenging for teachers. It should be noted that we did not include the "lack" of alignment of the CS curricular model with the NASPE standards as a limitation. We would argue this is an important addition to the standards, not a limitation of the model.

Sample Unit of the Cultural Studies Model

The following Cultural Studies block plan (see Table 12.4) was designed for a high school physical education class. We studied the impact of the CS curriculum unit on these urban high school students (Kinchin, 1997). The physical education teacher helped design and pilot the initial ideas for this curricular approach. This was a second time for her to teach a CS module, but the first time for the students to experience this approach to teaching.

The goals of the 20-day integrated unit of volleyball incorporating both physical activity and Cultural Studies component were designed to:

1. Provide students opportunities to perform fundamental skills pertinent to volleyball (Standard 1).
2. Help students carry out appropriate volleyball strategy and tactics during game play, and exercise leadership through use of correct game rules, court etiquette, and non-playing roles such as referee, coach, and statistician (Standards 2 and 5).
3. Allow students opportunities both individually and as a group to gather information, share, and critique the position and role of volleyball within their immediate families, school, community, and wider society (Standard 6+[3]).
4. Expose students to unique events and customs associated with sport as a participatory activity organized on many levels, by using volleyball as an exemplar (Standard 6).
5. Address issues in contemporary sport such as the impact of sport media, gender, and how the sport body is portrayed by different entities, using the game of volleyball as the central focus for such discussions (Standard 6+).

Learning Activities and Assessments for Use with the Model

Here we outline some examples of **assessments** that have been used during the CS unit and offer some examples of work completed by the high school students and physical education teacher candidates.

> **assessments** Gathering information about students' abilities and understanding.

---

[3] Extends Standard 6 in ways not necessarily envisioned or endorsed by NASPE.

TABLE 12.4

Unit Plan for a Cultural Studies Unit Using a Sport Education Volleyball Season

Practical (Sport Education) Element	Theoretical (Cultural Studies) Element
Lesson One Welcome students Provide an overview of unit Form teams and determine student roles as in Sport Education curriculum	1. Students complete pre-unit survey instrument. 2. History and development of volleyball (slide show using Powerpoint). 3. Inform students of the final project: a 5-minute presentation on an element of sport of their choice. Students will be informed that the coming weeks will expose them to several issues in contemporary sport pertinent to volleyball. They may wish to apply one of these theoretical concepts to an activity of their choice. 4. Hand out worksheet with some helpful guidelines for the final presentation.
Lesson Two	1. Discuss geography of volleyball; where the game is played and who tends to play, and who is most successful. 2. World map activity: use pins to mark nations that play volleyball. Discussion: What do students notice about the distribution of the nations? 3. Rules, terms, strategies: give out teacher-produced handout for quiz on 11/19.
	4. Homework #1: "Volleyball in the Community": students will design a volleyball flyer to advertise a volleyball camp in their local communities. The flyer should include a description of its purposes, location, and how it will be organized to ensure all who attend can participate with enjoyment. Limit to one page of written accompanying text. Due 11/12 when students will present their flyers in class. Give out worksheet for students to help them complete this task.
Lesson Three Warm-up (stretching and circle drill) Beginning volleyball skills, bump, set and serve; 3v3 team practice	Remind students that flyers are to be brought to class tomorrow.

Continued

TABLE 12.4

Unit Plan for a Cultural Studies Unit Using a Sport Education Volleyball Season—Cont'd

Practical (Sport Education) Element	Theoretical (Cultural Studies) Element
Lesson Four	1. Students present their flyers to peers in 1-minute presentations. 2. The organization of volleyball: community, high school, college, and professional; provide data from the OSU Women's Volleyball Program 2009–2010 roster, and from the rankings of the top U.S. high school teams. Discussion: What are students' reactions to these data in terms of where volleyball is played and who plays? 3. Hand out "Family Multiple Choice Quiz," on the history, rules, and terms of volleyball. Students have a family member complete quiz, and bring the item to class on 11/14.
Lesson Five Warm-up: spike and the block 3v3 practice in teams	
Lesson Six Warm-up: dink and back set 3v3 practice in teams	
Lesson Seven	1. Teacher-constructed written quiz (30 minutes). 2. In teams, collate scores from family members' performance on the quiz. Use guiding questions worksheet to discuss and record responses. 3. For those who finished brainstorm, respond to the statement: "Why is participation in volleyball as popular as soccer as a global sport?" 4. Whole class discussion on family quiz reactions.
Lesson Eight	1. Volleyball in the Olympic games: history, discussion of medal winners, participating countries, and rise of success of the U.S. 2. Atlanta 1996: The introduction of beach volleyball. Discuss most successful teams and players, and patterns of sponsorship and development of professional code in the form of a timeline.

Continued

TABLE 12.4

Unit Plan for a Cultural Studies Unit Using a Sport Education Volleyball Season—Cont'd

Practical (Sport Education) Element	Theoretical (Cultural Studies) Element
Lesson Nine Warm-up: practice games 3v3; scrimmage 6v6 with other teams Offensive and defensive strategy	Watch segments of 1980 and 1996 Olympic volleyball videos.
Lesson Ten	1. Volleyball and the sport media: students complete newspaper assignment of the coverage of sport (including volleyball) during the Olympic games. 2. Discuss findings related to sports covered, athletes features by race, gender, and sporting activity. 3. Homework: find an article/advertisement connected with volleyball from books, magazines, or the Web, and write a reaction to the piece (1/2- to 1-page maximum). Submit by 12/2.
Lesson Eleven Scrimmage 6v6 Continue with offense and defense	Show Liz Masakayan performance tips video (10 minutes).
Lesson Twelve	1. Volleyball and the image of the body: show snippet of beach volleyball (5 minutes). Show selected items from the Bud Light Men's and Women's Volleyball League (10 minutes). Class discussion: What do we notice about the appearance of the players? How are the players' performances described? Who endorses the players and the event and why? 2. Refer to *Journal of Sport and Social Issues* 1992 article that summarizes differences in language used by commentators to describe men's and women's execution of volleyball skills in the Olympics. Were there differences or similarities in the data from the article and the earlier videos?
Lesson Thirteen Introduce refereeing and line-judging roles as in Sport Education Practice calls and appropriate signals Practice how to umpire a game Use of red and yellow cards Practice in 6v6 structure with "duty team"	

Continued

TABLE 12.4

Unit Plan for a Cultural Studies Unit Using a Sport Education Volleyball Season—Cont'd

Practical (Sport Education) Element	Theoretical (Cultural Studies) Element
Lessons Fourteen/Fifteen Preparation for tournament in teams, individuals drills, 3v3 within teams, and scrimmage against other teams 6v6.	
Lesson Sixteen	Guest speaker: "Women and Minorities in Sport"
Lessons Seventeen/Eighteen	Student final presentation
Lessons Nineteen/Twenty Final culminating event	Students complete post-unit questionnaire

The nature of these exemplar assignments most closely sit with Standard 6, although we do acknowledge that this alignment is, at best, moderate. The growing interest in student voice (see Thomson & Gunter, 2006) potentially offers opportunities for students to engage in either individual or group-based research (recognizing the persisting group emphasis) in their own setting and spaces on matters related to physical education, physical activity, and sport and use data as a means for promoting debate, stimulating action, and advocating change. We hope these activities illustrate the range of ways in which students can engage with specific issues of gender, race, age, disability, and so on.

Posters/Flyers

Students complete some projects, which are shared with peers either as individuals or as a team. In keeping with the theme of volleyball in the unit described earlier, students could design a flyer to advertise a volleyball camp in their local communities. The teacher provides the following prompts to support completion of the task and its assessment:

- When and where will the volleyball camp take place?
- What facilities are available?
- Who within your community can attend the volleyball camp? Why?
- What is the purpose of the camp? What will participants do at the camp?
- How will the camp be organized to ensure all who attend can play?
- What else can you include to make the camp appealing and attractive?

In the unit where this was done, the teacher gave credit to each student who completed and submitted a flyer with the basic components included. There is scope to offer extra credit in relation to appearance, creativity, use of technology, and when attention is given particularly to issues of equity and

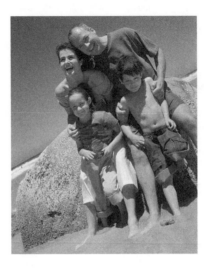

inclusion. A refinement of the assignment could be to have the students design a flyer to motivate other students who are alienated from physical activity to participate in a camp. They would discuss how to appeal to those students (e.g., older, special needs, non-athletic, low-fit).

Individual Presentations

High school students have also given short individual presentations during the CS unit. Students selected a particular aspect of sport within an activity of their choice, and discussed its position in their lives and society. The goal was to have students gather information about a topic and discuss, question, and critique the contribution of that aspect of sport/physical activity to their lives or to the local and national sport culture. This type of work could be viewed in support of Standard 6 of the NASPE content standards. Although the standard is focused on the intrinsic benefits of sport and physical activity, a Cultural Studies approach seeks to also look at some of the negative consequences of sport engagement or the lack of access for specific populations to parts of this infrastructure, and encourages students to do something about that in appropriate and practical ways. The following guidance was offered to students to assist in their preparation:

- What sporting issue did you choose to investigate?
- Why did you choose this particular activity? How does it relate to your life?
- Why did you choose this way of presenting?
- How did you react to what you found (positive and negative aspects)?
- What is the most interesting thing you found out and why?
- Does anything concern and/or surprise you? Why is this so?

In response to this task, students have given presentations on the following topics:

- Differential media coverage of men's and women's basketball
- The rules of basketball
- Women's gymnastics and the Olympics
- African-Americans and basketball
- Women's clothing and the Olympics
- The stresses of youth soccer
- Skateboarding

The task could not be revised to allow students to modify an existing game to appeal to "non-traditional" students (however one wanted to define this category of students), or to allow a new game to be created that would appeal to a broader range of students.

For purposes of assessment, Beach and Marshall's (1991) taxonomy was applied. This taxonomy represents a hierarchical framework setting out the range of responses that emerge when students engage in the reading and study of text (Carroll, 1994). Carroll indicated engaging with text suggests a reluctance among students to probe further, whereas judging the text points to a more complete critique where opinions are more sophisticated and analytical. The response levels by Beach and Marshall include: 1) Engaging, 2) Describing, 3) Explaining, 4) Interpreting, and 5) Judging, where writing can range from 'Engaging' (stating an emotional reaction in the absence of reasoning) to 'Judging' (critiquing action and thoroughly exploring issues with a view to hypothesis building). These 'levels' are more thoroughly set out in Table 12.5.

Beach and Marshall's taxonomy can allow a teacher to make some distinction between verbal presentations where students describe events and facts (e.g., the rules of a game) and those where students offer a more personal analysis and reflective critique of an issue (body image in sport). Here are some segments from high school student transcripts that illustrate the difference in the levels of analysis and critique:

I am going to be talking about the rules of football. Football is played by two teams of eleven players each. The idea is to move the ball across the opponents' goal-line. This results in a touchdown. The team then attempts to kick the ball across the goal-line over a crossbar and between the two up-rights. This is called a field-goal. It is worth three points. The football playing field is a rectangle. It can be played on grass or Astroturf. The distance between the two end lines is 100 yards. (High school male)

In contrast to this descriptive view of football rules, another student brought in a newspaper article, which set out efforts by one eastern state to curb inappropriate examples of competition within youth soccer. She provided a summary

TABLE 12.5

Beach and Marshall's (1991) Taxonomy of Verbal Presentations

Engaging (E)	Readers are engaging with the text whenever they articulate an emotional reaction . . . readers may simply state their initial emotional reaction without examining the reasons for that reaction (pp. 28–29).
Describing (D)	Readers describe a text when they restate or reproduce information that is provided in the text (p. 28).
Explaining (EX)	Why characters are behaving as they are (p. 30).
Interpreting (I)	When we make interpretations we are usually answering the question "What does this text say?" . . . a reader must first adopt a certain stance (pp. 32–33).
Judging (J)	We make judgments about characters . . . we may view their actions as appropriate/inappropriate, right/wrong . . . for a more thorough exploration of the issues involved that can lead to hypothesis building (p. 33).

of this article, and appraised the piece in light of her own experiences. The following transcript illustrates where the content of this presentation was more evaluative and reflective, and indicates some evidence of an ability to be an informed participant and critical observer of sport and physical activity:

> *I am going to talk about reducing the pressure on youth under 12 that play soccer because from experience . . . it is not like a recreational sport. It is, you win, win, win and if you don't then you practice, practice. I can remember I also ran track when I played soccer. I would go from running about three hours of track and straight to soccer. If you did not win, you would practice more . . . it was crazy. In Massachusetts there is a youth soccer association where the President and three other guys . . . they don't want to have this type of competition . . . they have high drop-out rates or poor instances of sportsmanship and they decided that the problem is too much pressure from adults. Adults really don't know how hard it is to play a sport unless they have played it themselves. The problem lies with parents that have not played soccer. Soccer is a game and for youth players it should be fun too. We would go to a tournament and would play four games in a day. After the second game there is no way that you can give your all and they [coaches] expect you to win. I was not even having fun. We were so drilled at running. We were not even friends on our team; we were more like enemies. (High school female)*

Beashel and Taylor (1992) published a series of active learning sport assignments for teachers to use with British middle and high school students. These assignments were designed to provide a series of active learning experiences to help students learn about sport. The activities help students question, discuss, explain, and clarify issues related to the management, administration, and vocational aspects of sports. One set of assignments focused on the price of excellence, as in the drive and dedication to be a first class athlete at a young age, and the stresses and strains associated with these goals for parents, athletes, and their siblings. They could be substituted for this assignment.

Journal Writing

INDIVIDUAL JOURNAL. Journals have been used to enable students to reflect upon and share their views, attitudes, and beliefs about learning experiences presented in class. High school students have completed individual journals in response to particular aspects within the sport studies component of the CS unit (reacting to sporting advertisements), and with the Sport Education component (working in a team and as a team). Some questions in the high school volleyball CS unit included:

1. Today we learned a little of the history of volleyball. What was the most interesting thing you learned, and why was this interesting for you?
2. What do you like or dislike about the volleyball team you are on? Explain.
3. What reasons do you have why volleyball appears to be such a popular sport played by friends and families in yards and parks, and during vacations/holidays?
4. Look at the photograph of the female beach volleyball player. Write a reaction to this picture.
5. What pleased you most about the volleyball culminating event? What encouragement did you get from your team?

Of course the focus of the journal might reflect particular local/regional physical activity issues and interests.

Using Beach and Marshall's (1991) taxonomy presented above, Kinchin (1998) analyzed the content of student journal entries to report the range of responses following prompts provided by a high school teacher on topics related to body image, sport media, and the status of women's sport (via advertisements, written text, and photographs). The content of students' journal entries suggested high school girls were generally troubled by the nature of these items. One high school female student wrote the following response to an advertisement calling for male basketball players to practice with women:

At first my reaction was anger because I thought they needed male basketball players to teach women how to play. Because of the unfairness and inequality between men and women, it causes some immediate anger because I am so used to seeing men viewed as more athletically inclined than women.

The extent to which boys acknowledged the challenges women face in sport was minimal. This was even more so from the higher-skilled male students. Indeed, the large majority of their comments reinforced some of the taken-for-granted assumptions about women in sport. One high school male student wrote on the issue of sport clothing and body image as follows:

I think wearing skimpy outfits and being males' sex objects, I think is alright with me. That is the only reason I watch beach volleyball and gymnastics. I think nobody would watch that stuff if women were wearing long stuff like the men did.

Group Journals. We have had high school students complete some journal items as a team. The following is a group journal task that was used in one session:

Group Journal Assignment: *In your sport education teams, huddle around and look at the following short article. The athletes in this article claim their sport is not viewed legitimately. Who perpetuates this image of beach volleyball in our society? Is it correct? What other sports seem to face similar problems? Why is this? Has anybody on your team confronted a situation where they felt they were not being taken seriously in their sport, or were looked at in an unacceptable way? What were the reasons for this?*
    Captains: *Write down a brief summary of the different reactions/experiences.*
    Equity officers: *Be prepared to provide a 2-minute summary for other teams in the class.*

With a college-level class of physical education teacher candidates, Table 12.6 provided a rubric for guidance on the assessment of individual journal writing. The table includes an example of what might be written at each level.

Team Portfolios

There is considerable potential for including student work produced during a Cultural Studies unit within a 'team portfolio.' Kinchin (2001) discussed how team portfolios were used in the context of a 15-day unit experienced by physical education teaching majors. These portfolios included many pieces of work (e.g., team philosophy statements, self-assessment of performance, player profiles, team emblems/shirt designs, sample journal entries, team photographs). As Kinchin (2001) indicates, teams can be assessed using a four-level rubric to set out the range of attainment in relation to key expected elements of the port-

---

TABLE 12.6

Modified Rubric for Assessment of Journal Items

Level	Criteria
0	The student does not write anything, or what is written does not make sense or is illegible. *I think that. *&^%$#@! It is OK. It is fun. ZZZZZZZZZ*
1	The student's writing is descriptive in nature in response to a particular journal prompt. *We are having fun playing volleyball.* *Our team is playing well together.* *I have no comment really.* *I do not care about it that much.*
2	The student's writing includes description, but expands to attempt some justification/rationale/explanation for their views or reactions, which might be accompanied by an example from class or personal experience if appropriate. *Our team is very supportive of one another. We regularly warm up together and follow the directions of our team leaders and captain. I believe that this is because of the responsibility each person has in order for the team to play and practice effectively.*
3	The student's writing shows evidence of description, justification, and evaluation where they make judgements about the issue or actions of others. The journal item is scrutinized and thoroughly explored with the intention of being reflective/critical and analytical in their reactions. *My role is that of the coach. I have the responsibility of leading drills and assisting the captain in his/her duties. Coaching and teaching are very similar and both require knowledge of the game and how to motivate players. Today nobody is an island. Inter-dependency is so crucial to success in sports and in other areas of the work force. This inter-dependency is particularly critical in how we learn. We can learn from each other and not just from the instructor, and such an arrangement makes the situation learner-centered.*

folio and where students have gone beyond the minimum expectations. For example,

- **Level 1** is awarded for the non-submission of a portfolio.
- **Levels 2 and 3** are differentiated by the overall organization of the portfolio, the level of generality and/or specificity of the expected contents such as journal responses, the number of additional artifacts presented, and the quality of the presentation (hand-written). Some information may be missing. The significance of the items presented is either absent or implicit.

- **Level 4** meets all criteria related to expected content plus the inclusion of a set number of additional artifacts and journal/diary elements. The portfolio is organized, simple to follow, and presented in a neat and creative manner where the significance of the items in relation to the team is outlined.

Personal Sport Autobiography Assignment

The task of this presentation is to allow students to take a critical look at their own personal sport history (or a small section of it in the form of a particular event), and write an account. The assignment would aim to be relatively brief in length (two to three double-spaced pages), and might be informed by the following guidelines:

1. As you consider your own sport history, what factors have supported your efforts to participate in physical activity/sports (home influence, school, etc.)?
2. What factors have prevented you from participating in certain sports that you would have liked to have played, and never got the chance (discuss your feelings about this)?
3. To what extent have the experiences set out within this mini-autobiography shaped your views on participating in physical activity?

This type of assignment is intended to help high school students "begin to understand how adult work and family roles and responsibilities affect their decisions about physical activity and how physical activity, preferences and opportunities change over time" (NASPE, 2004, p. 39). It goes beyond family to look at local and national infrastructure and polices that impact on such decisions. Such assignments add a different experience for students to achieve the NASPE content standards.

Community Mapping

Every school is located in a community, and that community has a history and current resources that can enhance the learning experiences in physical education. Too often, we miss the opportunity to incorporate the community in enhancing students' learning and their experience of active lifestyles. Physical education teachers should introduce students to the sport, fitness, and recreation programs and facilities that exist in and near the students' local community so students can learn about and access these amenities and services during non-school time. The resources of the community can be used at various times to support and complement the physical education program. Community mapping promotes increased interaction between the school and the community, engaging teachers and students in systematic information gathering about use of the community in the planning of your teaching and in optimizing the learning of your students (O'Sullivan, Tannehill, & Hinchion, in press).

Additional Learning Activities Appropriate for the Model

There are several other learning activities that would be appropriate for this curricular approach. Activities and assignments related to Sport Education have been described in Chapter 11, and are not the focus of this chapter. This section of the chapter will focus on activities that enhance students' sport literacy and critical consumer skills. The first is the analysis of sport coverage in the school. In this activity (see Table 12.1), students work in small groups (could be the Sport Education teams) to understand the role that physical activity plays in the life of their school, as portrayed in the school media outlets. The goal will be for students to develop an awareness of not only which sports and physical activities are featured in the students' media guides, but also how that presentation has changed over time, in terms of the types of physical activities that are allocated space and the interaction of race, ethnicity, and ability in these text and photographic representations. A second activity (see Table 12.7) has students review data from the Centers for Disease Control and Prevention data set (2003) on barriers to young children's participation in physical activity as perceived by their parents. Students are asked to summarize the key findings, to determine to what degree students in their class would agree with these barriers to activity, and make recommendations that could be implemented in their school to minimize these barriers. A third activity involves an analysis of the school sports program, in terms of the budget allocated to different physical activities at the school and the number of students who are participating in those activities (see Table 12.8). Students share their analysis of the school's physical activity budget with their peers.

Disadvantages and Cautions to Teachers in Development of the Model

For many physical education teachers, especially those who are not health teachers, the ideas presented here subscribe to a different role for the physical education teacher. Those teachers who would enjoy the opportunity to discuss contemporary issues of sport and physical activity with their students would be most quickly drawn to this curricular model. There are four cautions we suggest as you think about implementing some of the ideas presented in this chapter. First, develop and deliver one unit for one class initially. You need student buy-in to such a different model, so choose a class you feel would be most receptive to these experiences. Second, balance the class time with a focus on

TABLE 12.7

Percentage of Parents of Children Ages 9–13 Years Who Reported Barriers to Their Children's Participation in Physical Activities, by Barrier and Selected Characteristics (Youth Media Campaign Longitudinal Survey, United States, 2002)

Characteristic	Transportation Problems		Lack of Opportunities in Area		Expense		Lack of Parents' Time		Lack of Neighborhood Safety	
	%	(95% CI*)	%	(95% CI)	%	(95% CI)	%	(95% CI)	%	(95% CI)
Sex										
Female	26.9	(±2.7)	20.8	(±2.3)	47.5	(±3.2)	22.8†	(±2.2)	17.6†	(±2.3)
Male	24.4	(±2.6)	19.5	(±2.0)	45.8	(±2.7)	19.2†	(±2.4)	14.6†	(±1.9)
Age (yrs)										
9	25.6	(±3.7)	20.5	(±3.1)	46.3	(±3.3)	20.3	(±3.6)	16.9	(±2.9)
10	26.2	(±3.5)	19.2	(±3.5)	46.4	(±3.9)	21.6	(±3.4)	18.0	(±3.4)
11	26.1	(±4.3)	21.1	(±3.1)	46.0	(±4.6)	20.7	(±3.2)	16.9	(±3.6)
12	24.9	(±3.0)	20.0	(±3.7)	49.0	(±3.6)	20.8	(±3.2)	15.9	(±3.0)
13	25.2	(±3.1)	19.8	(±3.5)	45.4	(±4.2)	21.5	(±3.1)	12.4	(±2.7)
Race/Ethnicity§										
Black, non-Hispanic	32.6†	(±4.8)	30.6†	(±5.7)	54.9†	(±6.2)	23.3	(±5.6)	13.3†	(±3.3)
Hispanic	36.9†	(±5.8)	30.8†	(±3.6)	62.3†	(±5.5)	23.3	(±4.7)	41.2†	(±5.8)
White, non-Hispanic	18.9†	(±2.3)	13.4†	(±2.1)	39.5†	(±2.5)	19.1	(±2.1)	8.5†	(±1.5)
Parental education										
<High school	42.7†	(±7.2)	36.7†	(±6.2)	65.9†	(±7.7)	27.3	(±6.6)	42.9†	(±7.3)
High school	32.3†	(±3.6)	23.8†	(±3.7)	54.8†	(±4.3)	20.5	(±3.1)	18.2†	(±3.4)
>High school	19.3†	(±2.0)	15.4†	(±2.2)	39.2†	(±2.5)	20.0	(±2.4)	10.2†	(±1.5)
Parental income										
≤$25,000	44.5†	(±4.7)	35.6†	(±4.4)	70.6†	(±4.6)	25.6†	(±3.5)	29.4†	(±4.0)
$25,001–$50,000	28.9†	(±3.9)	21.9†	(±3.2)	53.6†	(±3.4)	20.4	(±3.1)	17.8†	(±3.1)
>$50,000	14.4†	(±2.1)	11.5†	(±2.3)	30.8†	(±2.6)	19.0†	(±2.6)	8.6†	(±1.6)
Total	25.6	(±1.9)	20.1	(±1.7)	46.6	(±2.0)	21.0	(±1.6)	16.1	(±1.4)

* Confidence interval.
† Statistically significant difference ($p < 0.05$).
§ Numbers for other racial/ethnic populations were too small for meaningful analysis.

Source: Centers for Disease Control and Prevention. (2003). Physical activity levels among children aged 9–13 years—United States, 2002. *Morbidity and Mortality Weekly Report, 52*(33), 785–788. Retrieved February 25, 2004, from http://www.cdc.gov/mmwr/preview/mmwrhtml/mm5233a1.htm

TABLE 12.8

Sport, Status, and Access

Purpose of assignment	Understand the relationship between physical activity and the economy.
Materials needed	Your school's athletic department's budget for a fiscal year; student participation data for school sports for same year.
Procedure to complete task	In small groups, review the budget and participation data for your school. Discuss your findings in small groups. Prepare graphs showing how the budget was distributed, and its relationship to enrollment. Discuss access to participation from an equity perspective.
Rubric	

physical activity and integrating a discussion of the topics with the specific physical activity content focus. Third, choose a sport you are familiar with, and that you view as one of your teaching strengths. We chose volleyball simply because it was a content our teaching colleagues felt most comfortable with, because they had been longtime coaches and/or participants in the sport. Fourth, be prepared with a clear rationale for this curricular approach to your students, especially high school students, who will want to know the value of this for them. Their ownership of the content ensures meaningful engagement with the content. We suggest that you begin with in-class work assignments and work up slowly to out-of-class assignments (homework). We would recommend work that engages with local and regional issues and allows students opportunity to examine and debate these issues from a range of viewpoints. There is certainly no reason why students couldn't be encouraged to locate particular sources/prompts and bring them to class (e.g., local newspaper articles). Don't overuse the journaling activity. We found that asking students to write in their journal once or twice a week in a 5-day-a-week unit was about the limit of what they were willing to do if we wanted quality and reflective entries.

Summary

In summary, we would like to suggest that students are interested in the diverse world around them, and in interacting with that world in constructive and meaningful ways, if we present materials and information to them in forms that connect to their lives. Educating students to see themselves as part of this diversity and to be critical and reflective of their health and the sporting culture is an important part of their education. We think this is an exciting curricular model to engage them with these issues.

References

Beach, R., & Marshall, J. (1991). *Teaching literature in the secondary school*. San Diego, CA: Harcourt, Brace Jovanovich.

Beashel, P., & Taylor, J. (1992). *Sport assignments*. Scarborough, Ontario: Nelson Canada.

Burrows, L. (2004). Understanding and investigating cultural perspectives in physical education. In J. Wright, D. Macdonald, & L. Burrows (Eds.), *Critical inquiry and problem-solving in physical education* (pp. 105–119). New York: Routledge.

Capel, S., & Blair, R. (2007). Making physical education relevant: increasing the impact of initial teacher training. *London Review of Education, 5*(1), 15–34.

Carroll, P. (1994). Metamorphosis: one teacher's change, one class's reaction. *English Journal, 83*(6), 22–28.

Centers for Disease Control and Prevention. (2003). Physical activity levels among children aged 9–13 years—United States, 2002. *Morbidity and Mortality Weekly Report, 52*(33), 785–788. Retrieved February 25, 2004, from http://www.cdc.gov/mmwr/preview/mmwrhtml/mm5233a1.htm

Centers for Disease Control and Prevention. (2004). *Adolescents and young adults*. Retrieved January 15, 2009, from http://www.cdc.gov/nccdphp/sgr/adoles.htm

Eisner, E. (1985). Aesthetic modes of knowing. In E. Eisner (Ed.), *Learning and teaching the ways of knowing: eighty-fourth yearbook of the National Society for the Study of Education* (pp. 23–36). Chicago: National Society for the Study of Education.

Ennis, C. D., Cothran, D. J., Davidson, K. S., Loftus, S. J., Owens, L., Swanson, L., et al. (1997). Implementing a curriculum within a context of fear and disengagement. *Journal of Teaching in Physical Education, 17*(1), 52–71.

Ennis, C. D., Solmon, M. A., Satina, B., Loftus, S. J., Mensch, J., & McCauley, M. T. (1999). Creating a sense of family in urban schools using the "Sport for Peace" curriculum. *Research Quarterly for Exercise and Sport, 70*, 273–285.

Enright, E., & O'Sullivan, M. (2007, September). *Can I do it in my pyjamas?: negotiating a physical education curriculum with teenage girls*. Paper presented at the British Educational Research Association Annual Conference, London, England.

Enright, E., & O'Sullivan, M. (2008, February). *"Cos that's what I thought ye wanted to hear": participatory methods and research agendas in physical education research*. Paper presented at the Researching Children's Worlds Conference, Galway, Ireland.

Enright, E., & O'Sullivan, M. (in press). Carving a new order of experience with young people in physical education: participatory action research as a pedagogy of possibility. In M. O'Sullivan & A. MacPhail (Eds.), *Young people's voices in physical education and youth sport*. London: Routledge.

Fernandez-Balboa, J. M. (Ed.). (1997). *Critical postmodernism in human movement, physical education, and sport*. New Albany, NY: SUNY Press.

Glasby, T., & Macdonald, D. (2004). Negotiating the curriculum: challenging the social relationships in teaching. In J. Wright, D. Macdonald, & L. Burrows (Eds.), *Critical inquiry and problem solving in physical education* (pp. 133–145). New York: Routledge.

Hastie, P. A., & Curtner-Smith, M. D. (2006). Influence of a hybrid Sport Education-Teaching Games for Understanding unit on one teacher and his students. *Physical Education and Sport Pedagogy, 11*(1), 1–27.

Jewett, A, & Bain, L. (Eds.). (1987). The purpose process curriculum framework: a personal meaning model for physical education. *Journal of Teaching in Physical Education, 6*, 195–366.

Kinchin, G. D. (1997). High school students' perceptions of and responses to curriculum change in physical education. Unpublished doctoral dissertation, The Ohio State University.

Kinchin, G. D. (1998). Secondary students' responses to issues of gender in sport and physical activity. *Journal of Sport Pedagogy, 4*(1), 29–42.

Kinchin, G. D. (2001). Using team portfolios in a sport education season. *Journal of Physical Education, Recreation and Dance, 72*(2), 41–44.

Kinchin, G., & O'Sullivan, M. (1999). Making physical education meaningful for high school students. *Journal of Physical Education, Recreation and Dance, 70,* 40–44, 54.

Kinchin, G., & O'Sullivan, M. (2003). Incidences of student support for and resistance to a curricular innovation in high school physical education. *Journal of Teaching in Physical Education, 22,* 245–260.

Kirk, D. (1997). Schooling bodies for new times: the reform of school physical education high modernity. In J. M. Fernandez-Balboa (ed.), *Critical aspects in human movement: rethinking the profession in the post-modern era.* Albany: SUNY Press.

Kirk, D. (2005). Model-based teaching and assessment in physical education: the tactical games model. In K. Green and K. Hardman (Eds.), *Physical education: essential issues* (pp. 52–67). London: Sage.

Kirk, D., & Tinning, R. (Eds.). (1992). *Physical education, curriculum and culture: critical issues in the contemporary crisis.* New York: Falmer Press.

Kirk, D., Burgess-Limerick, R., Kiss, M., Lahey, J., & Penney, D. (1999). *Senior physical education: an integrated approach.* Champaign, IL: Human Kinetics.

Knop, N., Tannehill, D., & O'Sullivan, M. (2001). Making a difference for urban youths. *Journal of Physical Education, Recreation and Dance, 72,* 38–44.

Laker, A. (2002). *Beyond the boundaries of physical education.* London: Routledge.

Locke, L. (1992). Changing secondary school physical education curriculum. *Quest, 44,* 361–372.

National Association for Sport and Physical Education. (2004). *Moving into the future: national standards for physical education* (2nd ed.). Reston, VA: Author

New Zealand Ministry of Education. (1999). *Health and physical education in the New Zealand curriculum.* Wellington, New Zealand: Author.

Oliver, K. (2001). Images of the body from popular culture: engaging adolescent girls in critical inquiry. *Sport, Education, and Society, 6,* 143–164.

Oliver, K., & Lalik, R. (2001). The body as curriculum: learning with adolescent girls. *Journal of Curriculum Studies, 33,* 303–333.

Oliver, K. L., Hamzeh, M., & McCaughtry, N. (in press). "Girly girls can play games/Las niñas pueden jugar tambien": Co-creating a curriculum of possibilities with 5th grade girls. *Journal of Teaching in Physical Education.*

Oliver, K. L., & Lalik, R. (2004). Critical inquiry on the body in girls' physical education classes: a critical poststructural analysis. *Journal of Teaching in Physical Education, 23*(2), 162–195.

O'Sullivan, M., Kinchin, G., Kellum, S., Dunaway, S., & Dixon, S. (1996). Thinking differently about high school physical education. Paper presented at the AAHPERD National Convention, Atlanta, Georgia.

O'Sullivan, M., Tannehill, D., & Hinchion, C. (in press). Teaching as professional enquiry. In R. Bailey (Ed.)., *Physical education for learning.* London: Routledge.

Oxford Cambridge and RSA. (2008). *Advanced GCE in physical education.* Oxford, UK: Oxford, Cambridge & RSA Examinations.

Queensland Board of Senior Secondary School Studies. (1998). *Physical education senior syllabus*. Brisbane, Australia: Author.

Rink, J. (1993). What's so critical? In J. Rink (Ed.), *Critical crossroads: middle and secondary school physical education*. Reston, VA: NASPE.

Siedentop, D. (1994). *Sport education: quality PE through positive sport experience*. Champaign, IL: Human Kinetics.

Siedentop, D. (2002). Sport education: a retrospective. *Journal of Teaching in Physical Education, 21*, 409–418.

Siedentop, D., Hastie, P. A., & van der Mars, H. (2004). *The complete guide to sport education*. Champaign, IL: Human Kinetics.

Sparkes, A. (1988). The micropolitics of innovation in the physical education curriculum. In J. Evans (Ed.), *Teachers, teaching, and control in physical education* (pp. 157–178). Lewes, England: Falmer Press.

Steinhardt, M. (1992). Physical education. In P. W. Jackson (Ed.), *Handbook of research on curriculum* (pp. 964–1001). New York: Macmillan.

Thomson, P., & Gunter, H. M. (2006). From "consulting pupils" to "pupils as researchers": a situated case narrative. *British Educational Research Journal, 32*(6), 839–859.

Tinning, R., & Fitzclarence, L. (1992). Postmodern youth culture and the crisis in Australian secondary school physical education. *Quest, 44,* 287–304.

Wright. J. (2004). Critical inquiry and problem solving in physical education. In J. Wright, D. Macdonald, & L. Burrows (Eds.), *Critical inquiry and problem-solving in physical education* (pp. 3–15). New York: Routledge.

Wright, J., Macdonald, D., & Burrows, L. (Eds.). (2004). *Critical inquiry and problem-solving in physical education.* New York: Routledge.

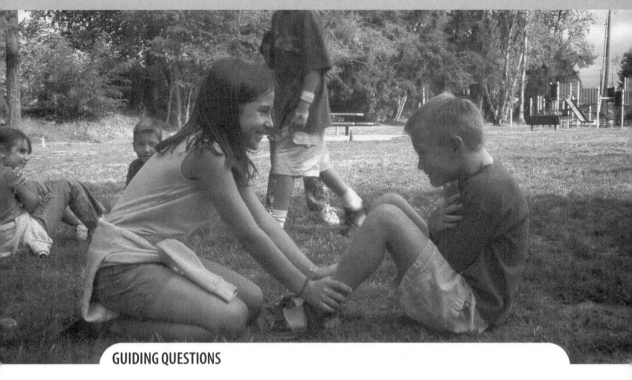

GUIDING QUESTIONS

1 What is fitness education?
2 What basic goals guide a concepts-based fitness education curriculum?
3 What is the philosophy of concepts-based fitness education?
4 What are the primary strengths and weaknesses of fitness education?
5 How can fitness education be used to meet national standards? Which NASPE content standards does this model best support?
6 What main components make up a fitness education curriculum, and what are some organizational options for incorporating these components into a course?
7 Why might there be an interest in this curriculum model for contemporary youth?
8 How might this curriculum model be incorporated into the physical education curriculum?
9 Describe assessment within this curriculum model.

Fitness Education

13

Karen McConnell, Pacific Lutheran University

Overview

Fitness education is a broad term that is frequently used to describe a number of different teaching scenarios. Courses that focus on traditional fitness activities such as weight training, jogging, aerobic dance, or swimming are often labeled as "fitness education." In other instances, teachers may infuse fitness activities into other common curriculum models by modifying drills, warm-up activities, or game rules. Teachers may also add an aerobic fitness activity to designated class sessions. The most common of such activities is running or jogging, which has been noted by students to be "boring" and "repetitive" (Rikard & Banville, 2006) and has been shown to be less effective at improving cardiovascular fitness than variable activity approaches that provide a combination of running, games, drills, and other aerobically centered activities (Wright & Karp, 2006). Although these scenarios may provide opportunities to engage in lifetime physical activity or develop elements of physical fitness, they often fail to provide students with the knowledge needed for decision making or independent activity. The most comprehensive approach to fitness education involves the use of **concepts-based fitness and wellness education**. In this curriculum model, the student is involved in classroom, laboratory, and physical activity experiences that are coordinated to emphasize both the how and why of physical fitness and wellness. In a concepts-based fitness model, the teacher maintains a focus on the process of physical activity rather than the product of physical fitness. Helping the student to develop the knowledge and skills necessary to maintain lifetime physical activity and fitness is paramount. Infusing fitness activities into other physical education courses, or

> **concepts-based fitness and wellness education**   A curriculum-based approach that focuses on one's knowledge and understanding of physical activity, physical fitness, and wellness.

offering specific fitness activity courses (such as weight training), are excellent ways to supplement a comprehensive concepts-based fitness course, but should not be considered the primary means of delivering fitness education. In essence, the concepts-based fitness course serves as the anchor of a more comprehensive fitness or wellness curriculum. Once a concepts-based course or courses are completed, a program could provide an offering of complementary fitness courses for students to select from (see Box 13.1). The remainder of this chapter is focused on the concepts-based fitness education model.

Fitness education is a highly relevant and useful curriculum model in today's society. The rates of physical inactivity among youth and adolescents are high (Centers for Disease Control and Prevention [CDC], 1996, 2002; Pate, Long, & Heath, 1994; Sallis, 1993), while indicators of premature death (such as hypertension, serum cholesterol levels, and obesity) are increasing (Nicklas, Web-

Box 13.1

Case Study: Lincoln Sudbury High School, Sudbury, Massachusetts

At Lincoln Sudbury High School, the fitness curriculum takes on a holistic wellness approach. Students are required to take 12 credits of wellness courses as part of a wellness curriculum that provides students with a comprehensive health and fitness education. The curriculum is designed to help students seek a balance of expression of individuality, a responsible concern for the needs of others, and the opportunity to examine and monitor personal wellness. Six of the 12 courses are required of all students. The required courses provide students with the foundation of wellness theories that assist them throughout their high school experience while fostering a lifelong commitment to health and fitness. The required courses are Introduction to Wellness, Cardiovascular Fitness, Muscular Fitness, Health Issues, Basic CPR/First Aid, and Outdoor Pursuits. Students then select six elective credits from an array of offerings including Fitness Games, Personal Fitness, Rocks and Ropes, Yoga, Cross Training, and an array of lifetime sport activities such as badminton, tennis, and golf.

The curriculum is spread over 3 years, with students taking two required courses and two elective courses each during their freshman, sophomore, and junior years. Courses are graded on an "A", "Pass", or "Fail" basis. In addition, the department maintains a health fitness assessment program that emphasizes the importance of the health-related components of fitness, motivates students to maintain good health, allows students to self-monitor their fitness levels, and provides individual assistance for students whose ratings fall below satisfactory levels. Students are monitored annually on muscular strength, flexibility, muscular endurance, and cardiovascular endurance. This type of comprehensive approach to fitness education supports the need to teach students key concepts and knowledge while allowing for ample opportunities to apply critical skills as well as exercise choice and individualized application.

Source: Susan Shields, Wellness Department Coordinator, Lincoln Sudbury High School.

ber, Johnson, Srinivasan, & Berenson, 1995; Troiano, Flegal, Kuczmarsksi, Campbell, & Johnson, 1995). Important parameters have been established regarding the adequate amounts of moderate and vigorous physical activity levels necessary for optimizing the health of children and youth (Corbin, Pangrazi, & Welk, 1994; Sallis & Patrick, 1994; U.S. Department of Health and Human Services [USDHHS], 2008) and research has repeatedly demonstrated that current practices in physical education classes fail to achieve these standards (Pate et al., 1995; USDHHS, 2008). Even under ideal circumstances, physical education alone cannot provide enough moderate or vigorous activity to meet the established standards (McGinnis, Kanner, & DeGraw, 1991; Pate et al., 1995; USDHHS, 2000), and research shows that the positive gains in fitness acquired in physical education during the academic year are transient and suffer from reversibility even during a single summer break (Carrel et al., 2007). As a result, physical education must do more to prepare and motivate students to engage in physical activity outside of school, and throughout their lives. Although a focus on fitness in physical education is not a new idea, current approaches to fitness education should be directed at developing lifetime physical activity habits, as opposed to "getting kids fit" by "doing fitness to kids." This is particularly important in light of the growing obesity epidemic and the temptation to utilize physical education as a sort of "fitness bootcamp," rather than as a mechanism for engaging students in developing the values, skills, and abilities necessary to pursue a lifetime of healthy physical activity regardless of body size. In doing so, this approach is rooted in achieving important public health outcomes and addressing behavioral training rather than exercise training. Fitness education provides an opportunity for students to develop healthy habits while gaining a value and appreciation of their importance throughout life. Concepts-based fitness courses have been shown to be effective at promoting positive improvements in knowledge, attitudes, and physical activity behaviors, in both the immediate and long term (Brynteson & Adams, 1993; Corbin & Dale, 2000; Slava et al., 1984) and have been shown to be more positively than negatively received by students (Jenkins, Jenkins, & Collums, 2006).

Model Philosophy

The philosophy of concepts-based fitness education is rooted in three primary needs (Strand, Scantling, & Johnson, 1997). First, students need the opportunity to engage in lifetime physical activities of sufficient intensity and duration necessary to help maximize health benefits. Second, students need to learn why it is important to develop and maintain adequate levels of physical activity and fitness. Finally, students must develop the knowledge base and skills necessary to plan and execute personal activity programs throughout their lives. This includes not only knowledge about programming (such as intensity, duration, and time), but also self-knowledge about attitudes, motivation, barriers, and abilities. In achieving these goals, the basic philosophy of moving the student from a state of dependence on external instruction and motivation to a state of independent motivation and decision making is achieved. Corbin's Stairway to Lifetime Fitness (Corbin & Lindsey, 2002) provides a schematic that demonstrates this progression (Figure 13.1). Corbin criticizes most physical education curricula for stopping at Level 1, and failing to guide students to the higher order objectives. A teacher who successfully moves his or her students up the stairway will begin to relinquish control over decision making, but will be available to help guide students in making realistic individual activity choices and in developing obtainable activity and fitness goals.

Concepts-based fitness education is best implemented at the secondary level. Focusing on general **health-related fitness** components (cardiovascular, muscular strength, muscular endurance, muscular flexibility, and body composition) through an introduction to self-assessments, short-term goal setting, and fitness activities would be an appropriate practice for the middle school level. Expanding upon these concepts, focusing on more long-term and lifetime goals, and developing comprehensive fitness and wellness programs (often including related planning around nutrition and stress management), is an appropriate focus at the high school level. Implementing a comprehensive concepts-based fitness course at the elementary level is both inefficient and developmentally inappropriate (McConnell et al., 2004). However, teaching basic fitness vocabulary and introducing basic concepts (such as introducing what cardiovascular fitness is, and how to take and interpret resting heart rate) are appropriate practices within a traditional elementary education program.

The overarching goal of concepts-based fitness is to provide students with all of the skills necessary to choose to be active for a lifetime. At the elementary level, one should maintain a focus on enjoyment, social development, and motor skill development through exposure to a wide variety of games, dance, sports, and activities. Ultimately, success at achieving these goals in the elementary years will provide the critical foundation necessary for the long-term success of a secondary fitness education program.

health-related fitness   Aspects of physical fitness that are known to positively impact overall health, such as cardiorespiratory fitness, muscular strength, muscular flexibility, muscular endurance, and body composition.

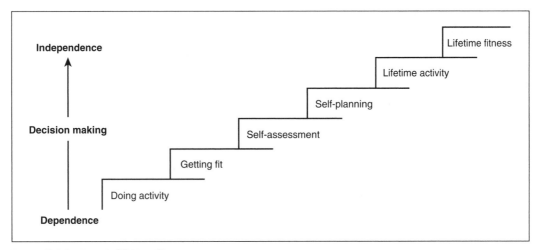

FIGURE 13.1 Stairway to lifetime fitness.
Source: Adapted from McConnell, K., Dale, D., & Corbin, C. (2004). *Fitness for life: teacher resources.* (5th ed.). Champaign, IL: Human Kinetics.

Model Characteristics

Concepts-based fitness education offers opportunities for experiential learning and application of knowledge through an integrated and evolving exposure to fitness, and health and wellness concepts and practices. Courses using this model are typically organized around general concepts (i.e., cardiovascular health, muscular strength, body composition, energy balance, etc.), and activities are focused primarily on lifetime sports and lifetime activities as opposed to traditional team sports or youth sports. Key terms and basic concepts are introduced in the classroom and applied through laboratory experiences and activity options. Examples of commonly taught concepts are found in Box 13.2. Fitness education places a stronger emphasis on the cognitive domain than traditional physical education models. Textbooks, worksheets, self-assessments, reflection activities, homework, and activity logs stimulate learning and help to move the student from a state of dependence upon the teacher to a state of self-directed, independent physical activity. Many concepts-based courses require students to demonstrate an ability to conceptualize, plan, execute, and evaluate personal fitness programs as a culminating project.

A typical week of a daily concepts-based physical education class might involve three activity-centered days (including one laboratory experience or self-assessment experience) and two classroom-focused lessons. Activity days may be designed and led by the teacher, or they may involve some degree of student selection of activities or student leadership of activities. Having students work in small groups to create an aerobic dance lesson to be taught to the class is an

---

Box 13.2

Commonly Addressed Fitness Education Concepts

Foundational base
Elements of health-related fitness.
Elements of skill-related fitness.
Importance of physical activity to lifetime health.
Importance of exercise to performance and fitness.
Importance of each health-related fitness component to lifetime health and fitness.
FIT principle (frequency, intensity, time) in relation to physical activity and exercise objectives.
Self-assessment of health and skill-related fitness.
Application of self-assessment results in goal setting and program planning.
Setting short- and long-term goals for physical activity and fitness.
Safety concerns pertaining to a variety of lifetime and fitness activities (clothing, hydration, environment, equipment, warm-up, etc.).
Consumer skills for fitness services and products, including Internet literacy.

Behavior change concepts
Understand common barriers to physical activity and the strategies used to overcome them. Examples include:
  Time management
  Performance anxiety
  Physique anxiety/image concerns
  Self-confidence
  Social support
  Changing attitudes about activity

Wellness concepts (advanced courses)
Stress and its effects on physical and emotional well-being.
Self-assessment of stressors and physical effects of stress.
Stress management and relaxation techniques (emphasis on physical activity and exercise for stress management).
Basic nutrition.
Dietary self-assessment.
Dietary planning (emphasis on energy balance and eating appropriately to support activity and exercise goals).

---

example of a typical activity. Circuits highlighting fitness activities are also common. **Laboratory experiences** are likely to include self-assessments such as a **fitness assessment** or dietary analysis, or other applied learning experiences such as comparing heart rate responses from activities of differing intensities. Laboratory experiences are designed to involve the student in active

laboratory experiences   Activities designed to provide an arena for cognitive concepts to be applied and understood within a fitness education approach; the experience usually involves some sort of personal awareness or application.
fitness assessment   Designed to provide individualized feedback regarding one's overall fitness status and/or physiological responses to physical effort.

learning and self-evaluation. The outcome of a laboratory experience should provide each student with useful information about his or her own health or fitness, and should reinforce concepts presented in class. Classroom days focus on cognitive learning and application. A traditional classroom is not essential for designated classroom days, but is preferred. The *Fitness for Life* curriculum employs this basic organizational scheme, and is one of the earliest and most widely recognized fitness education curricula (Corbin & Lindsey, 1997). The student textbook covers 18 chapters, and a wide variety of teacher's resources exist to aid in the delivery of content and organization of activities. An example of how one week of the *Fitness for Life* curriculum is organized is found in Table 13.1.

Other organizational strategies can be used to accommodate different scheduling options. When no classroom is available, a combination approach is often applied. In this organizational scheme, each class period includes a "mini-lecture" lasting 10 to 20 minutes, followed by an appropriate physical activity. Block plans and accelerated block plans can include a full classroom-based lesson and a full session of activity on each day the class meets (typically 2 to 3 days per week). Examples of how these organizational schemes might look are presented in Figure 13.2. Regardless of how a fitness education course is organized, the basic elements of the model (cognitive concepts, laboratory experiences, physical activity) should be included.

Fitness Education and the National Standards

Fitness education is able to address all of the national standards (to varying degrees) when well executed. Standards 2, 3, 4, and 6 are major components of the model, while Standards 1 and 5 are minor components. The Physical Education Curriculum Analysis Tool (PECAT) developed by the Department of Health and Human Services of the Centers for Disease Control and Prevention highlights critical markers of strong curriculum in light of each of the national standards set forth by NASPE.

The Major Components

Standard 2: Demonstrates understanding of movement concepts, principles, strategies, and tactics as they apply to the learning and performance of physical activities.

NASPE Content Standard 2 is focused on the ability of the learner to use cognitive information to understand and enhance motor skill development. Fitness education regularly applies important concepts from the disciplines of sport psychology and exercise physiology towards the analysis of, selection of, and participation in appropriate fitness activities. Students may be taught about the common barriers to physical activity; they then may assess the barriers in their own lives in order to be guided in establishing and applying strategies to

TABLE 13.1

Example Content and Organizational Layout for One Lesson of the *Fitness for Life* Curriculum

Monday	Tuesday	Wednesday	Thursday	Friday
Physical Activity Activity 1.1: Starter Workout	Classroom Lesson 1.1: Physical Activity: A Lifestyle	Physical Activity Self-Assessment 1: Exercise Basics	Classroom Lesson 1.2: Fitness Through Activity	Physical Activity Activity 1.2: Health- and Skill-Related Fitness Stunts
Description: An introductory workout involving 10 stations that students work through independently. A handout is available that describes each activity, and allows for the number of repetitions completed to be recorded.	Description: This lesson introduces basic concepts (physical fitness, health, wellness, physical activity, exercise), and presents some of the benefits of regular physical activity.	Description: Students practice basic warm-up stretches using appropriate technique. Instructions guide students through appropriately taking resting and exercise heart rate.	Description: Introduces the 11 components of fitness (5 health and 6 skill related), and presents the Stairway to Lifetime Fitness.	Description: Stunts designed to utilize each of the fitness components are completed by students. A worksheet allows students to record successes and to comment on their personal strengths and weaknesses.
Assessment Option: Place students in groups and have each group demonstrate one of the activities correctly.	Assignment Option: Self-management questionnaire on "self-confidence." Students evaluate their own self-confidence, and reflect on the results.	Assessment Option: Students complete worksheet that requires calculating heart rates using varying techniques and answering questions regarding heart rate responses to exercise. Worksheet is placed in portfolio or notebook.	Assignment or Assessment Option: Application worksheet that has students identify the health- and skill-related fitness components needed for a variety of recreation and job-related activities.	Assignment or Assessment Options: Chapter test, reinforcement worksheet (crossword puzzle on vocabulary), project (interview adults on health-related fitness practices).

Source: Adapted from Corbin, C. B., & Lindsey, R. (1997). *Fitness for life: teacher's edition* (4th ed., pp. T21–T22). Glenview, IL: Scott Foresman.

The Basic Plan—daily physical education, one-semester course

Monday	Tuesday	Wednesday	Thursday	Friday
Physical activity Activity 1.1	*Classroom* Lesson 1	*Physical activity* Self-assessment	*Classroom* Lesson 2 Chapter review	*Physical activity* Activity 1.2

The Combination Plan—daily physical education, one-semester course

Monday	Tuesday	Wednesday	Thursday	Friday
Classroom and Activity Begin Lesson 1 Activity 1.1	*Classroom and Activity* Finish Lesson 1 Additional activity	*Classroom and Activity* Self-management feature Self-assessment	*Classroom and Activity* Begin Lesson 2 Activity 1.2	*Classroom and Activity* Finish Lesson 1.2 Chapter review Additional activity

The Integrated Plan—daily physical education, combined with traditional physical education over two semesters

Monday	Tuesday	Wednesday	Thursday	Friday
Physical activity Regular physical education	*Classroom* Lesson 1 Self-management feature	*Physical activity* Self-assessment	*Physical activity* Regular physical education	*Physical activity* Activity 1.1

Monday	Tuesday	Wednesday	Thursday	Friday
Physical activity Regular physical education	*Classroom* Lesson 2 Chapter review	*Physical activity* Activity 1.2	*Physical activity* Regular physical education	*Physical activity* Regular physical education

FIGURE 13.2 Example organizational formats for the *Fitness for Life* curriculum.
Source: Adapted from Corbin, C. B., & Lindsey, R. (1997). *Fitness for life: teacher's edition* (4th ed., pp. T21–T22). Glenview, IL: Scott Foresman.

overcome these barriers. Understanding anxiety in terms of generalized stress, as well as how it pertains to performance or appearance, may also be included in the behavioral modification focus of this model. Students may also complete self-evaluations of their stress levels, their body image, or their performance anxiety in order to integrate successful coping mechanisms into their daily lives. Important exercise physiology concepts provide much of the foundation upon which the cognitive component of fitness education is established. Understanding how basic physiology concepts impact important training principles, such as specificity, overload, reversibility, and progression, is paramount to integrating such principles into lifetime activity program development. Applying this knowledge through self-assessments and laboratory experiences constitutes an essential component of fitness education.

Standard 3: Participates regularly in physical activity.

The intent of this standard is to establish regular participation in meaningful physical activity. Essential to this standard is the student's engagement in physical activity outside of the physical education environment. Achievement of this standard involves the demonstration of effective self-management skills, coupled with enjoyment and skill acquisition, which leads the student to achieve the recommendations regarding the type, frequency, duration, and intensity of activity necessary to promote a healthy lifestyle. The philosophy of fitness education is an ideal match for this standard. Providing adequate opportunities for students to engage in a variety of lifestyle activities in class, while teaching them how to plan, prepare, participate in, and evaluate a personal activity program outside of class, constitutes the basic philosophy of fitness education. Ultimately, the success of fitness education is the achievement of lifelong physical activity.

Standard 4: Achieves and maintains a health-enhancing level of physical fitness.

This standard addresses the student's ability and willingness to accept responsibility for personal fitness. In doing so, the student develops higher levels of basic fitness around the health-related components of cardiorespiratory endurance, muscular strength and endurance, flexibility, and body composition. The intent of this standard is not to achieve a single predetermined level of fitness for all students, but to work with students individually to establish and reach personal goals. Not only do students work to achieve individual levels of personal fitness, they engage in learning opportunities that allow them to understand individual differences and how they impact each element of fitness. External influences such as time management, social support, and intrinsic motivation are also explained in a concepts-based fitness course. Ultimately, a successful fitness education program will allow a student to achieve and maintain the expectations of Standard 4 throughout all of the unexpected circumstances and changes they may encounter in their lives.

Standard 6: Values physical activity for health, enjoyment, challenge, self-expression, and/or social interaction.

The intent of this standard is to place intrinsic value and personal meaning on the benefits of participating in physical activity. Guiding students through self-reflection and evaluation of activity interests and opportunities occurs in fitness education. Students are helped to identify their attitudes toward different activities, explore opportunities for activity participation in the community, seek out social support for their interests, and evaluate their own skills and health-related fitness in an effort to enhance their success and enjoyment in lifetime physical activity. Challenge is achieved through the development, assessment, and modification of both physical activity goals and physical fitness goals. Fundamental to fitness education is the notion of choice of activity selection. Allowing students the opportunity to choose which activity they will engage in helps to establish self-expression and enjoyment both inside and outside of the classroom setting. Goal setting and choice combine to maximize personal success and achievement for all students.

The Minor Components

Standard 1: Demonstrates competency in motor skills and movement patterns needed to perform a variety of physical activities.

Developing the necessary breadth of skill needed to enjoy a variety of activities is the intent of Standard 1. Because fitness education is best implemented at the secondary level, and the focus is on lifetime activities that often require less skill, the development of motor skills is not a primary focus of the model. Students do select relatively fewer activities to engage in during a fitness education course, and therefore opportunities for refinement of skill are present. However, refining skills is not deemed as important to the model as making appropriate selections based on personal strengths of existing skills. It should be noted that the lesser focus on skill development does not preclude the use of skill-oriented drills or sport drills and activities, and these can be used to enhance fitness and help students to perform at a higher level. However, the choice of activity should ultimately belong to the student, and sport skill competence should not be a required element of a fitness course. Preserving student choice is essential because it increases the likelihood of enjoyment and adherence.

Standard 5: Exhibits responsible personal and social behavior that respects self and others in physical activity settings.

The achievement of self-initiated behaviors that promote personal and group success in activity settings constitutes the intent of this standard. Safe practices, adherence to rules and procedures, etiquette, cooperation, ethical behavior, and positive social interactions are important to the achievement of this standard. Fitness education is clearly rooted in self-motivation and self-respect, and places a specific emphasis on safe practices for individual fitness, but does not place a focus on teamwork or social dynamics as a critical outcome. How a concepts-based course is taught will have more to do with the achievement of the social domain of this standard than the actual fitness education curriculum. Opportunities for group work abound in both the classroom and gym environment, and the intent of the individual instructor, or the makeup of a given class, may dictate how much focus is given to conflict resolution or character development issues. Diversity in individual fitness levels does present itself in a fitness course, and offers potential for addressing differences that occur as a result of heredity, gender, size, and maturation. However, because these issues are not direct outcomes for most fitness education courses, they remain a minor focus.

Benefits and Limitations of Fitness Education

The major benefits of this model include the cognitive focus, the inclusiveness that lifetime activities provide, and the individualized and personal approach to activity selection and achievement. The strong cognitive component of concepts-based fitness education teaches students to understand the why and how of physical activity and fitness, while guiding them to be informed and independent consumers of health and fitness information. Ultimately, this helps to develop critical self-responsibility skills related to behaviors and life choices. The cognitive element is also more easily justified to academic administration, thus helping to strengthen the position of physical education in the school curriculum. Additionally, teachers can utilize homework and numerous assessments such as tests, projects, and personal programs to provide objective evaluation of student comprehension. The emphasis on lifetime physical activities that typically require less skill development allows for a high likelihood of personal success for all students. Choice in activity selection and student involvement in activity design also enhances student interest and enjoyment. In addition, the individualized approach works well in co-educational settings and in diverse classes. Fitness education is also a natural match for integrating technology into physical education. Presentation software, pedometers, heart rate monitors, computer graphing and data analysis, interactive video gaming activities, and Internet research can all be used to enhance a fitness education course.

As with any curriculum model, limitations do exist. The limitations of this model include a variety of resource-related constraints, preparation and evaluation time demands, teacher readiness, and misuse of fitness objectives. Fitness education must be handled carefully and conducted thoroughly in order for the objectives to be met and the goals of the program to be achieved. Orchestrating a successful fitness education course requires considerable planning and evaluation time, and presents a real challenge when constraints limit the amount of time available. Conducting a comprehensive program that effectively addresses all of the fitness and wellness concepts in a single semester is a daunting, if not impossible, task. Teachers must carefully select the most relevant and necessary concepts for addressing their local standards, while providing the necessary core knowledge. Even if a commitment exists to expand a concepts-based course across multiple grade levels or semesters, coordinating and planning the scope and sequence within a district can be difficult. Physical education teachers who are not used to preparing handouts, worksheets, assignments, and tests might find these elements of preparation overwhelming or tedious. Similarly, evaluation of essay questions, student goals, student fitness programs, and other written work may be unwelcome or burdensome when combined with coaching or administrative responsibilities. Materials that help aid a fitness education curriculum, such as textbooks and photocopies, may not be budgeted for, and fitness equipment may not be available or cost-effective. Additionally, teachers trained primarily in physical education may not feel comfortable in a classroom setting, or have the necessary background in health, fitness, and wellness. Although not a specific weakness of the model itself, misunderstanding regarding fitness assessments abound, and often lead to inappropriate use of results within a fitness education program. Using student fitness assessment results in student, teacher, or program evaluations are examples of such misuses (Corbin, 2002) (see Box 13.3).

Box 13.3

PECAT Assessment Analysis Items Strongly Associated with a Concepts-Based Fitness Curriculum and Sample Assessment Items

Standard 1: Demonstrates competency in motor skill movement patterns needed to perform a variety of physical activities

PECAT Item 1.4: The curriculum includes protocols for assessing student's ability to apply a variety of locomotor, nonlocomotor, manipulative, combination, and specialized skills, such as asking students to demonstrate the ability to perform a routine using manipulative equipment to music.

Example fitness education assessment item: Students design and teach a 128-count step aerobic routine to music that maintains heart rate within the desired training zone.

Standard 2: Demonstrates understanding of movement concepts, principles, strategies, and tactics as they apply to the learning and performance of physical activities.

PECAT Item 2.1: The curriculum includes protocols for determining student's ability to describe and demonstrate the critical features of movement forms for all specialized skills taught in grades 9–12.

Example fitness education assessment item: Students analyze their ability to successfully engage in a selected lifetime activity, based on its associated movement patterns and requirements, in relation to their self-assessed levels of both health-related and skill-related fitness.

Standard 3: Participates regularly in physical activity

PECAT Item 3.1: The curriculum includes protocols for assessing students' knowledge (e.g., through written exams and quizzes) about patterns of physical activity participation and how they change over the lifespan.

Example fitness education assessment item: Students are given a case study to read that chronicles an individual's activity patterns across the lifespan and are asked to identify how the case study is similar to and different from lifespan physical activity trends.

PECAT Item 3.2: The curriculum includes protocols for determining students' ability to independently develop and implement a personal physical activity program, such as asking students to write a comprehensive program and identify reasons for their choice of physical activities.

Example fitness education assessment item: Students engage in weekly goal setting for individual activities, (both in and out of class), log activities, and reflect on their success in meeting their activity goals. Students then develop a comprehensive plan based on their observations and reflections throughout the course.

Continued

Box 13.3

PECAT Assessment Analysis Items Strongly Associated with a Concepts-Based Fitness Curriculum and Sample Assessment Items—Cont'd

PECAT Item 3.3: The curriculum includes protocols for determining students' ability to independently apply training principles to their own participation in their favorite activities and/or sports, such as asking students which principles of training are being utilized in basketball.

Example fitness education assessment item: Students learn basic training principles and are asked to explain each one using one sport example and one lifetime activity or recreation example.

PECAT Item 3.4: The curriculum includes protocols for determining students' capacity to monitor their own physical activity and use appropriate behavior change strategies to positively impact their activity patterns.

Example fitness education assessment item: Students complete a variety of behavior change questionnaires (such as those based on the Stages of Change model) and reflect on their own barriers to change, including identifying concrete strategies for overcoming identified barriers.

Standard 4: Achieves and maintains a health-enhancing level of physical fitness.

PECAT Item 4.1: The curriculum includes protocols for determining student knowledge about the appropriate activities for each component of fitness as well as the activities that will help students meet their personal goals.

Example fitness education assessment item: Students work in groups to develop three to five training activities that develop one of the components of fitness. Each group leads the class in its activities and students reflect on their level of mastery and enjoyment of each training activity.

PECAT Item 4.2: The curriculum includes protocols for knowledge about the basic concepts of exercise physiology, such as asking students to identify and explain two or more principles of training that influence their own personal activity program.

Example fitness education assessment item: Students are asked to utilize the basic training principles as part of the development of a personalized fitness plan.

PECAT Item 4.3: The curriculum includes protocols for determining students' knowledge about fitness testing standards and their ability to monitor and interpret personal fitness data.

Example fitness education assessment item: Students engage in comprehensive health-related fitness testing at multiple points in the curriculum and are asked to interpret their results and reflect on changes in relation to their lifestyle patterns.

PECAT Item 4.4: The curriculum includes protocols for analyzing students' personal health-related fitness programs, including an analysis of their personal fitness goals.

Example fitness education assessment item: Students develop a personalized fitness plan that is aligned to their personal fitness goals. Plans are evaluated on how well the activities align with stated goals.

Continued

Box 13.3

PECAT Assessment Analysis Items Strongly Associated with a Concepts-Based Fitness Curriculum and Sample Assessment Items—Cont'd

Standard 5: Exhibits responsible personal and social behavior that respects self and others in physical activity settings.

PECAT Item 5.3: The curriculum includes protocols for assessing students' knowledge, skills, and ability to set up safety procedures for a variety of physical activities, fitness testing, games, and sports.

Example fitness education assessment item: Students are asked to identify three risks of a given activity and provide one safety precaution for each potential risk.

Standard 6: Values physical activity for health, enjoyment, challenge, self-expression, and/or social interaction.

PECAT Item 6.2: The curriculum includes protocols that ask students to identify and analyze characteristics of sports and physical activities they enjoy, and explain their reason for enjoyment.

Example fitness education assessment item: Students are asked to select two sports or activities they enjoy and two they don't enjoy, and explain the reasons for their selections.

PECAT Item 6.4: The curriculum includes protocols for assessing students' ability and willingness to pursue new challenges and competition in physical activity, such as asking students to participate in a new activity outside of physical education class and provide a brief overview of the experience.

Example fitness education assessment item: Students engage in a class project in which they identify all of the community-based opportunities to participate in sport or activity during the given term. Students then select one activity from the list to try, and report back to the class what they experienced.

Source: Centers for Disease Control and Prevention. (2006). *Physical education curriculum analysis tool* (PECAT). Atlanta: Author.

Student Assessment in Fitness Education

Assessments of student learning may take numerous forms within a concepts-based fitness curriculum. Essential to the objectives is the attainment of knowledge about physical activity and fitness. Both formative and summative assessments that are traditionally used in other academic areas may be applied to assess the cognitive component of the course. These include quizzes and exams, presentations, projects, journals, papers, demonstrations, laboratory reports, and learning games, as well as informal feedback through class discussion, question and answer sessions, and other similar interactions (see Table 13.2). Activity competence can be assessed through demonstrations, activity leadership,

---

TABLE 13.2

Sample of Select Assessment Items

Journal/Reflection Questions	Use personal reflection questions to practice writing skills or to spark class conversation. An example question might be: "What is the difference between being physically active and being athletic?" or "When are you most comfortable exercising, and why?" Have students keep their answers in a journal to be collected and evaluated on thoughtfulness and completion.
Group Projects	Have groups of 3 to 4 students develop 32 counts of an aerobic dance routine (traditional, hip-hop, kick-boxing, etc.). Have each group teach the class, and build the segments together into a single class routine. Have students give a short presentation on a lifestyle disease (e.g., heart disease, diabetes, or cancer), and explain how physical activity/inactivity relates to it.
Individual Projects	Create a Risk Factor Family Tree. Identify lifestyle risks for heart disease (smoking, fatty diet, sedentary lifestyle, etc.) that run in the family and present them on a poster. Include a statement on how to avoid these negative family traditions. Interview someone who works in a career or profession of interest. Find out what a typical day involves. Write a paragraph that evaluates which components of fitness are important for the job.
Demonstrations	Have each student demonstrate an appropriate activity for a given objective and body part. For example "demonstrate an exercise for building muscle endurance in the quadriceps" or "demonstrate a flexibility exercise for the trapezius muscle." Have students demonstrate how to correctly conduct a fitness assessment or portion of a fitness assessment. For example, "show me how to set up a step test, and explain how you would do it," or "perform a flexibility assessment of your choosing."

---

and active participation. In addition, integration of both the knowledge base and activity competence can be assessed through personal program development, which includes goal setting, program planning, program participation, and program evaluation.

Many options exist for translating assessments of student learning to evaluation and grading in a concepts-based fitness course. An important consideration to remember is that grades should not be tied to fitness levels as determined by fitness assessments. The important outcome is not the student's fitness levels, but his or her understanding of what the results mean, and how to go about improving the results if desired. The student should ultimately know how to assess his or her own fitness levels, interpret the results, and develop a personal program that is centered around the results and his or her personal goals. Comprehensive personal program development is not necessary or advised for all situations. Using several specific, short-term planning opportunities is sufficient for introductory courses (for example, planning one week of muscular strength activities, completing and logging the activities, and reflecting on them in order to change or improve the plan).

Fitness Education in Practice

The practice of fitness education in schools varies widely. Facilities and equipment often dictate the specific approach that is taken. The fitness education program at Lake Park High School in Illinois is recognized as a Blue Ribbon Award winner by the Illinois Association of Health, Physical Education, Recreation, and Dance. The commitment to fitness education at Lake Park High School began in the late 1960s, and has progressed ever since. Fitness education is considered the thread that runs through all elements of the program, and the entire curriculum is aligned with national goals and standards. The curriculum is fully developed, and available for all teachers to utilize. Written schematics and assessments for each course show the alignment with goals and standards. Students are not graded on fitness levels or improvement on fitness tests, but are evaluated on knowledge and participation. Deb Vogel, a 26-year veteran teacher at the school, acknowledges that first-year students often struggle with the academic approach to physical education until they fully understand what is trying

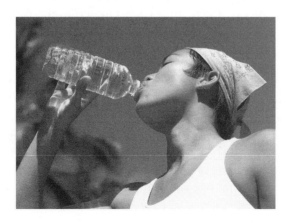

to be accomplished. According to Vogel, a credible and enthusiastic instructor helps to quickly diffuse student struggles.

The campus at Lake Park High School is equipped with two fitness centers, gymnasiums, balcony spaces, and two weight rooms. Computers and heart rate monitors are also available for downloading and tracking exercise data. The one-semester course for 9th grade students includes the following five units of instruction: 1) aerobic training and conditioning, 2) strength and endurance training, 3) first aid, 4) coordination and flexibility, and 5) spatial awareness. Program objectives require students to demonstrate competency in a variety of leisure and work-related activities; know and apply the principles and components of health-related fitness; assess individual fitness levels; set goals based on fitness data; develop, implement, monitor, and improve individual plans; explain the basic principles of health promotion, illness prevention, and safety; and explain the health-related actions of body systems. A second, semester-long course is offered for grades 11–12. The Personal Wellness: Nutrition and Exercise course integrates family and consumer sciences with health and physical education. Students alternate weeks between the classroom and the gym, and participate in nutrition and fitness assessments, while learning about nutrition and exercise. Each student maintains a diet and activity log that includes a requirement of 30 minutes of physical activity outside of school on days when students are in the classroom. In the physical activity portion of the course, heart rate responses to exercise are recorded. Students maintain all of their data in an electronic portfolio, and use their information to develop and implement a personal nutrition and activity plan.

Lake Park High School benefits from a well-established program with strong facilities and equipment. However, as Vogel states, ". . . funding is a non-issue. The issue is what should we be teaching and how teachers deliver the information being taught." In central Washington, an individual high school teacher implements a strong standards-based program on a limited budget, and without the aid of fitness specific equipment or advanced technology. Drawing from the *Fitness for Life* curriculum materials, the teacher provides mini-lectures in the gymnasium at the beginning of each class. Each day starts with a short reflection question to engage the students on the topic to be covered. The cognitive focus is on basic fitness concepts, goal setting, program planning, safety, nutrition, and stress management. Each student collects self-assessment data from a variety of fitness assessments and other health assessments; maintains a journal with answers to the reflection questions; writes and evaluates weekly activity goals; evaluates their level and quality of physical activity participation; and completes a variety of worksheets and handouts designed to enhance the learning and application of key concepts.

All of the student's information and work are maintained in a Wellness Port-folio, and a comprehensive wellness plan is completed by each student as a final culminating project.

Summary

The term "fitness education" is often used casually to describe a variety of ap-proaches to a fitness-centered curriculum. However, concepts-based fitness edu-cation encompasses a specific approach to fitness education that is designed to emphasize both the how and why of physical activity and fitness. Corbin's Stair-way to Lifetime Fitness serves as a visual to reinforce the importance of moving students from a state of dependence upon the teacher to a state of independent decision making and activity. Teaching is done in both the classroom and the gym in order to incorporate cognitive learning opportunities, self-evaluations, and participation in moderate amounts of lifetime physical activities. The goal of a strong fitness education curriculum is to provide students with all of the tools and skills they will need in order to choose to be active now and through-out their lives.

References

Brynteson, P., & Adams, T. M. (1993). The effects of conceptually based physical education programs on attitudes and exercise habits of college alumni after 2- and 11-year follow-up. Research Quarterly for Exercise and Sport, 64(2), 208–212.

Carrel, A. L., Clark, R. R., Peterson, S., Eickhoff, J., & Allen, D. B. (2007). School-based fitness changes are lost during the summer vacation. Archives of Pediatrics and Adolescent Med-icine, 161 (6), 561–564.

Centers for Disease Control and Prevention. (1995). Youth risk behavior surveillance—United States. Morbidity and Mortality Weekly Report, 45(SS-4).

Centers for Disease Control and Prevention. (2002). Physical activity levels among children aged 9–13 years—United States. Morbidity and Mortality Weekly Report, 52(33), 785–788.

Centers for Disease Control and Prevention. (2006). Physical education curriculum analysis tool (PECAT). Atlanta: Author.

Corbin, C. B. (2002). Physical activity for everyone: what every educator should know about promoting lifelong physical activity. Journal of Teaching in Physical Education, 21(2), 12.

Corbin, C. B., & Dale, D. (2000). Physical activity participation of high school graduates fol-lowing exposure to conceptual or traditional physical education. Research Quarterly for Exercise and Sport, 71(1), 61–69.

Corbin, C. B., & Lindsey, R. (1997). Fitness for life teacher's edition (4th ed.). Glenview, IL: Scott Foresman.

Corbin, C. B., & Lindsey, R. (2002). Fitness for life (4th ed., updated). Champaign, IL: Human Kinetics.

Corbin, C. B., Pangrazi, R. P., & Welk, G. J. (1994). Toward an understanding of appropriate physical activity levels for youth. *Physical Activity and Fitness Research Digest, 1*(8), 1–8.

Jenkins, J. M., Jenkins, P., & Collums, A. (2006). Student perceptions of a conceptual physical education activity course. *Physical Educator, 63*(4), 210–221.

McConnell, K., Dale, D., & Corbin, C. (2004). *Fitness for life: teacher resources.* Champaign, IL: Human Kinetics.

McGinnis J. M., Kanner L., & DeGraw C. (1991). Physical education's role in achieving national health objectives. *Research Quarterly for Exercise and Sport, 62*(2), 138–142.

Nicklas, T. A., Webber, L. S., Johnson, C. C., Srinivasan, S. R., & Berenson G. S. (1995). Foundations for health promotion with youth: a review of observations from the Bogalusa Heart Study. *Journal of Health Education, 26*(2 suppl), S18–S26.

Pate, R. R., Long, B. J., & Heath, G. (1994). Descriptive epidemiology of physical activity in adolescents. *Pediatric Exercise Science, 6*, 434–447.

Pate R. R., Pratt M., & Blair S. N., et al. (1995). Physical activity and public health: a recommendation from the Centers for Disease Control and Prevention and the American College of Sports Medicine. *Journal of the American Medical Association, 273*(5), 402–407.

Pate, R. R., Small, M. L., Ross, J. G., Young, J. C., Flint, K. H., & Warren, C. W. (1995). School physical education. *Journal of School Health, 65*(8), 312–318.

Rickard, L .G., & Banville, D. (2006). High school students' attitudes about physical education. *Sport, Education and Society, 11*(4), 385–400.

Sallis J. F. (1993). Epidemiology of physical activity and fitness in children and adolescents. *Critical Review of Food and Nutrition Science, 33*(4/5), 403–408.

Sallis, J. F., & Patrick, K. A. (1994). Physical activity guidelines for adolescents; consensus statement. *Pediatric Exercise Science, 6*(4), 302–312.

Slava, S., Laurie, D., & Corbin, C. B. (1984). Long-term effects of a conceptual physical education program. *Research Quarterly for Exercise and Sport, 55*(2), 161–168.

Strand, B. N., Scantling, E., & Johnson, M. (1997). *Fitness education: teaching concepts-based fitness in the schools.* Scottsdale, AZ: Gorsuch Scarisbrick.

Troiano, R. P., Flegal, K. M., Kuczmarksi, R. J., Campbell, S. M., & Johnson, C. L. (1995). Overweight prevalence and trends for children and adolescents. *Archives of Pediatric Adolescent Medicine, 149*, 1085–1091.

U.S. Department of Health and Human Services. (2000). *Healthy people 2010* (CD-ROM ed.). Atlanta: Centers for Disease Control and Prevention.

U.S. Department of Health and Human Services. (2007). School health policies and programs study. *Journal of School Health, 77*(8). Retrieved November 21, 2008, from http://www.cdc.gov/shpps

U.S. Department of Health and Human Services. (2008). Chapter 3: active children and adolescents. *Physical activity guidelines for Americans.* Atlanta: Centers for Disease Control and Prevention. Retrieved November 21, 2008, from http://www.health.gov/paguidelines/guidelines/Chapter3.aspx

Wright, R. W. & Karp, G. C. (2006). The effect of four instructional formats on aerobic fitness of junior-high school students. *Physical Educator, 63*(3), 143–153.

Keeping Your Curriculum Dynamic

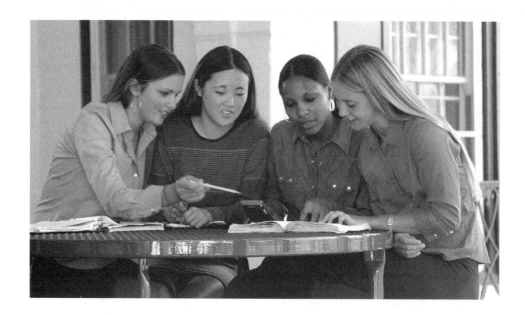

After reading this book, one should have a sense of how to "build a house" or, in this case, how to build a quality physical education curriculum using the main theme curriculum models designed to give the curriculum unique characteristics that appeal to philosophic desires and students' needs. It is the little things that make a good house great—decorations, upkeep, and the landscaping—as owners look for ways to improve the house and make the house a home.

In Section III, the book concludes with some ideas about moving a program from good to great. We borrowed from the words of our friend and men-

tor, Daryl Siedentop, when we titled Chapter 14 "It's Not Business as Usual."
This chapter challenges physical education teachers and curriculum designers
to dare to be great by doing things differently. All too often, physical education programs try to be everything to everyone, and this chapter encourages
educators to stay focused by limiting what they do to what they can do well.
There are many factors that are important in a great physical education program, including advocacy with parents and school boards; staying current by
reading relevant professional materials and attending conferences; and being
a role model for students and others. Developing a curriculum is hard work,
and leaders must roll up their sleeves to complete the task.

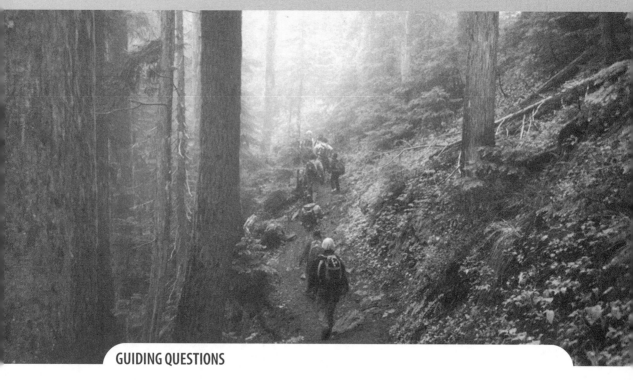

GUIDING QUESTIONS

1 What are key elements that can elevate a good program to a great one?

2 How might attending conferences and reading professional journals impact the design and delivery of a meaningful physical education program?

3 How can you share your passion for physical activity with your students?

4 What methods might you employ to extend your physical education program beyond the school's walls?

5 How might you involve parents and the community in your physical education program?

6 What types of technology might you be able to incorporate into the teaching and learning process in your program?

7 How would you design an advocacy campaign to promote what you do in the name of physical education?

It's Not Business as Usual

14

Deborah Tannehill, University of Limerick
Jacalyn Lund, Georgia State University

Our goal for writing this book is to help preservice and practicing teachers develop a standards-based curriculum in physical education. As you have undoubtedly discovered by now, standards-based curriculum design involves change, it is about doing things differently, or as Daryl Siedentop has repeatedly suggested, "it's not business as usual." We recognize that for most, this will be a departure from what has become routine and easy, and that change can be both frightening and exciting at the same time. In this final chapter, we challenge you to step outside your comfort zone, try new things, and seek the knowledge and tools necessary to develop innovative and coherent curricula to meet the physical education standards and the needs and interests of young people today.

Developing a Great Curriculum

On the first page of his best-selling book, *Good to Great*, Jim Collins (2001) makes the following statement, "We don't have great schools primarily because we have good schools." Collins and his research team selected several top performing companies that had been good, but then transformed into companies that were great with greatness being defined by the following: financially, the company's profits exceeded the gains of the stock market; the company made an impact on society; and the company was concerned about employee welfare. Although schools cannot be measured by their increase in financial worth, financial prudence, especially in times of economic downturns, is a necessary component of a well-run school. Several of the qualities identified in the book have relevance to a school curriculum, moving a good curriculum to greatness. Very briefly, these qualities to move from good to great are as follows:

- Leaders roll up their sleeves and work hard, but don't require recognition and accolades for their efforts. They do the right things because they care about the end results.
- The right people are "on the bus," and then those people figure out where they are headed.
- The hedgehog principle is followed: they define what they are really good at doing, narrow down the scope of activities, and become really good at doing a few of them. Some innovations that seem like a good idea might not be adopted in favor of focusing on fewer ideas and doing them well.
- The process of improvement begins with a really hard look at the current status of things—what is working and what needs to change. A healthy dialogue about the issues occurs and things are evaluated from a variety of perspectives. During this discourse emotions are kept out of the discussion and a hard look at the facts produces a fair and accurate evaluation.
- There is a discipline to stay focused on what needs to be accomplished— an eye is always kept on the final outcome or ultimate goal.
- Technology that will help achieve the goal is embraced, but every new trend is not adopted.
- There is slow and steady progress toward the final goal—continued momentum rather than sudden bursts followed by periods of low activity.
- The ultimate purpose is for the greater good of society—money is a factor, but the achievement of the ultimate goal is the final factor guiding all decisions.

These qualities have relevance for building a quality curriculum. As identified in Chapter 2, a great curriculum starts with a purpose or a vision about what is excellent. Too many people begin the process without taking time to develop a vision for what "could be" and instead settle for "what we are currently doing." Developing a vision requires a really hard look at what is working and what should change. Too many physical education teachers are "doers" and are reluctant to take the time necessary to discuss this vision.

When developing curriculum, we need to stay focused on this vision and avoid our attention deficit tendencies to hop from one idea to the next. After completing the unpacking process we must focus on carefully selecting the content that will move us forward to that next level. Getting the right people on the bus is often not an option in the public schools, but we can make sure that the people on the bus have the adequate resources and skills to make a great curriculum come to life. In many school districts, it is more about being willing to get on the bus rather than having the luxury of selecting new riders.

Rome wasn't built in a day, and similarly your curriculum will develop over time. All members of the team must be willing to roll up their sleeves and work hard to make it happen. As with Collins's companies, steady progress (like the tortoise, not the hare) will eventually lead to success. This final chapter is devoted to helping people think outside of the box during the curriculum development process.

Challenges for Change

Dealing with change can be achieved, but we know it is not easy; it is hard and involves feelings of being "out on a limb" with nowhere to go but down. However, if as a group of colleagues we move toward meaningful change, the road is less difficult because there is support and camaraderie along the way. As you move forward to design innovative, challenging, and coherent curricula to meet the needs of children and youth in today's world, we challenge you to take some of the steps outlined in this chapter. Although many of you are already doing many of these and more, there are some who are stuck in a rut that results from years of teaching the same thing in the same way, with the outcome being boredom for both you and the learners. Adding a little challenge to your professional career is an excellent way to help you grow and achieve a greater good.

Challenge 1: Go to Professional Conferences

For novice teachers fresh out of college, veterans who have been attempting to implement new ideas, and those who have remained at status quo, conferences are an excellent resource and can provide a motivational boost. Within the past few years, conference sessions have focused on strategies for reaching the NASPE content standards, assessment tools to measure student success, and implementing various curriculum models across K–12. These sessions have been delivered by K–12 practitioners who want to share their experiences, university professors in teacher education sharing applied research ideas, teams of teachers reporting on grant activity through the federally funded Physical Education for Progress initiative (PEP grants), and those working to design state assessment systems. Local, state, district, and national conferences give teachers the opportunity to participate in the professional physical education community, interact with fellow teachers from different areas, keep current on what is happening in the field, and have an opportunity to see creative ways to implement various issues and topics. Conferences are also a great opportunity to catch up with old friends and make new ones; some of the best ideas gained from conferences come while talking informally with professionals.

Challenge 2: Read Professional Journals

Reading professional journals is another way to keep up with what is happening in the field, and gain ideas on how to make positive and innovative changes to your program. There are many quality applied professional journals devoted exclusively to physical education. These journals typically have in-depth feature editions that focus on specific topics. In the past, the *Journal of Physical Education, Recreation, and Dance (JOPERD)* has featured Teaching Games for Understanding (Volume 67, February & March 1996) and Sport Education (Volume 69, April & May 1998). Also, the *Journal of the Wilderness Education Association* (Volume 72, August & September 2003) published articles worth looking into. In addition there have been separate articles on social responsibility, adventure, and fitness. *Strategies* contains useful articles that will stimulate new thinking, and help you become a more effective teacher. There are additional professional journals outside of physical education that provide important resources for us, as well. The Association for Supervision and Curriculum Development (ASCD) publishes articles to keep the reader informed about what is happening in education in general. Additionally, ASCD has an online daily newsletter that highlights happenings in education. Subscribing to journals and reading them is part of being a professional. Although expensive, the costs can be shared with a colleague, become a part of your school budget, or even be purchased by your school or school district to support your professional development.

Challenge 3: Share Your Passion for Physical Activity with Your Students

Most physical education teachers have an activity for which they have a passion and in which they love to participate. That activity may be one of the reasons that they chose to enter the field of physical education and become a teacher. For some, this passion developed through years of experience as an athlete; for others, a coach may have inspired them, and for still others, it might be the camaraderie of being part of a team. There are some teachers who may have been dancers and enjoy the feeling of moving to the beat, mountain climbers who risk life and limb just to experience the thrill of conquering new challenges, golfers who started participating because it was a family tradition. Imagine if everyone had a physical activity about which they were passionate. Physical education teachers have the potential to inspire that passion. As we develop programs to meet the standards, we have the opportunity to design what is meaningful, relevant, and worthwhile for students. As we design learning experiences to help students achieve success, we need to keep in mind that success is something that can inspire and encourage everyone. By offering challenging activities, and teaching in such a way that students have an opportunity to experience success, physical education teachers have an opportunity to inspire this love of movement in others. Teach with passion, and give others the same gift that was given to you.

Challenge 4: Be a Role Model to Others

In a letter to the editor in the May/June 2004 *Journal of Physical Education, Recreation, and Dance,* a fitness consultant noted that the credibility of a physical education teacher was compromised when the teacher lacked the personal commitment to live a healthy lifestyle. To "sell" physical education, teachers should buy into it as well. It is much easier to convince others about the value of fitness when one eats healthy meals and works out on a regular basis. This does not mean that physical education classes are workout sessions for teachers. Although some teachers do participate with students, they must remember that their primary function is to teach, not play. In other words, your daily physical activity session or fitness workout should not be at the expense of instruction. Time often gets in the way of working out and eating right. Many physical education teachers coach several sports, and it is difficult to squeeze time into the day for a personal physical activity session. Being a role model is hard work, and as such, it must be planned. Time for physical activity must be scheduled—biking, jogging, kayaking, kickboxing, or whatever. Students enjoy knowing about their teachers' choices of physical activity and that they are participating in physical activity—it makes students much more willing to "buy into" a physically active lifestyle. A 2008 issue of *Update* describes ways that you can be a role model to others by participating regularly in physical activity, by staying fit, and by engaging in professional development activities (Bell, 2008; Lund, 2008; Mears, 2008).

Challenge 5: Invite Guest Speakers to Your Class

Students enjoy variety, and so do teachers. Perhaps you have a coach, another teacher, or a community member with expertise in an area. Invite them in for the day to teach your class or to team teach with you. Talk with students' parents and family members and you may find some who have skills they are willing to share, or a willingness to take part in supervising physical activity field trips. Not only will this enhance the content for the students, and help them see how it fits with everyday life, it will let others know what you are doing in physical education, and help them realize that learning takes place both in the gym and on the field. There are more groups willing to share and interact with your classes than you might realize. For example, local fishing clubs, the Audubon Society, orienteering clubs, and hiking groups have expressed an interest in talking to young people in some areas, which will certainly impact an Outdoor Education program. Other teachers have noted that golf courses have offered used clubs to schools for physical education, so perhaps they could also be enticed into sharing their expertise for a day as well. Attempt to think beyond what you have become used to and surprises may occur that impact your work with young people.

Challenge 6: Expand the Physical Education Program Beyond the School Day

Time spent in physical education is probably not sufficient for students to fully develop all of the standards and the skills, knowledge, and fitness they demand. Keep in mind that the more skilled we are the more successful we will be, and that typically we choose to participate in activities in which we find success and achievement. There is no reason why our curricula must be restricted to physical education within the confines of the school day. Facilities can be made available to students at other times so that they have the opportunity to enjoy extended participation, practice skills and strategies, or work out. Perhaps it is possible to have an open gym before or after school or during lunch. When classes are not using the weight lifting facilities, they could be available for other students or groups. Access to facilities, intramurals, or sports clubs are additional ways to extend the physical education program. Let's think about going beyond these examples. Utilize the community resources of those that have an interest in the physical activity patterns of young people. Foster these relationships, and work collaboratively to extend your program and provide additional outlets for students to be physically active. Off campus offerings are an option, especially at the high school level, and need not reduce the quality of instruction. Do fitness clubs in the area have special rates for students, does the dance studio offer after school programs that might be linked to your curriculum, or can the parks department work with you to offer an activity for young people on weekends that supports their participation in class? All of these activities are part of Standard 3 and will enhance the quality of your program.

Challenge 7: Build Authentic Field Trips into Your Program

Providing students experience in an activity in its authentic setting could be an important bridge for reaching Standard 3, developing lifelong participants in physical activity. Making connections within the community as a means of obtaining access to authentic sites can be useful and benefit both the physical education program and the organization with which you collaborate. Most physical activity facilities are willing to cooperate with schools, making their facilities available at no or very low cost. When teaching a Sport Education season of target games, developing a partnership with the local golf course or bowling lanes might provide several opportunities for student participation. Golf courses are usually willing to let students hit on the driving range during off peak hours, or offer reduced rates for rounds of golf, thus offering an incentive for parents or guardians to participate in the activity with their child. This might also hold true for bowling lanes, skate parks, and swimming pools

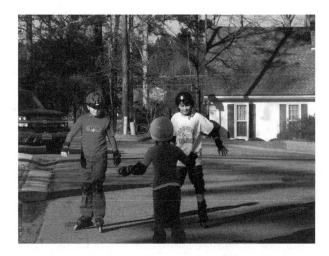

in your community. When teaching Adventure or Outdoor Education, developing connections with the local parks department will be beneficial. They have climbing walls, kayaking equipment, and often camps with low- and high-level initiative challenges. We have found them eager to collaborate with schools in these programs because it allows them to "get in" with the kids who they want to attract to summer opportunities. It ends up being a partnership that is a plus for everyone.

Challenge 8: Invite Parents to Visit Your Classes

Although we mentioned earlier that some parents may have skills and knowledge in an area that they might be willing to share, there are other ways to involve parents in your program. Many are interested in what their children are doing in school and out, and would value the opportunity to come and observe your classes. Parents are curious to see if physical education has changed since their experiences in school and in many cases may be pleasantly surprised. Invite parents to either participate with or instead of their child: the student might become a co-teacher for the day, which would provide the parent with a new perspective of the child. This is a great public relations tool for getting support from parents, but be sure you ask the student first, as this could cause either a positive or negative reaction. Waiting until a program is in jeopardy is not the only time to advocate for it. In fact, this work should be done on a regular basis. Be proactive, and let parents know what your physical education program entails.

Challenge 9: Use Technology in Your Classes

Advances in technology are widespread in our society, and schools are no exception. In fact, students are becoming more skilled using technology than their parents, and in some cases, their teachers. Instead of looking at technology as having a negative impact on or for physical education (students are spending too much time on the computer), turn it into a positive. Students can access the Internet and do research on many topics related to physical education and physical activity. A number of excellent physical education websites have been developed in recent years, and provide a wide variety of resources for our field. There are discussion groups for teachers and students, sites for students to maintain fitness logs, ideas on innovative teaching strategies, sample assessment tools, video clips of sport performance, and on and on. Pelinks4U and PE Central are the two most frequently accessed websites in our field, and provide an abundance of useful ideas and tools for physical educators.

Technology is not limited to the Internet, and there are many applications that can be used to help children and youth be more active. Pedometers and heart rate monitors can encourage students to increase their activity levels during physical education or after school, and are motivating for them to measure their progress. Video cameras are great learning devices where students can videotape a performance, and then analyze it for tips on where they need to improve. Being able to see themselves perform provides excellent feedback to students and teaches them to self-assess and reflect on their developing skills. Using digital cameras, students can create bulletin boards about what they are doing in class, take team pictures in Sport Education, and collect photos of their progress for an assessment portfolio. Desktop publishing can be used to send newsletters home or promote a special event in physical education.

Challenge 10: Integrate Physical Education with Other Content Areas

Physical education is a science laboratory. Almost every time a student performs a skill, some principle of physics is applied. Ask teachers what they are doing in their classes, and incorporate supporting activities in your class or work together to design a joint unit of study. Square dancing might accompany a unit on westward expansion or a shop teacher might have the students make stations for a fitness trail designed in physcial education class. Linking Sport Education team names to countries being studied in social studies has been an effective strategy, and even brought other teachers to the door wondering why their content was not the focus. Stations set up on a fitness course might reinforce themes on Alaska (running the Iditarod), the Underground Railroad, mythology, or gladiators. Using baseball cards, one classroom teacher taught geography (birthplaces of the players, and teams that they played for) and math (various statistics on the cards), while teaching a softball season during a Teaching Games for Understanding program.

A teacher in Maple Valley, Washington, has developed what has been named the Adventure Academy. The academy is composed of physical education, literature, and science, all of which focus their content on adventure and the out-of-doors. For example, in science students may study the environment and how to care for it, in literature readings are focused on experiences in nature, and in physical education kayaking, hiking, camping, and climbing would be explored. Joint lectures are featured and students come to understand and appreciate the interconnectedness of the content. When learning is reinforced in several different areas, more depth of knowledge is possible, and students seem to "get into" the unit of study.

Challenge 11: Advocate for Physical Education

Every physical educator should be an advocate for physical education and physical activity. It can be as small as being a role model to others by working out and staying fit, having a message on your answering machine asking people whether they exercised today, or developing an advocacy campaign to promote your program. Several state AHPERDs have public relations committees that talk about advocacy and public affairs committees to promote physical education at the state legislature. NASPE's website has several public relations ideas that are updated monthly. In addition, the following are public relations ideas to promote a physical education curriculum:

- An open house for parents is not new; liven it up with novel ideas, such as parents being invited to participate in the latest dances that students have learned in their class, and even having students teach their parents.
- Offer youth sport programs during summer months to support and promote physical activity year round. Teachers might charge a modest fee to run them, or seek support from the local parks department.
- Fundraisers can be a nuisance, yet catch the eye of the community. One preservice teacher planned to bring in former college teammates who had made it into the pros to put on an afternoon clinic, followed by a dinner banquet and auction. Another planned a judo tournament as a fundraiser for the local hospital. Parents, participants, and the community could be invited with auction items donated from the community, and could include signed equipment or memorabilia from pro players/clinicians.
- Participants in a Sport Education season might organize a tournament for youth teams. This would give them the opportunity to use the skills learned through their Sport Education season to organize, officiate, keep score, keep statistics, run the clock, announce, and generally create festivity.
- A fitness class might offer a jog-a-thon or bike-a-thon as a fundraising idea, or merely an event to link to the community. Before an event, a running clinic or bike safety clinic might be offered by students who had researched and developed the skills to deliver this information.

- Development of activity calendars for the summer months with daily suggestions for activities for children would be useful. Parents are receptive to these calendars to address the "we're bored" syndrome that children often go through when school is out during the summer months. The NASPE website has a Teachers' Toolbox that features new ideas and activity calenders each month.
- Physical education t-shirts are always popular, and those that promote physical education are seen frequently. With iron-on transfers that can be printed from the computer, they are relatively inexpensive to produce, and students love to design them. Mottos for physical education might be used; one student came up with a version of the top 10 reasons for participating in physical education. Recently, a teacher-in-training used camouflage shirts for printing his Adventure Education motto. Another student developed a character education program for her school named STARS, which stands for Students Taking Active Roles, and promoted respect for others, cooperation, compassion, and self-discipline. Other items that students have made include socks, headbands, and tote bags for carrying physical education clothes to and from school.

Challenge 12: Get Involved on School Governance Committees

Schools are changing the way they are governed. Principals used to make all the decisions for the school. Recent trends have been to increase the importance of getting input from others, and letting school councils have a voice in what happens in the school. Some states have instituted site-based management teams to share in school governance, with teams consisting of administrators, teachers, parents, staff, and students. Issues impacting the school are brought before the group, and the group decides what action to take. Physical education teachers involved with coaching responsibilities that prevent active involvement in school governance need to stay connected so their voices are heard on school issues. If schools are developing school improvement plans, pushing for increased physical education time and physical activity initiatives is important from both a health and social standpoint.

In a recent *Strategies* article (January/February 2009, Stephen Jeffries outlines 10 steps for effectively advocating with school boards that we found informative and appropriate (Figure 14.1). Each step is outlined below.

1. *Understand school board responsibilities*: Know and understand school board responsibilities, which usually include vision, structure, accountability and advocacy.
2. *Connect health to academics*: Schools are about students achieving academic success, so it is up to us to help them see the relationship between health and academic achievement.

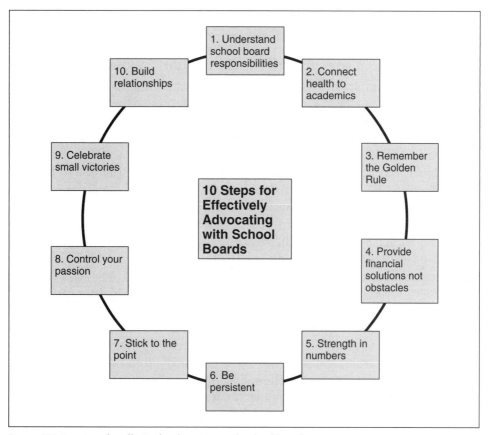

FIGURE 14.1 Ten steps for effectively advocating with school boards.
Source: Adapted from Jeffries, S. (2009). School boarding 101: winning friends and influencing people. *Strategies, 22*(3), 35–36.

3. *Remember the Golden Rule:* Board members work with students' interests at heart and deserve to be treated with respect.

4. *Provide financial solutions, not obstacles:* If you have a proposal to put before the school board, attempt to include ideas on how to fund what you are suggesting.

5. *Strength in numbers:* Strong interest is represented by strong support, which board members will see through numbers of potential participants showing interest in a topic.

6. *Be persistent:* Don't give up; commit to an issue and let the board see this.

7. *Stick to the point:* Be clear, concise, specific, and focused.

8. *Control your passion:* As Jeffries says, "passion and enthusiasm will undo you if not tempered with patience and respect" (p. 37).

9. *Celebrate small victories:* Don't expect to do it all, and be willing to compromise.

10. *Build relationships*: It is important to build trust and respect with the board; they must know you as well as you know them.

Challenge 13: Keep the Dust Off the Curriculum Guides

This last suggestion comes from a district health and physical education coordinator. It is a lot of hard work to develop a comprehensive standards-based curriculum. Despite the meaningful and relevant resources contained within it, too many teachers leave curriculum guides on the shelf to gather dust. One way to avoid this is for school districts to provide regularly scheduled inservice meetings for physical educators to talk about implementation issues, curricular decisions, what is working well, and how to adapt problematic areas. This is consistent with what we know about teacher learning not ending when leaving school, and we hope that most teachers are, in fact, lifelong learners. In recent years we have come to realize the importance of providing teachers with continuing professional development (CPD) opportunities where they can share ideas, seek collegial support, draw links between new and existing knowledge, evaluate what is happening in the name of physical education, and explore ways of improving practice. Another option for CPD is to provide teachers guidance in designing district assessments that are given at certain junctures across the physical education program. This provides accountability for the program, and teachers must follow the curriculum if their students are going to experience success on these assessments. Working together to plan such initiatives involves teachers as active consultants who will be more likely to take ownership of plans that are developed.

These are our ideas for making change. What can you add to the list? Don't try to do them all at once—start with two or three of your favorites, and gradually make change. Change by choice is always preferred to forced change. By becoming an advocate for physical education and your program, you will have control over the direction you are going to head. Bea Orr, a former AAHPERD president, was a district physical education supervisor. She directed all of her teachers to identify 10 parents who were strong advocates of physical education. When any votes concerning physical education (positive or negative) came before the school board, these parents were called, and cared enough about the program to attend the meeting where the vote would be taken. Can you identify 10 parents who would support your program in this way?

Summary

Developing a curriculum for a K–12 school district requires insight and thoughtful planning on the part of those in charge. Standards provide focus and guidance for the process. The opening quote for this book asked, "What makes a program good?" We hope that we have provided an outline for developing a good program, one that can accomplish tangible outcomes for those involved. A good curriculum must be seen as a journey, rather than a destination. It must remain dynamic, receptive to change, and responsive to those whom it serves. It must also reflect the needs and context of the community in which it is implemented. Above all, a curriculum must accomplish what it stands for. We wish you the best with your journey of curriculum development. We hope the information contained in this book will help you with the decisions you make, and result in a great physical education program.

References

Bell, M. (2008, November/December). Advocating for fitness: walking the talk. *AAHPERD Update Plus*, 5–6.

Collins, J. (2001). *Good to great*. New York: Harper Collins.

Jeffries, S. (2009). School boarding 101: winning friends and influencing people. *Strategies, 22*(3), 35–36.

Lund, J. (2008, November/December). How to be a great role model: practice what you teach! *AAHPERD Update Plus*, 4.

Mears, D. (2008, November/December). Leading by example: physical educators as role models. *AAHPERD Update Plus*, 5.

Siedentop, D., & Tannehill, D. (2000). *Developing teaching skills in physical education* (4th ed.). Mountain View, CA: Mayfield.

Additional Resources

Cothran, D., & Ennis, C. (1999). Alone in a crowd: meeting students' needs for relevance and connection in urban high school physical education. *Journal of Teaching in Physical Education, 18*, 234–247.

Dyson, B. (2006). Students' perspectives of physical education. In D. Kirk, D. Macdonald, & M. O'Sullivan (Eds.), *The handbook of physical education* (pp. 326–346). London: Sage Publications.

Ermler, K., Mehrhof, J., Brewer, J., & Worrell, V. (2007). *Roadblocks to quality physical education*. Reston, VA: National Association for Sport and Physical Education.

Graham, G. (1995). Physical education through students' eyes and in students' voices: introduction. *Journal of Teaching in Physical Education, 14*, 364–371.

McCullick, B., Metzler, M., Cicek, S., Jackson, J., & Vickers, B. (2008). Kids say the darndest things: PETE program assessment through the eyes of children. *Journal of Teaching in Physical Education, 27*, 4–20.

O'Sullivan, M., & Deglau, D. (2006). Principles of professional development. *Journal of Teaching in Physical Education, 25*, 441–449.

Glossary

Adventure-Based Learning An alternate term to describe Adventure Education in the physical education curriculum.

Adventure Education Involves activities that encourage holistic student involvement (physical, cognitive, social, and emotional) in a task that involves challenges and an uncertainty of the final outcome. Activities are carefully sequenced to ensure student safety while allowing them to take ownership of their learning.

affiliation Being a member of a team; in sports, this can come out in team names, uniforms, mascots, and working together to achieve a common goal.

anchors Main protection points in a roped safety system.

application Using a skill in a new or more complex environment or using a skill in a dynamic (rather than a practice) and controlled situation.

assessment Gathering information about a student's abilities and understanding.

athletic privilege A form of elitism whereby those who are more athletically inclined are accorded higher status and privilege, socially, economically, and politically. For example, the athletic achievements of schools often are more recognized (i.e., trophy case at the school entrance) than are achievements of debate teams, music ensembles, or foreign language clubs.

authentic (more complete) sports experiences Experiences that reflect all of the key characteristics generally seen in institutional versions of sport.

backward design Intentional planning in which the teacher begins with the exit goals and designs the curriculum toward those goals; from high school down to elementary school.

bearings The direction one wants to travel.

belaying Using the system for—or the act of—managing the ropes to protect the climber.

bias   A predisposition or prejudice, such as holding inappropriate and/or incorrect assumptions about people who are different.

bouldering   Climbing without ropes close to the ground.

challenge by choice   Students have options to choose from, depending upon their comfort levels related to physical and emotional safety, and students are unable to opt out of participation before beginning the activities.

checklists   A list of elements or descriptors that are present or not present in the performance being evaluated.

cognitive and performance understanding   The combination of 1) the ability to demonstrate mental understanding for recall and verbalization and 2) the ability to translate cognitive understanding into performance/movement.

competent sportspersons   People with sufficient skills to 1) participate in games at a satisfactory level, 2) be knowledgeable players, and 3) execute strategies appropriate to their levels and the complexity of the game.

concepts-based fitness and wellness education   A curriculum-based approach that focuses on one's knowledge and understanding of physical activity, physical fitness, and wellness.

consumers of sport and physical activity   Students are educated not only to appreciate the intrinsic benefits of participation in health-enhancing physical activity but also to exercise critical judgment when evaluating the role and function of sport and physical activity in their lives.

contexts   Experiencing the skill in a variety of environments and situations, rather than experiencing the skill in only one setting (e.g., jumping and landing in its many forms), and in different settings, rather than in the singular, narrow setting of a particular sport.

contour lines   Lines on a map that connect points of equal elevation; each line indicates a constant elevation as it follows the shape of the landscape.

"cover the curriculum"   When teachers focus on teaching everything outlined in the curriculum guide rather than focusing on student learning.

crack climbing   Involves jamming or torquing your limbs or body inside of a rock's natural crack systems.

crampons   Steel-pointed attachments for mountain boots to help travel on steep snow and ice.

critical elements   The components determined to be the most critical pieces for attainment of the performance outcomes and mastery of the skill.

cues   The simple phrases—the 2 to 3 words—that give children the cognitive reminder of what is needed to perform the skill correctly (e.g., pads, pads, push, push—push, don't slap the ball).

culminating activity   The ending activity for the lesson, the series of lessons, or the study of the theme; the activity that brings together the skill components and concepts that were the focus of the lesson or theme.

culminating events   Festive, exciting, and appropriate conclusions to sport seasons, which involve all participants.

cultural content knowledge   Having an in-depth appreciation and understanding of multiple cultures and how individuals' cultures influence their perspectives and behaviors.

culturally responsive teaching   Both a frame of mind and actual teaching practice in which teachers are responsive to the culture, needs, interests, learning preferences, and abilities of each student.

Cultural Studies connoisseurs   Students who have heightened awareness or educated perceptions of the nuances; educated perceptions allow students to illuminate, interpret, and appraise physical activity, sport infrastructure, and sport cultures.

Cultural Studies (CS) curriculum   Involves the practical and cognitive involvement of students in learning not only how to participate in sport and physical activity but also in learning how sport and physical activity contributes positively and negatively to individual well-being and to group, community, and national cultures.

curriculum   Includes all knowledge, skills, and learning experiences that are provided to students within the school program.

curriculum guide   A formal document that identifies the objectives that students are to achieve in a subject area and the activities that will make up the content of the program.

deadpointing   When a climber makes a move for a handhold that appears out of reach, but he/she is able to complete the move with his/her feet still on holds (fully extended with four points of contact).

decision making   The process of deciding what to do, particularly when selecting and executing skills during game play.

developmentally appropriate experiences   Matching the curricular experiences to the developmental level of the child (cognitive, social, physical, and emotional).

dominant culture   In the United States (and specifically in education), the dominant culture is the white culture. Those within the dominant culture create rules and policies that often privilege those within the dominant culture. For example, given that 82–84% of teachers and administrators are white, they can be considered the dominant culture of education.

draw strokes   Stroke to move a canoe laterally.

edging   Pressing the edge and side of your climbing shoe into a hold and then standing on it.

educational climate   The emotional ambience or feeling of the gymnasium.

ego- or ability-oriented   A person (and learning environment) who references his or her skill or ability against his or her peers; the constant comparison to others instead of self-referencing improvement over time.

enthusiastic sportspersons   People who find additional outlets (outside of class) to participate in that provide meaning to sport experiences and actively support the sport culture.

essays   A performance assessment representative of what someone in the field would do, such as writing a dialogue, creating a brochure, or writing an article to demonstrate knowledge of a topic.

evaluation   The systematic appraisal of worth based on a thorough and detailed examination of data.

event tasks   Performance tasks that can be completed within a single class period.

everybody plays   A playing requirement of Sport Education where everyone is a participant; in Sport Education, sport should be developmentally appropriate so all players can take part and feel valued.

exit expectations   What learners are expected to know and be able to do when they exit a series of lessons, or, in the case of the national standards, when they exit a particular grade range.

experiential education   Involves the purposeful planning and implementation of direct experiences coupled with the facilitation of reflection and responsibility.

fair play   Behaving in positive and cooperative ways so that all participants can enjoy the sport experience.

festivity   A celebration that is present in sport of all levels; Sport Education encourages making sport festive by building the team spirit, publicizing records, creating team cheers, taking pictures, and holding culminating events that are meaningful to all learners.

fitness assessment   Designed to provide individualized feedback regarding one's overall fitness status and/or physiological responses to physical effort.

fitness tests   Assessments used to measure the components of fitness, often including assessments of cardiovascular endurance, muscular endurance, muscular strength, flexibility, and body fat composition.

formal competitions   Reflected by a schedule that lays out all of the competitions that will make up the season.

formative assessments   Assessment that is on-going, largely informal, and appears throughout the instructional process.

formative evaluation   An evaluation that occurs while a project is in progress.

frontloading   Emphasizes the key learning points of an activity before beginning, rather than simply reviewing after the activity is completed.

full value contract (FVC)   A social contract that members of a group adhere to in regards to their behavior/actions both as individuals and in their interactions with others. The essence of FVC is built on three commitments: 1) to work together as a group toward individual and group goals; 2) to adhere to safety and behavior guidelines; and 3) to give and receive feedback to help change behavior (Schoel, Prouty, and Radcliffe, 1988).

fundamental movement patterns   Two or more basic and fundamental skills combined for a movement pattern with a progression from basic motor skills to fundamental skills to movement patterns.

game-like experiences   Experiences designed by the teacher to move students beyond the practice-in-isolation to dynamic, unpredictable situations; designed by the teacher to control the number of variables and the complexity of the movement experience.

game performance   A student's ability to play in game situations.

generalized rubrics   Universal rubrics that can be used to evaluate many different types of related performances.

"goods" of physical education   What a teacher believes to be of the most importance in physical education.

"graded" competition   Based on levels of performance—novice or advanced, minor leagues or major league, and recreational or competitive.

group processing (debriefing)   The practice of encouraging students to reflect on and communicate with other group members about their feelings, observations, and experiences during an activity.

health-enhancing level of physical fitness   The fitness and level of fitness needed to be "healthy" in each of the categories considered critical for good health: muscular strength and endurance, flexibility, cardiovascular efficiency, and body composition; criteria are referenced as compared to norm-referenced physical fitness.

health-related fitness   Aspects of physical fitness that are known to positively impact overall health, such as cardiorespiratory fitness, muscular strength, muscular flexibility, muscular endurance, and body composition.

heel hook   Hanging by the heel.

holistic rubrics   Rubrics that look at the performance as a whole and make a single determination of worth; each level contains descriptions or criteria for the various traits or characteristics being evaluated in a single paragraph.

inclusive practices   A term adapted from physical education literature. For the purposes of this text, inclusive teaching is about providing physical education experiences for all children and youth in the regular classroom setting and access to rich curriculum and instruction as well as supporting each student's persistence toward excellence regardless of ability/disability, body size/type, or ethnicity/socioeconomic status.

instructional alignment   Alignment of what we intend for students to learn (goals), how we determine student success (assessment), how we teach, and how students practice (instructional strategies).

instructionally appropriate experiences   Matching instruction to the developmental levels of the children being taught in physical education.

jam   A cramming action that requires expanding a part of the body into a crack.

journals   An assessment that provides students opportunities to reflect and write on events or topics in class.

J-strokes   Forward-steering strokes that end with an outward hook.

laboratory experiences   Activities designed to provide an arena for cognitive concepts to be applied and understood within a fitness education approach; the experience usually involves some sort of personal awareness or application.

leave-no-trace   A widely accepted code of outdoor ethics and minimum-impact principles designed to shape a sustainable future for wildlands.

lieback   A move that involves pulling with the hands while pushing with the feet.

literate sportspersons   People who understand and appreciate the rules, rituals, and traditions that surround sport and are able to distinguish between good and bad sport practices.

logs   Lists of activities or practice trials completed by the students.

mantle   Boosting into a hold or onto a ledge by locking the elbows and bringing the feet up.

marginalized   Specific to those students who do not receive the full benefits (if any), those who are negatively impacted, and/or left out as a result of biased or indifferent teaching.

movement analysis framework   A framework developed by Rudolph Laban for the classification of the components of movement (i.e., skills and concepts) and divided into four categories: body awareness, space awareness, effort, and relationships.

movement concepts   Concepts that are the enhancers and the enrichers of the skill; they tell us how, where, and in what relationships the movement is going to take place.

movement culture   The infrastructure, norms, practices, policies, and values associated with sport, recreation, and physical activity at the local, national, and international levels.

multiactivity program   A program characterized by a wide variety of activities intended to expose students to physical activity options. Units are short in nature, often as many as 10–12 per year, with little time for students to become proficient in any one activity. The focus tends to be on students being active rather than on learning.

multiple independent questions   Open response question that ask a series of questions that are related, but are not dependent on the response given to the previous question of the series.

national content standards   The standards developed by NASPE (2004) to specify the curricular content for physical education—what students should know and be able to do in physical education.

"normal"   Typically defined by the dominant group. For example, the construction of "normal" in the United States is typically the following: white, heterosexual, male, middle class, able-bodied, Christian. Those who fail to conform to this social construction of "normal" are viewed as different and, possibly, deficient.

off-width   A crack that one can get his/her arms or legs into but not his/her entire body.

open response questions   Present problems and then require students to respond. The students' responses typically begins with "it depends."

opposition   Pushing in two different directions.

overhang   A rock that is farther away at the top than at the base (requires tilting the head back to see the top of the wall or climb).

palming   Placing the entire hand over a rounded hold.

performance-based assessments   Assessments used to measure higher levels of student learning, such as a student's ability to apply knowledge while doing a meaningful or worthwhile task (one that is representative of work done in the field).

performance outcomes   Student behaviors that demonstrate progress toward achieving the standards.

philosophy   What a person believes and values.

point system   A list of characteristics to be evaluated that has an assigned point value for each characteristic; if the characteristic is present, then the designated number of points is awarded.

portfolios   Collections of artifacts that typically are used to show students' competency or mastery of a subject area.

positively interdependent   Group members depend on each other, as each individual's part is essential to the entire group completing its task.

positive pull   A handhold on which one can pull downward.

preformative evaluation   An evaluation that is done prior to beginning a project or process.

process of learning   Involves active learners posing questions, problem solving possible answers using their knowledge and skills, and transferring the new knowledge to other content and settings.

"progressive" competition   Becomes more complex as the season progresses, from 1v1 to 3v3 to 4v4, depending on how the game performance develops.

Project Adventure (PA)   A student-centered curriculum that integrates adventure in physical education.

projects   Assessments that require student to create something that demonstrates their knowledge of a topic.

pry strokes   Deep, powerful strokes used in whitewater to move the canoe away from the side of the paddler (also termed pryaways).

psychological and emotional safety nets   Developed to help students psychologically and emotionally manage their way through the physical education environment. Analogous to how teachers create safe physical environments, teachers are ever mindful of each student's need to feel psychologically and emotionally safe.

push-off   Pushing upward off of a hold.

qualitative analytic rubrics   Rubric that use verbal descriptions of the various levels for each descriptor being evaluated.

quality programs   Programs that mean something; are built on a philosophy that reflects the values and beliefs of teachers; and have important goals, assessments aligned with those goals, and instructional practices that move students from the goal to a demonstration of learning.

quantitative analytic rubrics   Rubrics that use numbers to indicate how each descriptor is evaluated against pre-determined criteria; the numbers are anchored with a word or phrase to indicate the level of performance that the number represents.

rappelling   Descending a rope while controlling speed with friction.

records   Provide feedback to players, can be used as an assessment for the teacher, or can help as a goal setting tool for players; tracking student performance can vary from shots on goal to gymnastics event scores.

reliability   The degree of consistency with which a test measures what it is designed to measure.

responses to provided information questions   Open response questions that provide information (e.g., data, picture, article) to which a student must respond.

role play   An assessment in which students present a scenario and then demonstrate how they would react in that situation; role plays are useful as affective domain assessments.

roles   Help students gain a more complete understanding of sport by assigning students to experience roles beyond that of just a participant.

rubric   The criteria by which a performance, portfolio, or product is evaluated.

scaffolded questions   Open response questions that contain a sequence of questions, each dependent upon a previous answer and each more difficult than the previous question.

scope   Traditionally refers to the content being taught, its focus, and the activities selected within the content.

seasons   Length of time a sport is played; in sport education, seasons are longer than what is typical in physical education.

sequence   Refers to the order or progression in which learning activities are presented.

side pull   A hold that faces away from the climber (requires pulling sideways with fingers).

single dimension questions   Open response questions that usually require students to evaluate information, draw conclusions, and then justify their responses.

skill tests   Assessments of student psychomotor ability, usually done in a closed environment.

skill theme   The selection of a skill and all of the variables that accompany that skill for a study; the variables that accompany the skill (e.g., concepts, contexts, combinations) provide enrichment, breadth, and depth.

smearing   Pressing as much of a shoe's rubber sole as possible into a rock to create friction.

social construction of bias   Prejudice that develops as a result of social networks or interchanges or that is learned from others. For example, we come to form opinions and make assumptions about other people from family, peers, friends, and media.

specialized skills   The skills of a particular sport or activity (e.g., dig or bump in volleyball).

sport culture   The collective beliefs, customs, practices, and behaviors of people in the context of sport; a healthy sport culture contributes to a healthy society.

stakeholders   Those who have an interest in the evaluation process.

standardized examination courses   Rigorous tests that analyze students' practical and cognitive knowledge of sport, health, and fitness as well as the natural sciences (e.g., physiology, anatomy, biomechanics) and the social sciences (e.g., psychology, sociology).

standards   Curriculum goals established at the national, state, or district level that identify the skills, knowledge, and dispositions that students should demonstrate. Also, what students will know and be able to do as a result of participating in a quality physical education program.

standards-based curriculum   A curriculum that is developed by looking at the standards (district, state, or national); identifying the skills, knowledge, and dispositions that students should demonstrate to meet these standards; and identifying activities that will allow students to reach the goals stated in the standards.

stem   Pressing both feet against opposite holds.

student choice questions   Open response questions in which students are presented with several questions that assess similar knowledge and are given the option of selecting which question to answer.

summative assessments   Assessments given at the conclusion of the instructional process.

summative evaluation   An evaluation done at the conclusion of a project to measure the success of the project and to determine what has been accomplished.

sweep   Used for a major turn of the bow or for a complete pivot originating from the stern.

tactical frameworks   Ways of thinking about games based on the problems that need to be solved in order to be successful.

tactics   Decisions about what to do in response to problems that arise during a game.

task- or mastery-oriented   Self-referencing improvement in skill and ability instead of peer comparison; focuses on the process of mastering the task.

T-charts   Help students visualize appropriate behavior by asking students to write down what a certain behavior "sounds like" and what a certain behavior "looks like."

top-rope   A belay that is above the climber (where the rope is attached to an anchor above the climber).

undercling   Grabbing the underside of a hold with the palm up.

unpack the standards   Define the standards to clarify what they mean, what skills students will be able to demonstrate, how they might best be achieved, and how to measure student success.

validity   The degree to which a test measures what it is designed to measure.

value orientation   Teachers' beliefs on what students should learn, how they should learn it, and how it should be assessed.

Index

Photo Credits

SECTION I

Opener © Scott T. Baxter/Photodisc/Getty Images

CHAPTER 1

Opener Courtesy of Deborah Tannehill; **page 10** Courtesy of Rachel Gurvitch

CHAPTER 2

Opener Courtesy of Deborah Tannehill; **page 46** © iofoto/ShutterStock, Inc.

CHAPTER 3

Opener Courtesy of Rachel Gurvitch; **page 62** © Photodisc

CHAPTER 4

Opener Courtesy of Deborah Tannehill; **page 104** Courtesy of Rachel Gurvitch

CHAPTER 5

Opener Courtesy of Deborah Tannehill; **page 130** © Keith Brofsky/Photodisc/Getty Images; **page 148** © AbleStock

SECTION II

Opener © Photodisc

CHAPTER 6

Opener Courtesy of Deborah Tannehill; **page 165** © Photodisc; **page 176** Courtesy of Barbara Adamcik

CHAPTER 7

Opener Courtesy of Nancy Carow; **page 197** © LiquidLibrary; **page 207** © LiquidLibrary; **page 213** © Photos.com

CHAPTER 8

Opener Courtesy of Deborah Tannehill; **page 231** Courtesy of Michelle Dillon; **page 234** © michaeljung/ShutterStock, Inc.; **page 239** Courtesy of Michelle Dillon

CHAPTER 9

Opener Courtesy of Deborah Tannehill; **page 249** © Photodisc; **page 256** © Creatas/age fotostock

CHAPTER 10

Opener Courtesy of Deborah Tannehill; **page 277** Courtesy of Karin McKenna; **page 284** Courtesy of Karin McKenna; **page 289** © Photodisc

CHAPTER 11

Opener Courtesy of Deborah Tannehill; **page 304** © SW Productions/Photodisc/Getty Images; **page 311** © Jorge Felix Costa/ShutterStock, Inc.

CHAPTER 12

Opener Courtesy of Deborah Tannehill; **page 337** © Terrie L. Zeller/ShutterStock, Inc.; **page 352** © Photos.com

CHAPTER 13

Opener Courtesy of Deborah Tannehill; **page 383** © LiquidLibrary

SECTION III

Opener © LiquidLibrary

CHAPTER 14

Opener Courtesy of Deborah Tannehill; **page 397** Courtesy of Laura Strickland

Unless otherwise indicated, all photographs and illustrations are under copyright of Jones and Bartlett Publishers, LLC.

VERMONT STATE COLLEGES

0 0003 0852681 3

DATE DUE

APR 11 2012

DEMCO, INC. 38-2931

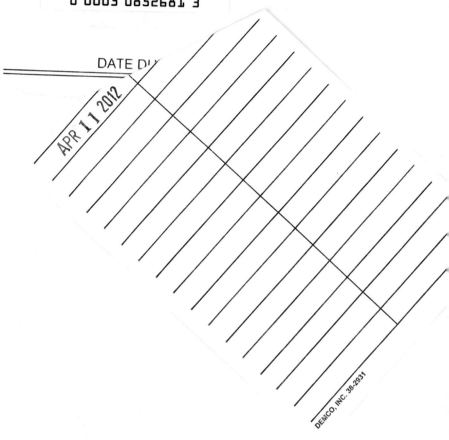

DISCARD